Food Allergy in Children

Guest Editors

HEMANT P. SHARMA, MD, MHS
ROBERT A. WOOD, MD
MAX J. COPPES, MD, PhD, MBA

PEDIATRIC CLINICS OF NORTH AMERICA

www.pediatric.theclinics.com

April 2011 • Volume 58 • Number 2

SAUNDERS an imprint of ELSEVIER, Inc.

W.B. SAUNDERS COMPANY
A Division of Elsevier Inc.

1600 John F. Kennedy Boulevard • Suite 1800 • Philadelphia, Pennsylvania 19103-2899

http://www.theclinics.com

THE PEDIATRIC CLINICS OF NORTH AMERICA Volume 58, Number 2
April 2011 ISSN 0031-3955, ISBN-13: 978-1-4557-0786-7

Editor: Kerry Holland
Developmental Editor: Donald Mumford

The Pediatric Clinics of North America (ISSN 0031-3955) is published bimonthly by Elsevier Inc., 360 Park Avenue South, New York, NY 10010-1710. Months of issue are February, April, June, August, October, and December. Periodicals postage paid at New York, NY and additional mailing offices. Subscription prices are $179.00 per year (US individuals), $423.00 per year (US institutions), $243.00 per year (Canadian individuals), $563.00 per year (Canadian institutions), $289.00 per year (international individuals), $563.00 per year (international institutions), $87.00 per year (US students and residents), and $149.00 per year (international and Canadian residents and students). To receive students/resident rare, orders must be accompanied by name of affiliated institution, date of term, and the signature of program/residency coordinator on institution letterhead. Orders will be billed at individual rate until proof of status is received. Foreign air speed delivery is included in all *Clinics* subscription prices. All prices are subject to change without notice. **POSTMASTER:** Send address changes to *The Pediatric Clinics of North America*, Elsevier Health Sciences Division, Subscription Customer Service, 3251 Riverport Lane, Maryland Heights, MO 63043. **Customer Service: 1-800-654-2452 (US and Canada). From outside of the US and Canada: 1-314-447-8871. Fax: 1-314-447-8029. For print support, E-mail: JournalsCustomerService-usa@elsevier.com. For online support, E-mail: JournalsOnlineSupport-usa@elsevier.com.**

Reprints. For copies of 100 or more, of articles in this publication, please contact the Commercial Reprints Department, Elsevier Inc., 360 Park Avenue South, New York, NY 10010-1710. Tel.: 212-633-3812; Fax: 212-462-1935; E-mail: reprints@elsevier.com.

The Pediatric Clinics of North America is also published in Spanish by McGraw-Hill Inter-americana Editores S.A., Mexico City, Mexico; in Portuguese by Riechmann and Affonso Editores, Rua Comandante Coelho 1085, CEP 21250, Rio de Janeiro, Brazil; and in Greek by Althayia SA, Athens, Greece.

The Pediatric Clinics of North America is covered in *MEDLINE/PubMed (Index Medicus), Excerpta Medica, Current Contents, Current Contents/Clinical Medicine, Science Citation Index, ASCA, ISI/BIOMED*, and *BIOSIS*.

Printed in the United States of America.

GOAL STATEMENT

The goal of the *Pediatric Clinics of North America* is to keep practicing physicians and residents up to date with current clinical practice in pediatrics by providing timely articles reviewing the state-of-the-art in patient care.

ACCREDITATION

The *Pediatric Clinics of North America* is planned and implemented in accordance with the Essential Areas and Policies of the Accreditation Council for Continuing Medical Education (ACCME) through the joint sponsorship of the University Of Virginia School Of Medicine and Elsevier. The University Of Virginia School of Medicine is accredited by the ACCME to provide continuing medical education for physicians.

The University of Virginia School of Medicine designates this educational activity for a maximum of 15 *AMA PRA Category 1 Credits*™ for each issue, 90 credits per year. Physicians should only claim credit commensurate with the extent of their participation in the activity.

The American Medical Association has determined that physicians not licensed in the US who participate in this CME activity are eligible for a maximum of 15 *AMA PRA Category 1 Credits*™ for each issue, 90 credits per year.

Credit can be earned by reading the text material, taking the CME examination online at http://www.theclinics.com/home/cme, and completing the evaluation. After taking the test, you will be required to review any and all incorrect answers. Following completion of the test and evaluation, your credit will be awarded and you may print your certificate.

FACULTY DISCLOSURE/CONFLICT OF INTEREST

The University of Virginia School of Medicine, as an ACCME accredited provider, endorses and strives to comply with the Accreditation Council for Continuing Medical Education (ACCME) Standards of Commercial Support, Commonwealth of Virginia statutes, University of Virginia policies and procedures, and associated federal and private regulations and guidelines on the need for disclosure and monitoring of proprietary and financial interests that may affect the scientific integrity and balance of content delivered in continuing medical education activities under our auspices.

The University of Virginia School of Medicine requires that all CME activities accredited through this institution be developed independently and be scientifically rigorous, balanced and objective in the presentation/discussion of its content, theories and practices.

All authors/editors participating in an accredited CME activity are expected to disclose to the readers relevant financial relationships with commercial entities occurring within the past 12 months (such as grants or research support, employee, consultant, stock holder, member of speakers bureau, etc.). The University of Virginia School of Medicine will employ appropriate mechanisms to resolve potential conflicts of interest to maintain the standards of fair and balanced education to the reader. Questions about specific strategies can be directed to the Office of Continuing Medical Education, University of Virginia School of Medicine, Charlottesville, Virginia.

The faculty and staff of the University of Virginia Office of Continuing Medical Education have no financial affiliations to disclose.

The authors/editors listed below have identified no financial or professional relationships for themselves or their spouse/partner:

Lee A Bricker, MD; Joseph L. Calles Jr, MD; L. Lee Carlisle, MD; Madeline A. Chadehumbe, MD; Bantu Chhangani, MD; Cynthia L. Feucht, PharmD, BCPS (Guest Editor); Neville H. Golden, MD; Donald E. Greydanus, MD, Dr HC (ATHENS) (Guest Editor); Carla Holloway, (Acquisitions Editor); Iliyan Ivanov, MD; Ian Kodish, MD, PhD; Jon McClellan, MD; Ahsan Nazeer, MD; Dilip R. Patel, MD, FAACPDM, FAAP, FSAM, FACSM (Guest Editor); Helen D. Pratt, PhD; Karen Rheuban, MD (Test Author); Ruqiya Shama Tareen, MD; Libbie Stansifer, MD; and Tiffany Thomas, MD.

The authors/editors listed below identified the following professional or financial affiliations for themselves or their spouse/partner:

Evelyn Attia, MD is an industry funded research/investigator for Eli Lilly & Co.

Robert L. Findling, MD receives grant/research support, is a consultant, and is on the Speakers' Bureau for Bristol-Myers Squibb, Johnson & Johnson, and Shire; receives grant/research support and is a consultant for Abbott, Addrenex, AstraZeneca, Forest, GSK, Lilly, Otsuka, Pfizer, Schering-Plough, Supernus Pharmaceuticals, and Wyeth; is a consultant for Biovail, KemPharm, Lundbeck, Novartis, Noven, Organon, Sanofi-Aventis, Sepracore, Solvay, and Validus; and receives grant/research support from Neuropharm.

Manmohan K. Kamboj, MD is on the Speakers' Bureau for Pfizer.

Gabriel Kaplan, MD is on the Speakers' Bureau for Shire, is a consultant for Commonhealth Hoboken, and is employed by University Medical Center.

Jeffrey H. Newcorn, MD is an industry funded research/investigator for Shire, Ortho McNeil Janssen, and Eli Lilly, and is a consultant and is on the Advisory Committee/Board for Shire.

Carol Rockhill, MD, PhD, MPH is an industry funded research/investigator for Seaside Therapeutics.

Sheryl Ryan, MD is on the Speaker's Bureau for Merck Pharmaceuticals.

Chris Varley, MD is on the Speaker's Bureau for Novartis.

Disclosure of Discussion of Non-FDA Approved Uses for Pharmaceutical Products and/or Medical Devices

The University of Virginia School of Medicine, as an ACCME provider, requires that all faculty presenters identify and disclose any off-label uses for pharmaceutical and medical device products. The University of Virginia School of Medicine recommends that each physician fully review all the available data on new products or procedures prior to clinical use.

TO ENROLL

To enroll in the Pediatric Clinics of North America Continuing Medical Education program, call customer service at 1-800-654-2452 or visit us online at www.theclinics.com/home/cme. The CME program is available to subscribers for an additional fee of $223.00

Contributors

GUEST EDITORS

HEMANT P. SHARMA, MD, MHS
Associate Chief, Division of Allergy and Immunology, Center for Cancer and Blood Disorders, Children's National Medical Center; Assistant Professor of Pediatrics, George Washington University, Washington, DC

ROBERT A. WOOD, MD
Chief, Division of Pediatric Allergy and Immunology, The Johns Hopkins Hospital; Professor of Pediatrics, The Johns Hopkins University School of Medicine; Professor of International Health, The Johns Hopkins Bloomberg School of Public Health, Baltimore, Maryland

MAX J. COPPES, MD, PhD, MBA
Senior Vice President, Center for Cancer and Blood Disorders, Children's National Medical Center; Professor of Oncology, Medicine and Pediatrics, Georgetown University; Clinical Professor of Pediatrics, George Washington University, Washington, DC

AUTHORS

SEEMA S. ACEVES, MD, PhD
Assistant Professor, Pediatrics and Medicine; Director, Eosinophilic Gastrointestinal Disorders Clinic, Division of Allergy and Immunology, Departments of Pediatrics and Medicine, University of California, San Diego, Rady Children's Hospital, San Diego, California

S. HASAN ARSHAD, DM, FRCP
Professor of Allergy and Clinical Immunology, III Research Division, University of Southampton, Southampton; Director, The David Hide Asthma and Allergy Research Centre, Newport, Isle of Wight, United Kingdom

KIRSTEN BEYER, MD
Klinik für Pädiatrie (Pneumo/Immunol), Charité, Campus Virchow-Klinikum, Berlin, Germany

A. WESLEY BURKS, MD
Chief, Division of Pediatric Allergy and Immunology, Department of Pediatrics; Kiser-Arena Professor of Pediatrics, Duke University School of Medicine, Durham, North Carolina

JEAN-CHRISTOPH CAUBET, MD
Division of Pediatric Allergy and Immunology, Pediatrics Mount Sinai School of Medicine, New York, New York; Department of Child and Adolescent, University Hospitals of Geneva and Medical School of the University of Geneva, Geneva, Switzerland

STACY CHIN, MD
Fellow, Division of Pediatric Allergy and Immunology, Department of Pediatrics, Duke University School of Medicine, Durham, North Carolina

RENATA R. COCCO, MD
Clinical Researcher, Division of Allergy, Clinical Immunology and Rheumatology, Department of Pediatrics, Federal University of São Paulo, São Paulo, Brazil

GEORGE DU TOIT, FRCPCH (UK)
Division of Asthma, Allergy and Lung Biology, Guy's and St Thomas' National Health Service Foundation Trust, the Medical Research Council and Asthma UK Centre in Allergic Mechanisms of Asthma, King's College London, London, United Kingdom

PHILIPPE A. EIGENMANN, MD
Pediatric Allergy Unit, Children's Hospital, University Hospital of Geneva, Geneva, Switzerland

KIRSI M. JÄRVINEN, MD, PhD
Assistant Professor, Division of Pediatric Allergy and Immunology, Department of Pediatrics, Jaffe Institute for Food Allergy, The Mount Sinai School of Medicine, New York, New York

JACOB D. KATTAN, MD
Clinical Fellow, Division of Pediatric Allergy and Immunology, Department of Pediatrics, Jaffe Institute for Food Allergy, The Mount Sinai School of Medicine, New York, New York

CORINNE KEET, MD
Assistant Professor of Pediatrics, Division of Pediatric Allergy and Immunology, Department of Pediatrics, Johns Hopkins School of Medicine, Baltimore, Maryland

JENNIFER S. KIM, MD
Assistant Professor of Pediatrics, Division of Allergy and Immunology, Mount Sinai School of Medicine, New York, New York

GIDEON LACK, FRCPCH (UK)
Division of Asthma, Allergy and Lung Biology, Guy's and St Thomas' National Health Service Foundation Trust, the Medical Research Council and Asthma UK Centre in Allergic Mechanisms of Asthma, King's College London, London, United Kingdom

DARLENE K. MANSOOR, MD, MS
Attending Physician, Division of Allergy and Immunology, Center for Cancer and Blood Disorders, Children's National Medical Center; Assistant Professor of Pediatrics, George Washington University, Washington, DC

KIM MUDD, RN, MSN
Research Nurse/Program Coordinator, Johns Hopkins Division of Pediatric Allergy and Immunology, Johns Hopkins Hospital, Baltimore, Maryland

ANTONELLA MURARO, MD, PhD
Professor, Department of Pediatrics, Food Allergy Centre, Veneto Region, University of Padua, Padua, Italy

ANNA NOWAK-WEGRZYN, MD
Associate Professor, Department of Pediatrics, Jaffe Food Allergy Institute, Mount Sinai School of Medicine, New York, New York

JONATHAN O'B HOURIHANE, MB, DM, FRCPI
Professor, Department of Paediatrics and Child Health, Clinical Investigations Unit, Cork University Hospital, University College Cork, Wilton, Cork, Ireland

JAE-WON OH, MD, PhD
Department of Pediatrics, Hanyang University Kuri Hospital, Seoul, Korea

HEMANT P. SHARMA, MD, MHS
Associate Chief, Division of Allergy and Immunology, Center for Cancer and Blood Disorders, Children's National Medical Center; Assistant Professor of Pediatrics, George Washington University, Washington, DC

SCOTT H. SICHERER, MD
Professor of Pediatrics, Division of Allergy and Immunology, Mount Sinai School of Medicine, New York, New York

CARINA VENTER, PhD, RD
NHIR Post Doctorate Research Fellow, University of Portsmouth, Portsmouth; Senior Allergy Dietitian, The David Hide Asthma and Allergy Research Centre, Newport, Isle of Wight, United Kingdom

BRIAN P. VICKERY, MD
Instructor, Division of Pediatric Allergy and Immunology, Department of Pediatrics, Duke University School of Medicine, Durham, North Carolina

JULIE WANG, MD
Division of Pediatric Allergy and Immunology, Pediatrics Mount Sinai School of Medicine, New York, New York

ROBERT A. WOOD, MD
Chief, Division of Pediatric Allergy and Immunology, The Johns Hopkins Hospital; Professor of Pediatrics, The Johns Hopkins University School of Medicine; Professor of International Health, The Johns Hopkins Bloomberg School of Public Health, Baltimore, Maryland

JAIME LIOU WOLFE, MD
Division of Gastroenterology, Department of Surgery, Children's National Medical Center, Washington, DC

Contents

Preface: Food Allergy in Children xv

Hemant P. Sharma, Robert A. Wood, and Max J. Coppes

Clinical Presentations of Food Allergy 315

Darlene K. Mansoor and Hemant P. Sharma

Food allergies are immune-mediated responses to food proteins. Because of differences in the underlying immunologic mechanisms, there are varying clinical presentations of food allergy. This article discusses the manifestations of IgE-mediated disorders, including urticaria and angioedema, rhinoconjunctivitis, asthma, gastrointestinal anaphylaxis, generalized anaphylaxis, food-dependent exercise-induced anaphylaxis, and oral allergy syndrome. It also reviews the presentations of mixed IgE- and cell-mediated disorders, including atopic dermatitis and eosinophilic gastrointestinal disorders. Finally, the manifestations of cell-mediated food allergies are discussed, including dietary protein-induced proctitis and proctocolitis, food protein-induced enterocolitis syndrome, celiac disease, and food-induced pulmonary hemosiderosis.

Epidemiology of Food Allergy 327

Carina Venter and S. Hasan Arshad

Food allergy (FA) is perceived as a common problem, especially during childhood. Accurate assessment of incidence and prevalence of FA has been difficult to establish, however, due to lack of universally accepted diagnostic criteria. Although many foods are reported to cause IgE-mediated FA, most studies focus on 4 common food groups: cow's milk, hen's egg, peanut/tree nuts, and fish/shellfish. There may be variation in the prevalence of FA in regions of the world and a likely increase in prevalence has been observed in recent decades. This cannot be stated with confidence, however, without the use of consistent methodology and diagnostic criteria.

Diagnostic Testing in the Evaluation of Food Allergy 351

Philippe A. Eigenmann, Jae-Won Oh, and Kirsten Beyer

Food-related symptoms are frequent in childhood, and pediatricians are often requested to initiate a food allergy diagnostic workup. A careful history is the cornerstone for assessing whether tests are needed and which diagnostic procedures are most appropriate. Skin prick tests should be performed only according to standard procedures by a skilled health professional. Determining serum IgE levels (in vitro tests) are available for a wide range of foods. Of utmost importance is the need to correlate test results to the clinical picture. When a conclusion cannot be reached, oral food challenges should be performed for a definite diagnosis.

Pathophysiology of Food Allergy 363

Brian P. Vickery, Stacy Chin, and A. Wesley Burks

In this article we review the pathophysiology of food allergy, which affects 4% of US children and 2% of adults, and is increasing in prevalence. Most

food allergens share certain specific physicochemical characteristics that allow them to resist digestion, thus enhancing allergenicity. During allergic sensitization, these allergens are encountered by specialized dendritic cell populations in the gut, which leads to T-cell priming and the production of allergen-specific IgE production by B cells. Tissue-resident mast cells then bind IgE, and allergic reactions are elicited when mast cells are reexposed to allergen. Adjacent IgE molecules bound to the surface of the mast cell become cross-linked, causing mast cell degranulation and release of powerful vasoactive compounds that cause allergic symptoms.

Recognition and Management of Food-Induced Anaphylaxis **377**

Corinne Keet

Food-induced anaphylactic reactions are common and increasing in frequency. Despite the existence of a consensus definition of anaphylaxis, many cases are missed, recommended treatments are not given, and follow-up is inadequate. New aspects of its pathophysiology and causes, including atypical food-induced causes, are still being uncovered. Epinephrine remains the cornerstone for successfully treating anaphylaxis; H1 and H2 antihistamines, glucocorticoids, and β-agonists are ancillary medications that may be used in addition to epinephrine. Early recognition of anaphylaxis, appropriate emergency treatment, and follow up, including prescription of self-injectable epinephrine, are essential to prevent death and significant morbidity from anaphylaxis.

Gastrointestinal Manifestations of Food Allergies **389**

Jaime Liou Wolfe and Seema S. Aceves

The rates of eosinophilic gastrointestinal disorders appear to be increasing. The most common of these is eosinophilic esophagitis (EoE) which is a clinicopathologic condition consisting of characteristic symptoms and endoscopic features accompanied by a pan-esophageal, acid resistant epithelial eosinophilia of greater than equal to 15 per high power field. Typical symptoms include dysphagia and abdominal pain. Typical endoscopic features include pallor, plaques, furrows, concentric rings. Complications include food impactions and strictures. EoE resolution with food elimination diets provides evidence that EoE is a food-antigen driven process. In vitro and microarray studies have identified specific immunologic factors underlying EoE pathogenesis. Other gastrointestinal manifestations of food intolerances/allergy include food protein induced enterocolitis syndrome.

Milk and Soy Allergy **407**

Jacob D. Kattan, Renata R. Cocco, and Kirsi M. Järvinen

Cow's milk allergy (CMA) affects 2% to 3% of young children and presents with a wide range of IgE and non-IgE–mediated clinical syndromes, which have a significant economic and lifestyle effect. It is logical that a review of CMA would be linked to a review of soy allergy because soy formula is often an alternative source of nutrition for infants who do not tolerate cow's milk. This review examines the epidemiology, pathogenesis, clinical features, natural history, and diagnosis of cow's milk and soy allergy. Cross-reactivity and management of milk allergy are also discussed.

Can Food Allergy Be Prevented? The Current Evidence **481**

George Du Toit and Gideon Lack

Food allergy is a recognized public health concern, for which preventative strategies are required. Although an intervention that adequately protects against the development of food allergy has still to be identified, limited benefits have been shown for the prevention of related allergic conditions such as eczema, and to a lesser extent asthma and rhinitis; these benefits are usually limited to at-risk populations. Prevention strategies need to be tested using randomized controlled study designs that account for the numerous methodological challenges, safety concerns, and necessary ethical limitations.

Food Allergy Therapy: Is a Cure Within Reach? **511**

Anna Nowak-Wegrzyn and Antonella Muraro

There is an unmet medical need for an effective food allergy therapy; thus, development of therapeutic interventions for food allergy is a top research priority. The food allergen-nonspecific therapies for food-induced anaphylaxis include monoclonal anti-IgE antibodies and Chinese herbs. The food allergen-specific therapies include oral, sublingual, and epicutaneous immunotherapy with native food allergens and mutated recombinant proteins. Diet containing heated milk and egg may represent an alternative approach to oral immunomodulation. Oral food immunotherapy remains an investigational treatment to be further studied before advancing into clinical practice.

Index **531**

FORTHCOMING ISSUES

June 2011

Pediatric Sleep Medicine Update
Judith Owens, MD, MPH, and
Jodi A. Mindell, PhD, *Guest Editors*

August 2011

Pediatric Endocrinology
Robert Rapaport, MD, *Guest Editor*

RECENT ISSUES

February 2011

Pediatric Psychopharmacology in the 21st Century
Donald E. Greydanus, MD, Dr HC (Athens),
Dilip R. Patel, MD, and Cynthia Feucht,
PharmD, BCPS, *Guest Editors*

December 2010

Pediatric Chest Pain
Guy D. Eslick, PhD, MMedSc(Clin Epi),
MMedStat and Steven M. Selbst, MD,
Guest Editors

October 2010

Birthmarks of Medical Significance
Beth A. Drolet, MD and
Maria C. Garzon, MD,
Guest Editors

Preface

Food Allergy in Children

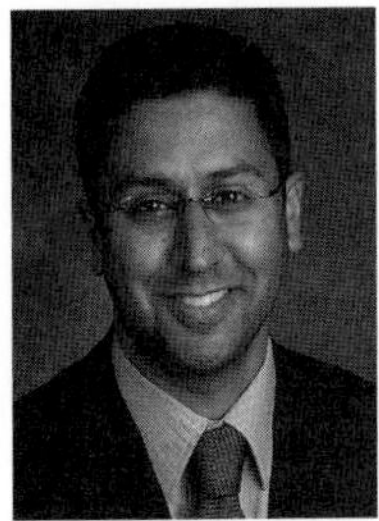
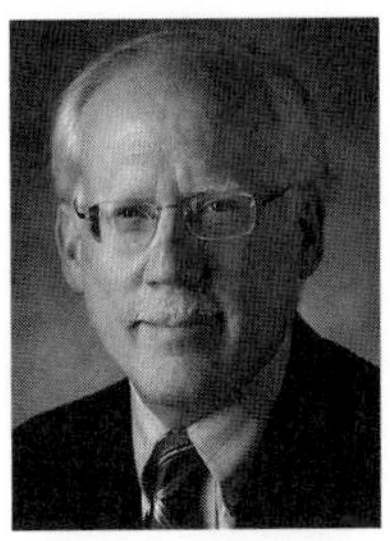
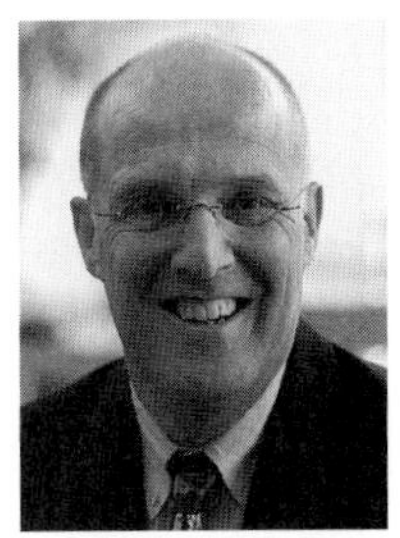

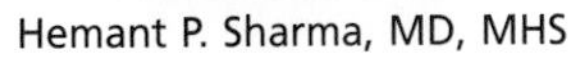

Hemant P. Sharma, MD, MHS   Robert A. Wood, MD   Max J. Coppes, MD, PhD, MBA
Guest Editors

Food allergy has become a serious health concern in the United States and around the world, particularly for children and young adults. This immune-mediated condition is estimated to affect 5% of children in the United States, and its prevalence is likely increasing worldwide.[1] Since no therapies yet exist to prevent or cure food allergies, management involves the avoidance of food allergens and treatment of reactions, which can range in severity from mild to life-threatening. Given the magnitude of this public health problem, pediatric practitioners of all kinds are now faced with the challenge of appropriately diagnosing and caring for children with food allergies. The purpose of this issue of *Pediatric Clinics of North America* is to provide clinicians with a comprehensive and practical review of the current food allergy literature. The timeliness of this topic is underscored by the recent release of guidelines for the diagnosis and management of food allergy by an Expert Panel sponsored by the National Institute of Allergy and Infectious Diseases.[2] This issue of *Pediatric Clinics* summarizes much of the evidence used to inform the development of these guidelines. There are articles addressing the diverse clinical presentations of food allergy, as well as, more specifically, gastrointestinal manifestations. Also discussed is our current knowledge regarding the underlying pathophysiology and its epidemiology across the globe. Other articles review the diagnosis of food allergy and treatment of food-induced anaphylaxis, and there are articles specifically dedicated to some of the more common food allergies, namely, allergies to cow's milk, soy, egg, peanut, and tree nuts. Issues of living with food allergies, such as allergen avoidance and school-based management, are also addressed. Finally, the future of this condition is examined by reviewing the current evidence for strategies to prevent and treat food allergies. As such, this

Pediatr Clin N Am 58 (2011) xv–xvi
doi:10.1016/j.pcl.2011.02.013

issue provides a comprehensive review of the current literature and can serve as a useful aid for practitioners as they care for children with food allergies.

Hemant P. Sharma, MD, MHS
Division of Allergy and Immunology
Center for Cancer and Blood Disorders
Children's National Medical Center
111 Michigan Avenue NW
Washington, DC 20010, USA

Robert A. Wood, MD
Division of Pediatric Allergy and Immunology
The Johns Hopkins Hospital
CMSC-1102
600 North Wolfe Street
Baltimore, MD 21287, USA

Max J. Coppes, MD, PhD, MBA
Center for Cancer and Blood Disorders
Children's National Medical Center
111 Michigan Avenue NW
Washington, DC 20010, USA

E-mail addresses:
hsharma@cnmc.org (H.P. Sharma)
rwood@jhmi.edu (R.A. Wood)
mcoppes@cnmc.org (M.J. Coppes)

REFERENCES

1. Branum AM, Lukacs SL. Food allergy among children in the United States. Pediatrics 2009;124(6):1549–55.
2. Expert Panel Report. Guidelines for the Diagnosis and Management of Food Allergy in the United States: report of the NIAID-sponsored expert panel. J Allergy Clin Immunol 2010;126(6):S1–58.

Clinical Presentations of Food Allergy

Darlene K. Mansoor, MD, MS, Hemant P. Sharma, MD, MHS*

KEYWORDS

• Food allergy • Symptoms • Classification

The clinical presentations of food allergy are diverse. In addition to symptoms of immediate hypersensitivity, there are other more subacute or chronic ways in which food allergy may manifest. In this article, the authors first distinguish food allergy from nonimmunologic adverse food reactions and then discuss the diverse clinical presentations of food allergies as categorized by their underlying immunopathology.

DEFINITION OF FOOD ALLERGY AND DIFFERENTIAL DIAGNOSIS

Food allergies or hypersensitivities are defined as adverse immune responses to food proteins.[1] It is important to distinguish food allergies from nonimmunologic adverse food reactions, which are considerably more common than true food allergies. Although 20% to 30% of the general population report food allergy in themselves or their children, the prevalence of true food allergy is only 6% to 8% in young children and 3% to 4% in adults.[2–5] Therefore, many nonimmune adverse food reactions are incorrectly assumed to be allergic.

Examples of nonimmunologic reactions to foods include host-specific metabolic disorders, such as lactose intolerance, galactosemia, and alcohol intolerance. In lactose intolerance, a deficiency in the enzyme lactase results in an inability to digest the carbohydrate lactose found in milk and dairy products. Characteristic symptoms include abdominal pain, bloating, gas, diarrhea, and nausea.[6] Responses to pharmacologically active components or toxins in foods constitute another group of nonimmune adverse food reactions. For example, in scombroid poisoning, histaminic chemicals found in spoiled dark-meat fishes, such as tuna, mackerel, and sardines, result in allergic symptoms on ingestion, including flushing, urticaria, angioedema, nausea, abdominal cramping, and diarrhea.[7] Although the symptoms resemble those of an allergic reaction, the underlying mechanism of scombroid poisoning is nonimmunologic. Another example of a pharmacologically active food component causing an adverse reaction is tyramine, found in aged cheeses and pickled fish, which can trigger migraine headaches because of the aromatic amine content. Finally,

The authors have nothing to disclose.
Division of Allergy and Immunology, Center for Cancer and Blood Disorders, Children's National Medical Center, 111 Michigan Avenue, North West, Washington, DC 20010, USA
* Corresponding author.
E-mail address: hsharma@cnmc.org

Pediatr Clin N Am 58 (2011) 315–326
doi:10.1016/j.pcl.2011.02.008 pediatric.theclinics.com
0031-3955/11/$ – see front matter

psychological disorders, such as anorexia nervosa, food aversions, and food phobias, may also cause nonimmunologic food reactions, as can neurologic disorders, such as auriculotemporal syndrome (facial redness or sweating after eating tart foods) and gustatory rhinitis (rhinorrhea after eating particularly hot or spicy foods). **Box 1** summarizes the differential diagnosis of nonimmunologic adverse food reactions.

CLASSIFICATION OF FOOD ALLERGIES

Given that food allergies are immunologically mediated, it is helpful to conceptualize them into 3 categories based on their underlying immunopathology: (1) IgE-mediated reactions, (2) mixed IgE- and cell-mediated reactions, and (3) cell-mediated reactions (**Table 1**). The following sections of this article discuss the clinical manifestations of the specific food-induced allergic disorders belonging to each of these 3 broad categories.

IgE-MEDIATED FOOD ALLERGIES

IgE-mediated food allergic reactions are characterized by the acute onset of symptoms, usually minutes to 2 hours after ingestion. The rapid time course is because of the

Box 1
Differential diagnosis of nonimmunologic adverse food reactions (conditions that are not food allergies)

- Host-specific metabolic disorders
  - Carbohydrate malabsorption
    - Lactase deficiency (lactose intolerance)
    - Sucrase-isomaltase deficiency (sucrose intolerance)
  - Galactosemia
  - Alcohol intolerance
- Response to pharmacologically active food component
  - Scombroid poisoning (fish: tuna, mackerel, mahi mahi, sardines, anchovies)
  - Caffeine
  - Tyramine (aged cheeses, pickled fish)
  - Theobromine (tea, chocolate)
- Toxic reactions (food poisoning)
  - Fish: ciguatera poisoning (grouper, snapper)
  - Shellfish: saxitoxin
  - Fungal toxins: aflatoxins, trichothecenes, ergot
- Psychological reactions
  - Anorexia nervosa
  - Food aversions
  - Food phobias
- Neurologic reactions
  - Auriculotemporal syndrome
  - Gustatory rhinitis

presence of food-specific IgE on the surfaces of tissue mast cells and circulating basophils after initial sensitization. On reexposure to the food antigen, IgE cross-linking results in a cascade of intracellular events, which lead to the rapid release of preformed allergic mediators that are responsible for immediate symptoms. Newly synthesized mediators may later be released, resulting in a delayed symptom phase as well.

IgE-dependent reactions to carbohydrate allergens in meats are a potential exception to this usual acute time frame, as well as to the traditional definition of food allergy as being protein driven. Recent reports suggest that this reaction, which is caused by the presence of IgE antibody to galactose-alpha-1,3-galactose, is typically delayed, 4 to 6 hours after ingestion.[8] The delay in symptom onset is likely due to digestion and/or processing of the antigen. The following sections focus on the more common IgE-mediated reactions to food proteins.

Potential clinical manifestations of IgE-mediated food allergy include urticaria and angioedema, rhinoconjunctivitis, asthma, gastrointestinal anaphylaxis, and generalized anaphylaxis. In addition, food-dependent exercise-induced anaphylaxis and oral allergy syndrome (OAS) are distinct conditions with IgE-mediated mechanisms.

Urticaria and Angioedema

After ingestion or contact exposure to a food allergen, food-specific IgE on cutaneous mast cells may cross-link, leading to the release of allergic mediators, such as histamine, which cause pruritus, and vasodilatory mediators, which cause local swelling. In urticaria, this reaction primarily occurs in the superficial dermis, whereas in angioedema, the deep dermis and subcutaneous tissues are involved. Urticarial lesions, or hives, are erythematous, raised, and well-demarcated plaques, often with central pallor and blanching on pressure. Angioedema presents as asymmetric swelling in non–gravitation-dependent areas because of the leakage of plasma into subcutaneous or mucosal tissues.[9]

Food allergy seems to be a common cause of acute urticaria. Although the exact prevalence is uncertain, it is estimated that 20% of cases of acute urticaria are caused by food allergy.[10,11] In contrast, chronic urticaria, defined as hives persisting for more than 6 weeks, is less commonly caused by food allergy. Although as many as 50% of adults with chronic urticaria think that foods are associated with their hives, only 2% to 10% actually have food-induced symptoms in placebo-controlled challenges.[11,12]

Among the skin manifestations of food allergy, acute urticaria and angioedema are likely the most common. The skin findings may be triggered by ingestion of the food allergen or by direct contact, which causes acute contact urticaria, in which hives are localized only to the areas of food contact. The most common foods to cause acute urticaria and angioedema are cow's milk, egg, peanut, tree nuts, soy, wheat, fish, and shellfish. With regard to foods that cause a reaction on contact with the skin (causing contact urticaria), some are thought to be more common than others, including raw meats, fish, and raw fruits and vegetables.[13,14]

Although hives and swelling are common signs of food allergic reactions, it should be noted that their absence does not preclude the possibility of a food allergy. Up to 20% of cases of anaphylaxis do not involve any skin symptoms.[15] The lack of skin symptoms may result in delayed recognition of an allergic reaction, as suggested by the observation that 80% of fatal food-induced anaphylaxis is not associated with skin findings.[15]

Rhinoconjunctivitis

Rhinoconjunctivitis is frequently a part of systemic food allergic reactions, although rarely the only presenting symptom. Ocular and nasal symptoms that may be

Table 1
Food-induced allergic disorders (classified based on underlying immunopathology)

Immunopathology	Disorder	Clinical Features	Typical Age	Most Common Causal Foods	Prognosis
IgE mediated	Urticaria/angioedema	Triggered by ingestion or direct contact	Children > adults	Major allergens	Depends on food
	Rhinoconjunctivitis/ asthma	Accompanies food-induced allergic reaction, but rarely isolated symptom May be triggered by ingestion of aerosolized food protein	Infant/child > adult, except for occupational disease	Major allergens (occupational: wheat, egg, seafood)	Depends on food
	Anaphylaxis	Rapidly progressive, multiple organ system reaction	Any age	Any allergen, but more commonly peanut, tree nuts, shellfish, fish, milk, and egg	Depends on food
	Food-dependent, exercise-induced anaphylaxis	Food triggers anaphylaxis only if ingestion is followed temporally by exercise	Onset in late childhood/ adulthood	Wheat, shellfish, celery	Presumed persistent
	Oral allergy syndrome	Pruritus, mild edema confined to oral cavity Uncommonly progresses beyond mouth (<10%) or anaphylaxis (1%–2%)	Onset after pollen allergy established (adult > young child)	Raw fruits/vegetables (cooked forms tolerated)	Might be persistent; might vary with seasons

Mixed IgE and cell mediated	Atopic dermatitis	Associated with food in 30%–40% of children with moderate/severe eczema	Infant > child > adult	Major allergens, particularly egg and milk	Usually resolves
	Eosinophilic gastrointestinal disorders	Symptoms vary on sites/ degree of eosinophilic inflammation	Any age	Multiple	Likely persistent
Cell mediated	Dietary protein–induced proctitis/ proctocolitis	Mucus-laden, bloody stools in infants	Infancy	Milk (through breastfeeding)	Usually resolves
	Food protein–induced enterocolitis syndrome	Chronic exposure: emesis, diarrhea, poor growth, lethargy Reexposure after restriction: emesis, diarrhea, hypotension 2 h after ingestion	Infancy	Milk, soy, rice, and oat	Usually resolves

Adapted from Sicherer SH, Sampson HA. Food allergy. J Allergy Clin Immunol 2010;125:S120,121; with permission.

observed include periocular pruritus, erythema, and tearing, as well as sneezing, pruritus, nasal congestion, and rhinorrhea. In a study of 480 children who underwent oral ingestion double-blind placebo-controlled food challenges (DBPCFC), 39% of the 185 children with positive reactions experienced ocular and respiratory symptoms. Only 5% had symptoms confined to the respiratory tract alone.[16]

Although cow's milk ingestion has been suggested as a cause of nasal congestion in infants, there is no evidence to support this notion. In 3 studies, only 0.08% to 0.2% of infants were observed to develop nasal symptoms following a milk challenge.[3,17,18]

Asthma

Asthma alone is a rare presentation of food allergy but may be part of a more systemic reaction. An exception is occupational asthma among workers in the food preparation and packaging industry. These individuals may present with isolated upper and/or lower respiratory tract symptoms on inhalation of the culprit food allergen, such as wheat flour in bakers' asthma.[19] However, the food is often tolerated on ingestion.

More characteristically, bronchospasm is a component of a more generalized food allergy reaction. In studies of children referred for evaluation of food allergy with DBPCFC, symptoms of acute bronchospasm, such as cough, wheezing, and dyspnea, have been observed.[20–22] For example, in a study of 88 children with asthma and food allergy, 15% developed symptoms of acute bronchospasm during DBPCFC, with 8% having a 20% or greater decrease in forced expiratory volume in the first second of expiration.[20] In addition to ingestion-induced symptoms, there have been case reports of asthma symptoms elicited by airborne food allergens, such as vapors generated during the cooking of eggs, fish, and shellfish.[23]

Gastrointestinal Anaphylaxis

Gastrointestinal anaphylaxis is characterized by symptoms of nausea, abdominal pain, cramping, vomiting, and/or diarrhea. It is usually accompanied by IgE-mediated symptoms in other organ systems.[24] Upper gastrointestinal tract symptoms typically occur within minutes to 2 hours after food allergen ingestion, whereas lower gastrointestinal tract symptoms (diarrhea) may be delayed, occurring 2 to 6 hours after ingestion.

Generalized Anaphylaxis

Generalized anaphylaxis refers to a rapidly progressive multiple organ system reaction, which in addition to the cutaneous, respiratory tract, and gastrointestinal tract symptoms noted earlier, may involve cardiovascular symptoms, such as hypotension, vascular collapse, and dysrhythmias. In approximately one-third of food-induced anaphylactic reactions, symptoms may follow a biphasic course, in which they recur hours after the initial presentation.[25] Food allergy is the most common cause of anaphylaxis treated in emergency departments, accounting for one-third to half of the cases.[26,27] The most common foods to cause anaphylaxis are peanut, tree nuts, shellfish, fish, milk, and egg.

Several risk factors seem to predispose to fatal food-induced anaphylaxis. In a recent case series of 32 food-induced anaphylactic fatalities, approximately two-thirds of the victims were adolescents or young adults, almost all (96%) had coexistent asthma, 94% had reactions because of peanut or tree nuts, and 90% had delayed or no administration of epinephrine.[28]

Food-Dependent Exercise-Induced Anaphylaxis

Food-dependent (or food-associated) exercise-induced anaphylaxis is a rare form of anaphylaxis that manifests only with physical exertion 2 to 4 hours after ingestion of the culprit food.[24] Affected individuals are able to tolerate the food without reaction if there is no exercise after ingestion. Although the underlying pathophysiology is not clearly understood, it seems to involve IgE-mediated mechanisms triggered after exercise has altered gut absorption, allergen digestion, or both.[29]

Case reports suggest that this form of anaphylaxis is more common in women, in the age range of late teens to midthirties, and among patients with other atopic diseases, such as asthma.[30] Patients usually react to 1 or 2 foods, and the most commonly implicated foods include wheat, shellfish, celery, fish, fruit, and milk. Food-specific IgE antibodies are generally detectable by skin prick testing or serum IgE testing. In addition, some patients seem to react after any food is consumed before exercise, regardless of what specifically they ate.

Oral Allergy Syndrome

OAS, also referred to as pollen-food allergy syndrome, is an IgE-mediated reaction observed in up to 50% of pollen-allergic patients after ingestion of certain fresh fruits and vegetables.[31] It occurs in individuals who are sensitized to pollen aeroallergens through the respiratory tract, which then predisposes them to clinical symptoms of OAS on ingestion of cross-reactive, heat-labile food proteins of plant origin.

Symptoms of OAS include immediate pruritus, tingling, and mild swelling of the lips, tongue, palate, and throat. Symptoms are almost always limited to the oropharynx and subside within minutes of ingestion; less than 10% of cases progress to more systemic findings and only 1% to 2% to anaphylaxis.[29] Cooking or heating of the culprit fruits and vegetables typically eliminates symptoms because of the heat-labile nature of the proteins.

Examples of cross-reactivity patterns in OAS[24] include the development of symptoms in a birch-allergic patient after eating apple, cherry, pear, potato, carrot, celery, or kiwi. A ragweed-allergic patient may show reaction after eating melons or bananas. Celery or mustard may provoke symptoms in a mugwort-allergic patient. Symptoms may be more prevalent during or after the relevant pollen season.

MIXED IgE- AND CELL-MEDIATED FOOD ALLERGIES

Food allergy may also play a role in more chronic diseases such as atopic dermatitis (AD) and eosinophilic gastroenteropathies, including eosinophilic esophagitis (EE) and eosinophilic gastroenteritis (EG), through mixed immune mechanisms involving both IgE- and non–IgE-mediated reactions. Patients with AD and eosinophilic gastroenteropathies may have detectable IgE antibody; however, the proposed pathophysiology of the diseases is related to homing of food-responsive T cells to the site of involvement, which is a non–IgE-mediated process.[29]

AD

AD is a chronic skin condition that usually begins in infancy. The features of AD include extreme pruritus, rash in a typical distribution, and a chronic relapsing course. In affected children, the rash is usually distributed in flexor surfaces, such as the antecubital and popliteal fossa, wrists, ankles, and neck. Food hypersensitivity may be a contributing cause in infants who have moderate to severe AD.

Approximately 30% to 40% of these infants and young children with moderate to severe AD have food hypersensitivity.[32–34] The relationship between AD and food allergy is evidenced by improvement in symptoms after the elimination of suspected foods, as well as the exacerbation of AD with repeat exposure to the foods. This relationship was demonstrated when 113 patients with severe AD underwent DBPCFC.[35] There were 101 positive food challenge results observed in 63 children (56%). Skin symptoms were observed in 84% of the food challenges. These patients were then placed on elimination diets based on the food challenge results, and most exhibited significant improvement in skin symptoms. Egg, milk, and peanut were the foods most commonly associated with eczema. Of the 63 patients with positive food challenge results, 40 were reevaluated, and 40% of them lost their hypersensitivity after 1 or 2 years, suggesting possible resolution of food allergy–associated eczema after a period of allergen elimination.

Another group examined 600 children with AD undergoing DBPCFC and found 40% of the food challenge results to be positive.[33] Approximately 75% of these resulted in skin manifestations such as macular, morbilliform, and/or pruritic rashes in the flexural areas characteristically affected in AD, again suggesting specific foods as triggers.

Eosinophilic Gastrointestinal Disorders

Similar to AD, eosinophilic gastroenteropathies including both EE and EG are thought to be caused by mixed immunologic mechanisms (IgE- and T-cell–mediated). Patients present with a wide range of chronic gastrointestinal symptoms that are experienced most commonly after eating. Biopsy specimens obtained by upper endoscopy showed increased eosinophil counts exclusively in the esophagus in patients with EE. If, on the other hand, eosinophils are found in other areas of the gastrointestinal tract, patients are diagnosed as having EG.

EE results in inflammation of the esophagus and can be seen in any age group. However, the clinical presentation of EE differs significantly based on the age of the affected child. Very young children (median age, 2 years) tend to present with feeding difficulties and failure to thrive. Older children may present with vomiting (median age, 8.1 years) and abdominal pain (median age, 12.0 years), whereas teenagers often have dysphagia (median age, 13.4 years) with possible food impaction (median age, 16.8 years).[36] Patients do not respond to treatment with antireflux medications, and this unresponsiveness is in fact one of the criteria used to diagnose EE. The other 2 diagnostic criteria include characteristic symptoms and presence of more than 15 eosinophils per high-powered field on esophageal biopsy. Many patients with EE have evidence of comorbid allergic disease, such as allergic rhinitis (57%) and IgE-mediated food allergy (46%).[36] Food allergens, and possibly aeroallergens, seem to play an integral role in the immunopathology of EE. A review of 381 children with EE found that the foods most commonly implicated were cow's milk, egg, soy, corn, wheat, and beef.[37] Targeted elimination of the culprit foods or complete elimination by using an elemental formula resulted in clinical and histologic improvement in most of the children in this series.

Patients with EG may also present at any age. Given that any segment of the gastrointestinal tract from the esophagus to the colon, including the bile ducts,[38] may be involved, the clinical symptoms vary depending on the location of inflammation within the gastrointestinal tract.[39] In general, symptoms consist of abdominal pain, nausea, diarrhea, and weight loss secondary to malabsorption. Infants may present with outlet obstruction with projectile vomiting after feeding. In adolescents, symptoms may be similar to those of irritable bowel syndrome.[38] Like EE, 50% of patients with EG also have other allergic diseases.[40,41]

CELL-MEDIATED FOOD ALLERGIES

A third group of food hypersensitivity disorders with delayed reactions and chronic course of the disease process are mediated primarily by T cells. These disorders include dietary protein–induced proctitis and proctocolitis; dietary protein–induced enterocolitis, also known as food protein–induced enterocolitis syndrome (FPIES); celiac disease; and food-induced pulmonary hemosiderosis (Heiner syndrome).

Dietary Protein–Induced Proctitis and Proctocolitis

Dietary protein–induced proctitis and proctocolitis are characterized by T-cell–mediated eosinophilic inflammation of the rectum as well as colon and rectum, respectively. These conditions are seen commonly in breastfed infants aged between 2 and 8 weeks.[42–45] These conditions are also seen, but less commonly, in infants fed cow's milk– or soy-based formulas. Affected infants may have mucus and blood in their stools but are otherwise healthy appearing. Some infants may be fussy or have increased bowel movements but not usually diarrhea. Removal of the culprit food, most commonly cow's milk, from the mother's diet results in improvement within 48 hours. The prognosis for dietary protein–induced proctitis and proctocolitis is good. The condition is thought to resolve after a period of allergen avoidance from 6 months to 2 years. There have been case reports of similar presentations in older children.[46] These children also have bloody stools with mucus, which resolves with the elimination of milk and recurs on milk challenge. It is not clear if this is the same disease as that seen in infants with a later presentation. About 25% of these children have other atopic diseases.

FPIES

FPIES is a more severe form of T-cell–mediated gastrointestinal food allergy than dietary protein proctitis. It is most commonly diagnosed in infants younger than 9 months, with a peak incidence between 1 week and 3 months of age. Unlike dietary protein proctitis, most infants with FPIES are fed cow's milk- or soy-based formulas, and it is rare in breastfed children. Although less common than cow's milk and soy, other foods may be implicated in FPIES, including grains (rice, oat, and barley), vegetables (sweet potato, squash, string beans, and peas), or poultry (chicken and turkey).[47,48] Patients with FPIES, if regularly ingesting the culprit food, may present with severe chronic gastrointestinal symptoms, such as vomiting, diarrhea, and malabsorption resulting in poor growth, anemia, and hypoproteinemia.[49–53] Symptoms typically resolve after the food is removed from the diet, although it may take weeks for the T-cell–mediated inflammation to resolve. If the causative food is reintroduced to the diet, a characteristic presentation results, consisting of profuse vomiting approximately 2 hours after ingestion. Affected children often present to the emergency department appearing quite ill, in shock with hypotension and lethargy secondary to dehydration from the profuse vomiting and third spacing of fluid. The prognosis for FPIES is good. Most children become tolerant of the culprit food by the age of 3 years. At that time, a hospital-based food challenge may be performed to confirm resolution and tolerance.[48]

Celiac Disease

A more common chronic disease that is mediated by non–IgE-mediated immune mechanisms is celiac disease. Celiac disease results from a T-cell–mediated inflammatory response to gluten in grains such as wheat, rye, barley, and oat. Patients present with symptoms of chronic diarrhea, failure to thrive, short stature, malabsorption, steatorrhea, or other signs of nutrient or vitamin deficiency.[54] The histologic changes (villous atrophy) of the small intestine and symptoms resolve when gluten-containing foods are removed from the diet within a few weeks to months.

Heiner Syndrome

Heiner syndrome, also known as food-induced pulmonary hemosiderosis, is a rare disorder seen in infants secondary to milk protein intolerance. Symptoms may include cough, recurrent fever, wheezing, dyspnea, and hemoptysis.[55] The milk protein may trigger recurrent pneumonia with infiltrates, pulmonary hemosiderosis, iron deficiency anemia, and failure to thrive. Heiner syndrome is associated with increased milk-specific IgG antibodies. This feature is in contrast to that of acute food allergy reactions, in which patients demonstrate IgE antibodies to the culprit foods. Detection of IgG antibodies to foods is not diagnostic in food allergy, except for the case of Heiner syndrome.[56] Elimination of milk protein results in the resolution of symptoms.

SUMMARY

The clinical manifestations of food allergies are varied and should first be distinguished from nonimmunologic adverse food reactions. It is helpful from a diagnostic and conceptual standpoint to delineate 3 broad categories of food allergy based on the underlying immunology: IgE-mediated, mixed IgE- and cell-mediated food allergies, and cell-mediated food allergies. Within each of these categories, the food-induced immunologic mechanisms result in the clinical symptoms of distinct food allergy disorders.

REFERENCES

1. Johansson SG, Bieber T, Dahl R, et al. Revised nomenclature for allergy for global use: report of the Nomenclature Review Committee of the World Allergy Organization, October 2003. J Allergy Clin Immunol 2004;113:832–6.
2. Young E, Stoneham MD, Petruckevitch A, et al. A population study of food intolerance. Lancet 1994;343:1127.
3. Bock SA. Prospective appraisal of complaints of adverse reactions to foods in children during the first 3 years of life. Pediatrics 1987;79:683.
4. Rona RJ, Keil T, Summers C, et al. The prevalence of food allergy: a meta-analysis. J Allergy Clin Immunol 2007;120:638–46.
5. Branum AM, Lukacs SL. Food allergy in U.S. children: trends in prevalence and hospitalizations. NCHS Data Brief 2008;10:1–8.
6. Suarez FL, Savaiano DA, Levitt MD. A comparison of symptoms after the consumption of milk or lactose-hydrolyzed milk by people with self-reported severe lactose intolerance. N Engl J Med 1995;333:1.
7. Hungerford JM. Scombroid poisoning: a review. Toxicon 2010;56:231–43.
8. Commins SP, Satinover SM, Hosen J, et al. Delayed anaphylaxis, angioedema, or urticaria after consumption of red meat in patients with IgE antibodies specific for galactose-alpha-1,3-galactose. J Allergy Clin Immunol 2009;123:426.
9. Baxi S, Dinakar C. Urticaria and angioedema. Immunol Allergy Clin North Am 2005;25:353–667.
10. Sehgal VN, Rege VL. An interrogative study of 158 urticaria patients. Ann Allergy 1973;31:279.
11. Champion RH, Roberts SO, Carpenter RG, et al. Urticaria and angio-oedema. A review of 554 patients. Br J Dermatol 1969;81:588.

12. Kobza Black A, Greaves MW, Champion RH, et al. The urticarias 1990. Br J Dermatol 1991;124:100.
13. Delgado J, Castillo R, Quiralte J, et al. Contact urticaria in a child from raw potato. Contact Dermatitis 1996;35:179.
14. Killig C, Werfel T. Contact reactions to food. Curr Allergy Asthma Rep 2008;8:209–14.
15. Simon FE. Anaphylaxis: recent advances in assessment and treatment. J Allergy Clin Immunol 2009;124:625–36.
16. Bock SA, Atkins FM. Patterns of food hypersensitivity during sixteen years of double-blind, placebo-controlled food challenges. J Pediatr 1990;117:561.
17. Host A, Halken S. A prospective study of cow milk allergy in Danish infants during the first 3 years of life. Allergy 1990;45:587–96.
18. Scrander JJ, van den Bogart JP, Forget PP, et al. Cow's milk protein intolerance in infants under 1 year of age: a prospective epidemiological study. Eur J Pediatr 1993;152:640–4.
19. Roberts G, Lack G. Relevance of inhalational exposure to food allergens. Curr Opin Allergy Clin Immunol 2003;3:211.
20. James JM, Eigenmann PA, Eggleston PA, et al. Airway reactivity changes in food-allergic, asthmatic children undergoing double-blind placebo-controlled food challenges. Am J Respir Crit Care Med 1996;153:597–603.
21. Bock SA. Respiratory reactions induced by food challenges in children with pulmonary disease. Pediatr Allergy Immunol 1992;3:188–94.
22. James JM, Bernhisel-Broadbent J, Sampson HA. Respiratory reactions provoked by double-blind food challenges in children. Am J Respir Crit Care Med 1994;149:59–64.
23. Crespo JF, Pascual C, Dominguez C, et al. Allergic reactions associated with airborne fish particles in IgE-mediated fish hypersensitive patients. Allergy 1995;50:257–61.
24. Sampson HA. Adverse reactions to foods. In: Adkinson NF, Yunginger JW, Buss WW, et al, editors. Middleton's allergy: principles and practice. 6th edition. St Louis (MO): Mosby; 2003. p. 1619.
25. Sampson HA, Mendelson LM, Rosen JP. Fatal and near-fatal anaphylactic reactions to food in children and adolescents. N Engl J Med 1992;327:380–4.
26. Sampson HA. Anaphylaxis and emergency treatment. Pediatrics 2003;11:1601.
27. Yocum MW, Khan DA. Assessment of patients who have experienced anaphylaxis: a 3-year survey. Mayo Clin Proc 1994;69:16–23.
28. Bock SA, Munoz-Furlong A, Sampson HA. Fatalities due to anaphylactic reactions to foods. J Allergy Clin Immunol 2001;107:191–3.
29. Sicherer SH, Sampson HA. Food allergy. J Allergy Clin Immunol 2010;125:S116–25.
30. Horan R, Sheffer A. Food-dependent exercise-induced anaphylaxis. Immunol Allergy Clin North Am 1991;11:757–66.
31. Bircher AJ, Van Melle G, Haller E, et al. IgE to food allergens are highly prevalent in patients allergic to pollen with and without symptoms of food allergy. Clin Exp Allergy 1994;24:367–74.
32. Eigenmann PA, Sicherer SH, Borkowski TA, et al. Prevalence of IgE-mediated food allergy among children with atopic dermatitis. Pediatrics 1998;101:E8.
33. Sicherer SH, Sampson HA. Food hypersensitivity and atopic dermatitis: pathophysiology, epidemiology, diagnosis, and management. J Allergy Clin Immunol 1999;104:S114.
34. Burks AW, James JM, Hiegel A, et al. Atopic dermatitis and food hypersensitivity reactions. J Pediatr 1998;132:132.

35. Sampson HA, McCaskill CM. Food hypersensitivity in atopic dermatitis. Curr Opin Allergy Clin Immunol 2003;3:211.
36. Noel RJ, Putnam PE, Rothenberg ME. Eosinophilic esophagitis. N Engl J Med 2004;351:940.
37. Liacouras CA, Spergel JM, Ruchelli E, et al. Eosinophilic esophagitis: a 10 year experience in 381 children. Clin Gastroenterol Hepatol 2005;3:1198.
38. Talley NJ, Shorter RG, Phillips SF, et al. Eosinophilic gastroenteritis: a clinicopathological study of patients with disease of the mucosa, muscle layer, and subserosal tissues. Gut 1990;31:54.
39. Klein NC, Hargrove RL, Sleisenger MH, et al. Eosinophilic gastroenteritis. Medicine (Baltimore) 1970;49:299.
40. Ureles AL, Alschibaja T, Lodico D, et al. Idiopathic eosinophilic infiltration of the gastrointestinal tract, diffuse and circumscribed; a proposed classification and review of the literature, with two additional cases. Am J Med 1961;30:899.
41. Leinbach GE, Rubin CE. Eosinophilic gastroenteritis: a simple reaction to food allergens? Gastroenterology 1970;59:874.
42. Patenaude Y, Bernard C, Schreiber R, et al. Cow's-milk-induced allergic colitis in an exclusively breast-fed infant: diagnosed with ultrasound. Pediatr Radiol 2000;30:379.
43. Anveden-Hertzberg L, Finkel Y, Sandstedt B, et al. Proctocolitis in exclusively breast-fed infants. Eur J Pediatr 1996;155:464.
44. Pittschieler K. Cow's milk protein-induced colitis in the breastfed infant. J Pediatr Gastroenterol Nutr 1990;10:548.
45. Lake AM, Whitington PF, Hamilton SR. Dietary protein-induced colitis in breast-fed infants. J Pediatr 1982;101:906.
46. Ravelli A, Villanacci V, Chiappa S, et al. Dietary protein-induced proctocolitis in childhood. Am J Gastroenterol 2008;103:2605.
47. Nowak-Wegrzyn A, Sampson HA, Wood RA, et al. Food protein-induced enterocolitis syndrome caused by solid food proteins. Pediatrics 2003;111:829.
48. Sicherer SH. Food protein-induced enterocolitis syndrome: case presentations and management lessons. J Allergy Clin Immunol 2005;115:149.
49. Kuitunen P, Visakorpi J, Savilahti E, et al. Malabsorption syndrome with cow's milk intolerance: clinical findings and course in 54 cases. Arch Dis Child 1975;50:351.
50. Iyngkaran N, Yadav M, Boey CG, et al. Severity and extent of upper small bowel mucosal damage in cow's milk protein-sensitive enteropathy. J Pediatr Gastroenterol Nutr 1988;7:667.
51. Walker-Smith JA. Cow milk-sensitive enteropathy: predisposing factors and treatment. J Pediatr 1992;121:S111.
52. Iyngkaran N, Robinson MJ, Prathap K, et al. Cow's milk protein-sensitive enteropathy. Combined clinical and histological criteria for diagnosis. Arch Dis Child 1978;53:20.
53. Yssing M, Jensen H, Jarnum S. Dietary treatment of protein-losing enteropathy. Acta Paediatr Scand 1967;56:173.
54. Rubin CE, Brandborg LL, Phelps PC, et al. Studies of celiac disease. I. The apparent identical and specific nature of the duodenal and proximal jejunal lesion in celiac disease and idiopathic sprue. Gastroenterology 1960;38:28.
55. Moissidis I, Chaidaroon D, Vichyanond P. Milk-induced pulmonary disease in infants (Heiner syndrome). Pediatr Allergy Immunol 2005;16(6):545–52.
56. Stapel SO, Asero R, Ballmer-Weber BK, et al. Testing for IgG4 against foods is not recommended as a diagnostic tool: EAACI task force report. Allergy 2008;63:793–6.

Epidemiology of Food Allergy

Carina Venter, PhD, RD[a,b], S. Hasan Arshad, DM, FRCP[b,c,*]

KEYWORDS

• Epidemiology • Food allergy • Prevalence • Incidence

Food allergy (FA) is perceived to be a common problem, especially during childhood. Accurate assessment of incidence and prevalence of FA has been difficult to establish, however, due to lack of universally accepted diagnostic criteria; hence, reported prevalence varies widely across the globe. Research has shown that perceived FA is 10 times higher than what can be confirmed by appropriate tests; hence, studies that rely on self-reports tend to show higher prevalence. The prevalence also depends on which foods or food additives were included and the type of adverse reaction considered. FA is defined as an immune-mediated adverse reaction to foods, and, if there is evidence of allergic sensitization (presence of immunoglobulin E) to a food, it is called IgE-mediated FA. Although many foods have been reported to cause IgE-mediated FA, most studies have focused on 4 common food groups. These are cow's milk, hen's egg, peanut/tree nuts, and fish/shellfish. There may be a true variation in the prevalence of FA in different regions of the world and a likely increase in prevalence has been observed in recent decades. This cannot be stated with confidence, however, without the use of consistent methodology and diagnostic criteria.

REPORTED FOOD ALLERGY

The natural history of FA is such that it is common in early childhood and becomes less common with age. Data from the United States showed that the annual incidence of doctor-diagnosed FA decreased from an average of 4.7% per year during the first 2 years of life to an average of 1.2% for the fifth and sixth years of age.[1] Thus, age is a major factor in determining FA prevalence. Even allowing for that, however, there

---

Financial disclosure: Dr C. Venter has given academic lectures or written educational articles for Danone, Mead Johnson, and GlaxoSmithKline. Prof. S. H. Arshad has been an advisor to the Phadia Ltd (UK).

[a] University of Portsmouth, 2 King Richard the 1st Road, Portsmouth, PO1 2FR, UK

[b] The David Hide Asthma and Allergy Research Centre, Parkurst Road, Newport, Isle of Wight, PO30 5TG, UK

[c] III Research Division, Southampton General Hospital, University of Southampton, MP: 810, Level F, South Block, Tremona Road, Southampton, SO16 6YD, UK

* Corresponding author. III Research Division, Southampton General Hospital, University of Southampton, MP: 810, Level F, South Block, Tremona Road, Southampton, SO16 6YD, UK.

E-mail address: S.H.Arshad@soton.ac.uk

Pediatr Clin N Am 58 (2011) 327–349

doi:10.1016/j.pcl.2011.02.011 **pediatric.theclinics.com**

0031-3955/11/$ – see front matter

remains considerable variation in the prevalence of FA in different populations. This is true for overall FA and also for allergy to individual foods. For example, maternally reported or doctor-diagnosed FA in early childhood was 6% in the United States[2] but only 1.7% in Israel.[3] A study from Germany, assessing doctor-diagnosed FA prospectively from 1 to 6 years of age, reported this to be 4.6% at age 1, 6.6% at age 2, and 3.9% from ages 3 to 6.[1] US data from the National Health Interview Survey in 2007 showed reported FA during childhood to be 3.9%.[4]

No two studies of FA prevalence have used the same methodology. Hence, data from the same geographic region often report widely varying prevalences. In France, Penard-Morand and colleagues[5] reported the prevalence of FA in children ages 9 to 11 to be 2.1%. In the same year, Roehr and colleagues[6] estimated FA prevalence to be 6.7% in children ages 2 to 14. In Germany, overall prevalence of reported FA was 20.8% in 1537 subjects,[7] whereas a telephone survey of 4477 adults in the United States showed self-reported FA to be 9.1%.[8] An overall view of FA prevalence was estimated by a meta-analysis of 51 studies. Self-reported FA varied between 3% and 35%, whereas confirmed FA was on average 1% to 10.8% in 6 studies using oral food challenges.[9] Only part of this variation reflects true variation in prevalence; the remainder likely relates to variation in how questions were formulated and which foods were included.

ALLERGIC SENSITIZATION

Allergic sensitization is defined by the presence of IgE antibodies to a specific food allergen. This may be assessed on skin prick test (SPT) or specific IgE as demonstrated in the serum using an immunoassay. The mere presence of IgE, however, does not necessarily mean that the subject will clinically react to the food. Thus, sensitization is often higher than true clinical FA. There is a direct correlation between the degree of sensitization and the likelihood of clinical FA. Previous studies have suggested various cutoffs, which might reliably predict FA while acknowledging that this may vary with the food and the age of the person. It has been suggested that specific IgE between 0.35 and 2 kilounits of allergen per litre (kU/L) indicates a low probability, between 0.7 and 5 kU/L moderate probability, and a high IgE level of greater than 5 kU/L a high probability of FA reaction.[10] Oral food challenge, however, may still be required in some cases to establish or exclude the diagnosis of FA.

In a birth cohort study from Germany, the prevalence of food sensitization was reported to be 9.2% in children age 2 and 11.7% in children age 6, using the ImmunoCAP (f × 5) (Phadia, Upsala, Sweden), which measures specific IgE to one or more of 6 common foods (cow's milk, hen's egg, peanut, wheat, cod fish, and soy).[1] In one of the largest multicenter studies, sera from 4522 individuals living in 13 countries were tested for IgE to at least one food allergen. Prevalence of sensitization to any of the 24 food allergens ranged from 7.7% in Reykjavik (Iceland) to 24.6% in Portland (Oregon, United States), with an overall prevalence of 16.2%.[11]

The natural history of food sensitization mirrors that of clinically reported allergy. In a large unselected study (n = 8203), the overall prevalence of food sensitization in the United States was 16.8%. The highest prevalence (28%) was observed in children 1 to 5 years old and declined steadily with age to 13.0% in adults. The prevalence of milk (22%) and egg (13.9%) sensitization was again highest in children ages 1 to 5. Peanut sensitization was most common in older children and young adults (6–19 years, 10.7%; 20–39 years, 8.7%).[10] Spontaneous remission of peanut and tree nut allergy is uncommon.[12] Savage and colleagues[13] recently reported that 50% of children with soy allergy outgrow their allergy by age 7.

INCREASING PREVALENCE OF FOOD ALLERGY

There is some support in the literature of increasing FA prevalence. The number of hospital discharges with a diagnosis of FA among children (<18 years) increased from approximately 2000 to 10,000 between 2004 and 2006, respectively.[4] A recent report from Boston suggests that food-induced anaphylaxis has been increasing in recent years, and, in addition to the classical 4 to 5 major foods, other food groups are increasingly associated with anaphylactic reactions. The report showed that the number of visits to a pediatric emergency department for food-induced anaphylaxis more than doubled from 14.9 per 10,000 visits in 2001 to 38.0 per 10,000 visits in 2006.[14]

COMMON FOOD ALLERGENS

Milk

Cow's milk protein allergy (CMA) is an immunologic reaction to the protein in cow's milk and can be IgE mediated, non–IgE mediated, or a mixture of both.[15] CMA is seen in both children[16,17] and adults.[18] The pattern of IgE-mediated and non–IgE-mediated allergies and the proportion of children suffering from IgE-mediated versus non–IgE-mediated CMA also seems to vary between countries, with higher rates of non–IgE-mediated allergy seen on the Isle of Wight (United Kingdom)[17] and in Denmark[19] than in Spain[20] and Australia.[21] Symptoms to cows' milk can also occur as a result of lactase deficiency (ie, lactose intolerance), which is a nonallergic food hypersensitivity reaction, because this indicates an inability or reduced ability to digest the carbohydrate in lactose.[22,23]

CMA usually develops in the first year of life[24] and is one of the most common allergies seen in childhood, with a documented prevalence of between 0.3% and 3.5% in young children under 5 years and less than 1% in older children (**Table 1**).

In adults, however, CMA is reported as rare, with less than 0.5% of adults suffering from cow's milk allergy (**Table 2**). The majority of data regarding CMA in adults report only sensitization data, which vary between 0.1% and 2.3%, depending on the population studied (see **Table 2**). In Australia, Woods and colleagues[33] found that only 0.7% of atopic adults had a positive SPT to cow's milk proteins and none of those patients reported symptoms associated with the consumption of cows' milk. In this population, however, a total of 4.8% reported adverse reactions when consuming dairy products but were not sensitized to cow's milk proteins.

Resolution of CMA

Several studies have looked at the remission rate of CMA. In an unselected Danish population studied by Host and Halken,[16] the overall prognosis of CMA, including both IgE-mediated and non–IgE-mediated CMA, was good, with a total recovery of 22 of 39 (56%) children at 1 year, 30 of 39 (77%) at 2 years, and 34 of 39 (87%) at 3 years. Venter and colleagues[17] reported a remission rate of 80% by age 3 in an unselected population studied in the United Kingdom. The natural history of CMA was also investigated in two centers that routinely investigated children with CMA for development of tolerance: approximately 45% to 50% of children at 1 year, 60% to 75% of children at 2 years, 85% to 90% of children at 3 years, 92% of children at 5 and 10 years, and 97% of children at 15 years of age developed tolerance.[34,35]

A recent study in the United States[18] challenged these high rates of clinical tolerance, which particularly may not be relevant for children seen in tertiary referral centers, because only 5% were tolerant at age 4 and 21% at age 8.

Table 1
Prevalence of cow's milk allergy in children

	Children (Age, y)	Prevalence of Sensitization (%)	Prevalence of Allergy (%)	Method of Diagnosis
United States				
United States (2004) Sampson[25]	Not specified		2.5	Not specified
United States (2009) Branum and Lukacs[4]	<18	12 2 (>90th percentile)	NA	NA
Europe				
France (2005) Rance et al[26]	2–14	NA	1.1	Reported cumulative incidence
France (2005) Rance et al[26]	2–5	NA	1.0	Reported
France (2005) Rance et al[26]	6–10	NA	0.6	Reported
France (2005) Rance et al[26]	11–14	NA	0.2	Reported
Norway (2001) Eggesbo et al[27]	2.5	NA	1.2	Food challenge
United Kingdom (2008) Venter et al[17]	1	0.3	1.8	Food challenge
United Kingdom (2008) Venter et al[17]	2	0.5	1.2	Food challenge
United Kingdom (2008) Venter et al[17]	3	0.5	0.45	Food challenge
United Kingdom (2008) Venter et al[17]	By 3	NA	2.3	Food challenge
United Kingdom (2008) Venter et al[28]	6	0.4	0.25	Food challenge
United Kingdom (2005) Pereira et al[29]	11	0.29	0.3	Food challenge
United Kingdom (2005) Pereira et al[29]	15	0.3	0.2	Food challenge
Denmark (1990) Host and Halken[16]	By 3	1.1	2.2	Food challenge
Denmark (2005) Osterballe et al[19]	3	NA	0.6	Food challenge
Rest of World				
Australia (1997) Hill et al[21]	2	4.1 (Cohort of infants from high-risk families)	2.02	Estimated/calculate
China (2010) Hu et al[30]	0–2	1999: 3.2 2009: 6.2	1999: 1.6 2009: 3.5	Food challenge
Israel (2002) Dalal et al[3]	0–2	NA	0.3 IgE mediated	History and sensitization

Abbreviation: NA, not available.

Table 2
Prevalence of milk allergy in adults and whole populations

	Adults (Age, y)	Prevalence of Sensitization	Prevalence of Allergy (%)	Method of Diagnosis	All Ages Sensitized (%)	All Ages Prevalence (%)
United States						
United States (2004) Sampson[25]	Not specified	—	0.3	Not specified	—	NA
United States (2009) Liu et al[10]	NA	2.3[a,11]	NA	NA	1–85 y: 5.7 sensitized	NA
United States (2007) Vierk et al[8]	18–>60	—	1.1	Self-reported doctor diagnosed	—	—
Europe						
France	20–40	0.1[a,11]	NA	NA	NA	NA
Norway	20–40	1.3[a,11]	NA	NA	NA	NA
United Kingdom	20–40	0.5[a,11]	NA	NA	NA	NA
Denmark (2009) Osterballe et al[31]	22	—	0.1	Food challenges	NA	NA
Denmark (2009) Osterballe et al[19]	Parents of a cohort of 3 y olds	—	0.3	Food challenges	NA	NA
Germany (2004) Zuberbier et al[32]	20–40	1.3[11]	NA	NA	NA (small sample)	4.5 of n = 104 with positive challenges (IgE mediated) 15.9 of n = 44 with positive challenges (non–IgE mediated)
Rest of World						
Australia (2002) Woods et al[33]	26–50	0.7 (Sensitized and tolerating milk)	4.8	Reported	NA	NA
	20–40	1.1[a,11]	NA	NA	NA	NA

[a] Random sample of adults who formed part of the European Community Respiratory Health Survey.

Several factors have been identified as playing a role in the development of tolerance, including (1) lower levels of cow's milk–specific serum IgE in the first 2 years of life than in those who remain allergic (median 1.8 kU/L vs 19.0 kU/L; $P<.001$)[18]; (2) absence of asthma or allergic rhinitis and never having been formula fed[18]; (3) the mechanisms involved in CMA, because individuals with delayed reactions have been shown to develop tolerance sooner than those with immediate reactions (In a Finnish study, 64% of those children with delayed symptoms developed tolerance at age 2, 92% at age 3, and 96% at age 4 vs 31% of those with immediate reactions developing tolerance at age 2, 53% at age 3, and 63% at age 4, respectively.)[36]; and (4) IgE sensitization to cow's milk in the first year of life, associated with an increased risk of persisting CMA by age 3.[37]

Egg Allergy

Egg allergy is, alongside milk, one of the most prevalent FAs in children. The estimated prevalence varies between 0.5% and 5% in early childhood (**Table 3**). Limited data available suggest that egg allergy is much less common in older children and adults, with an estimated prevalence in both cases of less than 0.5% (see **Table 3; Table 4**).

Resolution of Egg Allergy

In general, the prognosis for children with egg allergy is good.[39] Approximately half of egg-allergic children are tolerant by age 3 and 66% by age 5.[40,41] Egg allergy is considered mainly IgE mediated, although some non–IgE-mediated reactions, mainly related to eczema, have been reported.[17,42]

As with CMA, development of clinical tolerance may show reduced or delayed patterns when studying populations referred to tertiary centers. Retrospective data from the United States indicate that in these populations, only 11% of subjects develop clinical tolerance by age 4, 26% of subjects by age 6, 53% of subjects by age 10, and 82% of subjects by age 16.[13]

Risk factors identified for the persistence of egg allergy include (1) high levels of egg-specific serum IgE at diagnosis, (2) the presence of atopic disease, and (3) the presence of other FAs.[13]

Although several articles have reported peanut allergy recurring, only one case of egg allergy recurrence in adulthood after a period of tolerance (of approximately 23 years) has been reported. In this case, a 30-year old pregnant woman presented with egg allergy at the end of her pregnancy, which was characterized with immediate severe reactions and anaphylaxis.[43]

Wheat

Many people believe that they have a wheat allergy or intolerance, but research suggests that in reality, this is confirmed in only a few cases. In the United Kingdom, in a large nationwide survey conducted in 1994, 20.4% of people reported that they had an allergy to any food, of which 0.9% reported being allergic to wheat.[44] A more recent consumer survey in 2009 reported that 4.5% of the population then considered themselves wheat allergic or wheat intolerant.[45] The limited data in the literature however, suggest a prevalence of less than 0.5% to 1% (**Tables 5** and **6**). Studying the prevalence of wheat allergy is further complicated by deciphering the underlying mechanism involved and whether or not the wheat-induced adverse reactions are indeed caused by IgE immune-mediated reactions or non–IgE immune-mediated reactions, wheat intolerance to non-allergic food hypersensitivity,[46] or an inability to digest the poorly absorbed carbohydrates in wheat.[46] In addition,

Table 3
Prevalence of egg allergy in children

	Children (Age, y)	Prevalence of Sensitization (%)	Prevalence of Allergy (%)	Method of Diagnosis
United States				
United States (2004) Sampson[25]	Not specified	—	1.3	Not specified
United States (2009) Branum and Lukacs[4]	<18	7 Sensitized 2.2 Sensitized (>90th percentile)	NA	NA
Europe				
France (2005) Rance et al[26]	2–14	NA	0.8	Reported cumulative incidence
France (2005) Rance et al[26]	2–5	—	0.7	Reported
France (2005) Rance et al[26]	6–10	—	0.8	Reported
France (2005) Rance et al[26]	11–14	—	0.2	Reported
Norway (2001) Eggesbo et al[38]	2.5	NA	2.6	Food challenges
United Kingdom (2008) Venter et al[17]	1	1.8	1.8	Food challenges
United Kingdom (2008) Venter et al[17]	2	2.1	1.2	Food challenges
United Kingdom (2008) Venter et al[17]	3	1.4	0.45	Food challenges
United Kingdom (2008) Venter et al[17]	By 3	—	2.3	Food challenges
United Kingdom (2008) Venter et al[17]	6	0.9	0.25	Food challenges
United Kingdom (2005) Pereira et al[29]	11	0.29	0.26	Food challenges
United Kingdom (2005) Pereira et al[29]	15	0.15	0.13	Food challenges
Denmark (2005) Osterballe et al[19]	3	—	1.6	Food challenges
Rest of World				
Australia (2007) Hill et al[21]	2	16.4 (Cohort of infants from high-risk families)	3.2	Estimated/calculated
China (2010) Hu et al[30]	0–2	1999: 7.3 2010: 15.5	2.9 (1999) 5.0 (2009)	Food challenges
Israel (2002) Dalal et al[3]	0–2	—	0.5	History and SPT

Table 4
Prevalence of egg allergy in adults and whole populations

	Adults (Age, y)	Prevalence of Sensitization (%)	Prevalence of Allergy (%)	Method of Diagnosis	All Ages Sensitization (%)	All Ages Prevalence
United States						
United States (2004) Sampson[25]	Not specified	—	0.2	Not specified	NA	NA
	NA	0[a,11]	NA	NA	1–85 y: 3.9 sensitized[10]	NA
United States (2007) Vierk et al[8]	18–>60	—	0.3	Self-reported doctor diagnosed	—	—
Europe						
France	20–40	0.1[a,11]	NA	NA	NA	NA
Norway	20–40	1.5[a,11]	NA	NA	NA	NA
United Kingdom	20– 40	0.5[a,11]	NA	NA	NA	NA
Denmark (2005) Osterballe et al[19]	Parents of 3-y-old cohort	NA	0.1	Food challenges	NA	NA
Denmark (2009) Osterballe et al[31]	22	—	0	Food challenges	NA	NA
Germany (2004) Zuberbier et al[32]	20–40	0.3[11]	NA	NA	NA (small sample)	2.9% of n = 104 with positive challenges (IgE mediated)
Rest of World						
Australia (2002) Woods et al[33]	26–50	1.8 (Sensitized and 0.2 not tolerating egg)	1.3% (0.2% sensitised and not tolerating wheat + 1.1% not sensitised and not tolerating wheat)	History	NA	NA
	20–40	0.5[a,11]	NA	NA	NA	NA

[a] Random sample of adults who formed part of the European Community Respiratory Health Survey.

Table 5
Prevalence of wheat allergy in children

	Children (Age, y)	Prevalence of Sensitization (%)	Prevalence of Diagnosed Food Allergy (%)	Method of Diagnosis
United States				
—	NA	NA	NA	NA
Europe				
United Kingdom (2008) Venter[17]	1	0	0.3	Food challenges
United Kingdom (2008) Venter et al[17]	2	0.2	0.3	Food challenges
United Kingdom (2008) Venter et al[17]	3	0	0.2	Food challenges
United Kingdom (2008) Venter et al[17]	By 3	—	0.3	Food challenges
United Kingdom (2006) Venter et al[28]	6	0.4	0.4	Food challenges
United Kingdom (2005) Pereira et al[29]	11	0.57	0.0	Food challenges
United Kingdom (2005) Pereira et al[29]	15	1.2	0.1	Food challenges
Denmark (2005) Osterballe et al[19]	3	NA	0	Food challenges
France (2005) Rance et al[26]	2–14	NA	0.18	Reported
Rest of World				
Australia (1997) Hill et al[21]	2	NA	0.15	Estimated/calculated
China (2010) Hu et al[30]	0–2	1999: 0.3 2009: 0.5	NA	NA

Table 6
Prevalence of wheat allergy in adults and whole populations

	Adults (Age, y)	Prevalence of Sensitization (%)	Prevalence of Wheat Allergy (%)	Method of Diagnosis	All Ages Sensitization (%)	All Ages Prevalence
United States						
United States	20–40	6.1[a,11]	NA	NA	NA	NA
United States (2007) Vierk et al[8]	18–>60	NA	0.4	Self-reported doctor diagnosed	NA	NA
Europe						
United Kingdom	20–40	3.9[a,11]	NA	NA	NA	NA
Denmark (2005) Osterballe et al[19]	Parents of 3-y-olds cohort	NA	0	Food challenges	NA	NA
Denmark (2009) Osterballe et al[31]	22	—	0	Food challenges	NA	NA
Germany (2004) Zuberbier et al[32]	20–40	6.0[a,11]	—	—	NA (small sample)	14.9% Allergic to "flour" of n = 104 with positive challenges (IgE mediated) 6.8% Allergic to "flour" of n = 44 with positive challenges (non–IgE mediated/intolerance)
France	20–40	5.5[11]	NA	NA	NA	NA
Rest of World						
Australia (2002) Woods et al[33]	26–50	2.2 (Sensitized and tolerating wheat)	1.3	Reported	—	—
Australia	20–40	7.9[a,11]	NA	NA	NA	NA

[a] Random sample of adults who formed part of the European Community Respiratory Health Survey.

wheat-induced symptoms may also indicate the presence of celiac disease (a non–IgE immune-mediated reaction to gluten).[47]

Resolution of Wheat Allergy

Little is known about the natural history of wheat allergy, with only two studies available in the literature. A recent study from Finland[48] performed in children (n = 28) between 6 and 75 months of age, showed clinical tolerance in 59%, 69%, 84%, and 96% by ages 4, 6, 10, and 16 years, respectively. Both IgE-mediated and non–IgE-mediated symptoms were experienced by the children, presenting as skin symptoms (likely IgE mediated) and gut-related symptoms (likely non–IgE mediated). In a study from the United States,[49] 103 children with a history of reactions to wheat and sensitization to wheat were followed and the rates of tolerance noted were 29% by 4 years, 56% by 8 years, and 65% by 12 years. The median age of resolution of wheat allergy was approximately 6.5 years in this population. In both studies, only a minority of patients experienced ongoing wheat allergy into adolescence.

Factors that affected the development of clinical tolerance include (1) sensitization to gliadin with an SPT wheal of greater than or equal to 5 mm at the time of the diagnostic challenge, associated with a slower course of recovery from wheat allergy (P = .019),[48] and (2) higher wheat serum IgE levels, associated with poorer outcomes, although many children outgrew wheat allergy with even the highest levels of wheat-specific IgE.[49]

Fish and Shellfish

A wide range of seafood has been implicated in food-allergic responses, but the species identified usually reflects their availability and consumption. Regarding fish, cod, tuna, salmon, trout, and plaice have been involved in food-allergic reactions in the United States, United Kingdom, and Europe. Less well known species, such as sea urchin roe, boiled razor-shellclam, krill, bonita, yellowtail, saurel, skipper, pomfret, hilsa, and bhetki, are often eaten in other countries, such as Spain,[50,51] Japan,[52] and India.[53] The prevalence of fish allergy is low in children (≤0.2% [**Table 7**]) and adults (≤0.5% [**Table 8**]).

Although the prevalence of shellfish allergy is still lower in children (≤0.5% [**Table 9**]) than adults (≤2.5% [**Table 10**]), it is slightly higher than fish allergy.

Seafood allergy is usually only associated with immediate symptoms related to an IgE-mediated food hypersensitivity response and is not normally implicated in delayed reactions. Few of the children sensitized to cod fish were diagnosed with a clinical allergy to fish in a UK study, with the majority of the children consuming cod fish on a regular basis.[17] In this cohort, however, fish accounted for 11.4% of reported reactions, whereas shellfish accounted for only 3.8% of reactions.[29] A Danish study of a cohort of 3-year-old children and their older siblings reported they were unable to confirm any reported reactions to cod fish or shrimp in these children, although the actual prevalence of the same FAs in their parents was reported to be 0.2% to cod and 0.3% to shrimp (see **Tables 7–10**).[19]

Results from a US telephone survey suggest a prevalence of 0.2% for fish allergy in children and 0.5% in adults. Prevalence of an allergy to shellfish was 0.5% in children and 2.5% in adults. A more recent study suggests, however, that the prevalence of shellfish allergy is less than 0.3% for doctor-diagnosed allergy in adults. The reported fish allergy was higher than before (0.6% vs 0.5%).[8,54]

Seafood allergy is thought to be lifelong. Some studies and case reports suggest, however, that remission may be possible. Solensky[56] reported a case of resolution of fish allergy in an adult with a history of fish anaphylaxis and, in a study of 32 children

Table 7
Prevalence of fish allergy in children

	Children (Age, y)	Prevalence of Sensitization (%)	Prevalence of Diagnosed Food Allergy (%)	Method of Diagnosis
United States and Canada				
United States (2004) Sampson[25]	Not specified	NA	0.1	Not specified
United States (2004) Sicherer et al[54]	0–17	NA	0.2	Reported
Canada (2010) Ben-Shoshan et al[55]	>18	NA	0.18	Self-reported doctor diagnosed
Europe				
United Kingdom (2008) Venter et al[17]	1	0.3	0.1	Food challenges
United Kingdom (2008) Venter et al[17]	2	0.5	0	Food challenges
United Kingdom (2008) Venter et al[17]	3	0.5	0	Food challenges
United Kingdom (2008) Venter et al[17]	By 3		0.1	Food challenges
United Kingdom (2006) Venter et al[28]	6	1.0	0	Food challenges
United Kingdom (2005) Pereira et al[29]	11	1.3	0.0	Food challenges
United Kingdom (2005) Pereira et al[29]	15	1.4	0.1	Food challenges
Denmark (2005) Osterballe et al[19]	3	NA	0	Food challenges
Rest of World				
Australia (1997) Hill et al[21]	2	NA	0.07	Estimated/calculated
China (2010) Hu et al[30]	0–2	1999: 0.3 2009: 0.75	NA	NA
Israel (2002) Dalal et al[3]	0–2	—	0.1	History and SPT

Table 8
Prevalence of fish allergy in adults and whole populations

	Adults (Age, y)	Prevalence of Sensitization (%)	Prevalence of Fish Allergy (%)	Method of Diagnosis	All Ages Prevalence
United States					
United States (2004) Sampson[25]	Not specified	—	0.4	Not specified	NA
United States	20–40	0[a,10]	NA	NA	NA
United States (2004) Sicherer et al[54]	18–>61	NA	0.5	Reported	NA
United States (2007) Vierk et al[8]	18–>60	NA	0.6	Self-reported doctor diagnosed	NA
Canada (2010) Ben-Shoshan et al[55]	>18	NA	0.56	Self-reported doctor diagnosed	NA
Europe					
United Kingdom	20–40	0.2[10]	NA	NA	NA
Denmark (2005) Osterballe et al[19]	Parents of 3 y olds	NA	0.2	Food challenges	NA
Denmark (2009) Osterballe et al[31]	22	NA	0.1	Food challenges	NA
Germany (2004) Zuberbier et al[32]	20–40	0.9[a,10]	NA	NA	Food challenges 0–79 years: 0
France	20–40	0[10]	NA	NA	NA
Rest of World					
Australia	20–40	0[a,10]	NA	NA	NA

[a] Random sample of adults who formed part of the European Community Respiratory Health Survey.

Table 9
Prevalence of shellfish allergy in children

	Children (Age, y)	Prevalence of Sensitization (%)	Prevalence of Diagnosed Food Allergy (%)	Method of Diagnosis
United Kingdom and Canada				
United Kingdom (2004) Sampson[25]	Not specified	NA	0.1	Not specified
United Kingdom (2004) Sicherer et al[54]	0–17	NA	0.5	Reported
United Kingdom (2009) Branum and Lukacs[4]	<18	5.2	NA	NA
Canada (2010) Ben-Shoshan et al[55]	>18	NA	0.5	Self-reported doctor diagnosed
Europe				
United Kingdom (2008) Venter et al[17]	1	0	0	Food challenges
United Kingdom (2008) Venter et al[17]	2	0	0	Food challenges
United Kingdom (2008) Venter et al[17]	3	0	0	Food challenges
United Kingdom (2008) Venter et al[17]	By 3		0	Food challenges
United Kingdom (2008) Venter et al[28]	6	0	0.0	Food challenges
United Kingdom (2005) Pereira et al[29]	11	0.14	0.13	Food challenges
United Kingdom (2005) Pereira et al[29]	15	1.5	1.3	Food challenges
Denmark (2005) Osterballe et al[19]	3	NA	0	Food challenges
France (2005) Rance et al[26]	2–14	NA	1.4	Reported cumulative incidence
France (2005) Rance et al[26]	2–5	NA	0.2	Reported
France (2005) Rance et al[26]	6–10	NA	1.8	
France (2005) Rance et al[26]	11–14	NA	1.2	
Rest of World				
Australia	2	NA	NA	NA
China (2010) Hu et al[30]	0–2	1999: 0 2009: 0.3	NA	NA

Table 10
Prevalence of shellfish allergy in adults and whole populations

	Adults (Age, y)	Prevalence of Sensitization (%)	Prevalence of Shell Fish Allergy (%)	Method of Diagnosis	All Ages Prevalence (%)
United States and Canada					
United States (2004) Sampson[25]	Not specified	NA	2	—	Sensitization: 5.9 Allergy: 0.99[10]
United States	20–40	0 (Shrimp)[a,11]	NA	NA	NA
United States (2004) Sicherer et al[54]	18–>61	NA	2.5	Reported	NA
United States (2007) Vierk et al[8]	18–>60	NA	0.3	Self-reported doctor diagnosed	NA
Canada (2010) Ben-Shoshan et al[55]	>18	NA	1.69	Self-reported doctor diagnosed	NA
Europe					
United Kingdom	20–40	6.2 (Shrimp)[a,11]	NA	NA	NA
Denmark (2005) Osterballe et al[19]	Parents of 3 y olds	NA	0.3 (Shrimp)	Food challenge	NA
Denmark (2009) Osterballe et al[31]	22	NA	0.2 (Shrimp)	Food challenge	NA
Germany	20–40	4. 4 (Shrimp)[a,11]	NA	NA	0–79: 0[32]
France	20–40	7.0 (Shrimp)[a,11]	NA	NA	NA
Rest of World					
Australia (2002) Woods et al[33]	26–50	2002: 3.7 (0.9 Sensitized and not tolerating shrimp)	4.2 Reported a problem with ingesting shrimp (0.9 was sensitized and 3.3 not sensitized)	Reported	NA

[a] Random sample of adults who formed part of the European Community Respiratory Health Survey.

with fish allergy, 5 seemed to lose their allergy.[57] In contrast, this has yet to be reported for those who are allergic to shellfish, with no change in specific IgE antibody levels to shrimp reported in 11 shrimp-allergic subjects over a 2-year period.[58]

Peanut Allergy

Peanut allergy is the most common cause of food-induced anaphylaxis. In 1999, Sicherer and colleagues[59] reported that approximately 0.6% of the general population suffer from peanut allergy. Using the same methodology (random digit dialing), they reassessed the prevalence in 2002[60] and 2008.[61] There was a small increase in prevalence to 0.8% in 2008. Ben-Shoshan and colleagues[55] reported recently a 1% peanut and 1.22% tree nut allergy prevalence in Canada. As shown in **Table 11**, other studies indicate prevalences that vary from 0.06% (Israel) to 5.9% (Sweden).

Table 11
Prevalence of reported allergy to peanut

Country	Age Assessed (y)	N	Prevalence (%)	First Author
North America				
United States (2007)	18–85	4477	0.5	Vierk et al[8]
United States (1999)	1–65	12,032	0.6	Sicherer et al[59]
United States (2003)	1–65	13,493	0.6	Sicherer et al[60]
United States (2010)	1–65	13,534	0.8	Sicherer et al[61]
United States (2010)	1–85	8203	1.3	Liu et al[10]
Canada (2010)	1–65	3613	1.0	Ben-Shoshan et al[55]
Canada (2003)	7	4254	1.5	Kagan et al[62]
Europe				
France (2005)	9–11	6672	0.3	Penard-Morand et al[5]
France (2005)	2–14	2716	0.7	Rance et al[26]
Germany (2001)	25–74	1537	2.1	Schafer et al[7]
Sweden (2004)	13–21	1451	5.9	Marklund et al[63]
United Kingdom (1996)	4	1218	0.5	Tariq et al[64]
United Kingdom (2002)	3–4	1273	1.0	Grundy et al[65]
United Kingdom (2005)	11	775	1.8	Pereira et al[29]
United Kingdom (2006)	6	798	1.9	Venter et al[28]
United Kingdom (2005)	15	757	2.5	Pereira et al[29]
United Kingdom (2008)	4–18	3943	1.9	Du Toit et al[66]
Rest of the World				
Australia (2002)	20–45	1141	0.6	Woods et al[33]
Israel (2002)	0–2	9040	0.06	Dalal et al[3]
Israel (2008)	4–18	4657	0.2	Du Toit et al[66]
Singapore (2010)	4–6	4390	3.6	Shek et al[67]
Singapore (2010)	14–16	6450	1.18	Shek et al[67]
Philippines (2010)	14–16	11,322	1.29	Shek et al[67]
United Kingdom (2005)	15	649	2.6	Pereira et al[29]
United Kingdom (2002)	3–4	1246	3.3	Grundy et al[65]
United Kingdom (2005)	11	699	3.7	Pereira et al[29]

In a large US study, overall peanut sensitization in children and adults was 7.6%.[10] In the EuroPrevall study, peanut sensitization varied from 0.8% in Norway to 9.3% in the United States, with an overall prevalence of 2.6%.[11] Various other studies have reported prevalences of peanut sensitization between 1% and 11% in Europe (**Table 12**).

Peanut allergy often starts in early childhood but a late-onset group has also been identified in whom peanut allergy occurs for the first time in early adult life.[68] A small proportion (20%) of children with peanut allergy outgrow their allergy by adolescence or early adult life and occasionally a relapse may occur.[69] A low level of peanut-specific IgE or negative SPT indicates this possibility. In one study, however, both children and adults were shown clinically reactive to peanut despite negative skin test.[68]

Tree Nut Allergy

The prevalence of tree nut allergy in the United States has not changed much since 1997 and remained at approximately 0.5% (**Table 13**). The prevalence among children in European countries varied from 0.2% in France to 1.4% in the United Kingdom. In adolescents the prevalence was higher (2.2% to 4.1%) and in adults possibly even more so, with a reported 8.6% prevalence in one German study.

In a recent meta-analysis, the prevalence of perceived reactions to any tree nuts ranged from 0.03% to 1.4%, and the prevalence of sensitization was 0.02% to 0.7%.[71] The EuroPrevall study reported a sensitization to walnut in 2.2% and to hazel nut in 7.8% of 4220 adults.[11]

Allergy to tree nuts may start in childhood or occur for the first time in adult life. This allergy is usually persistent but approximately 10% of children grow out of tree nut allergy and among those with a low specific IgE (<5 kU/L), nearly 50% grow out.[69,72]

Allergy to Plant Food

Few studies have assessed allergy to foods, such as fruits, vegetables, legumes (except peanut), cereals, and meat. In children, the reported prevalence of food allergy to fruit or vegetables was 0.8% (56 of 6672).[5] In adults, however, perceived FA may be relatively high, as indicated by a study from Germany. This study showed a prevalence of reported allergy to vegetable of 3% and to fruits 6%.[7] Allergic symptoms to various fruits and some vegetables may be due to cross-reactive proteins in pollens, which is termed pollen-fruit syndrome or oral allergy syndrome. In this syndrome, IgE antibodies to pollen proteins react against similar proteins present in fruits and

Table 12
Prevalence of sensitization to peanut

Country	Age Assessed (y)	N	Sensitized (%)	First Author
North America				
United States (2010)	1–85	8203	7.6	Liu et al[10]
Europe				
Germany (2001)	25–74	4178	11.1	Schafer et al[7]
France (2005)	9–11	6672	1.1	Penard-Morand et al[5]
Sweden (2010)	2	1082	2.1	Schnabel et al[1]
Sweden (2010)	6	1982	5.2	Schnabel et al[1]
United Kingdom (1996)	4	981	1.1	Tariq et al[64]
United Kingdom (2008)	3	642	2.0	Venter et al[17]
United Kingdom (2006)	6	700	2.6	Venter et al[28]

Table 13
Tree nut allergy prevalence studies

	Age (y)	N	Reported Prevalence (%)	Sensitized (SPT or Specific IgE) (%)	History plus Sensitized (%)
North America					
United States (1999) Sicherer et al[59]	1–65	12,032	0.5	—	—
United States (2003) Sicherer et al[60]	1–65	13,493	0.6	—	—
United States (2010) Sicherer et al[61]	1–65	13,534	0.6	—	—
United States (2007) Vierk et al[8]	18–85	4477	0.5	—	—
Canada (2010) Ben-Shoshan et al[55]	1–65	3613	1.22	1	—
Europe					
France (2005) Penard-Morand et al[5]	7–9	6672	0.2	—	—
France (2005) Rance et al[26]	2–14	2716	0.7	—	—
Germany (2001) Schafer et al[7]	25–74	1537	8.5	17.8	—
Sweden (2004) Marklund et al[63]	13–21	1451	4.1	—	—
United Kingdom (1996) Tariq et al[64]	4	1218	—	0.2	0.2
United Kingdom (2008) Venter et al[17]	3	891	—	—	0.7
United Kingdom (2006) Venter et al[70]	6	798	1.4	—	0.4
United Kingdom (2005) Pereira et al[29]	11	775	1.2	—	—
United Kingdom (2005) Pereira et al[29]	15	757	2.2	—	—
Rest of the World					
Israel (2002) Dalal et al[3]	0–2	9040	0.03	—	0.02
Singapore (2010) Shek et al[67]	4–6 14–16	4339 6436	3.41 0.81	— —	— —
Philippines (2010) Shek et al[67]	14–16	11,071	0.72	—	—

vegetables, causing oral symptoms on ingestion. In a study from Sweden, 142 of 1451 (9.8%) adolescents ages 13 to 14 had oral allergy syndrome–like symptoms, such as itching and swelling of the lips and oral cavity.[63] Those sensitized to fruit and vegetable are often also sensitized to birch pollen (**Table 14**). In another study, however, the prevalence of self-reported FA to fruits and vegetables was 10% in early childhood and increased to 33% in the population above age 30.[73]

In a recent systemic review,[71,74] the prevalence of perceived allergy to any fruit varied from 0.4% to 11.5%. In adults, reported allergy to individual fruits was less

Table 14
Allergic sensitization to common plant origin foods in a multicenter study

Food	Sensitized (Specific IgE) (%)	Sensitized (Excluding Birch Positive) (%)
Apple	4.2	2.0
Peach	5.4	2.8
Melon	1.6	1.0
Tomato	3.3	2.3
Carrot	3.6	2.0
Celery	3.5	1.8
Sesame	3.7	2.8
Poppy seed	1.8	1.4
Sunflower	2.1	1.8
Mustard	0.9	0.8
Banana	2.5	2.4
Kiwifruit	3.6	2.7
Wheat	4.6	3.4
Buckwheat	2.8	2.2
Rice	2.9	2.2
Corn	3.3	2.6
Soya	2.1	1.4

Data from Burney P, Summers C, Chinn S, et al. Prevalence and distribution of sensitization to foods in the European Community Respiratory Health Survey: a EuroPrevall analysis. Allergy 2010; 65:1182–8.

than 1% in all studies and similarly, the prevalence of sensitization (assessed by SPT) to specific fruits was well below 1%. Overall, for fruits and vegetables, the prevalence based on perception was generally higher than that based on sensitization, but for wheat and soy, sensitization was higher. The prevalence of challenge-proved FA to fruits ranged from 0.1% to 4.3%.

SUMMARY

FA is commonly reported, but there is a large discrepancy between reported and diagnosed FA. The true prevalence of FA in adults particularly needs further investigation. In children, the prevalence of FAs depends on the food studied and the country involved. It seems that there may be pockets of higher and lower prevalence across the world and FA may be increasing in some countries, such as the United States. Many foods are reported to cause symptoms of FA, but only 6 to 7 foods and ingredients form the core components of FAs, although the number of foods increases dramatically if plant FAs are included.

REFERENCES

1. Schnabel E, Sausenthaler S, Schaaf B, et al. Prospective association between food sensitization and food allergy: results of the LISA birth cohort study. Clin Exp Allergy 2010;40:450–7.
2. Luccioli S, Ross M, Labiner-Wolfe J, et al. Maternally reported food allergies and other food-related health problems in infants: characteristics and associated factors. Pediatrics 2008;122(Suppl 2):S105–12.

3. Dalal I, Binson I, Reifen R, et al. Food allergy is a matter of geography after all: sesame as a major cause of severe IgE-mediated food allergic reactions among infants and young children in Israel. Allergy 2002;57:362–5.
4. Branum AM, Lukacs SL. Food allergy among children in the United States. Pediatrics 2009;124:1549–55.
5. Penard-Morand C, Raherison C, Kopferschmitt C, et al. Prevalence of food allergy and its relationship to asthma and allergic rhinitis in schoolchildren. Allergy 2005;60:1165–71.
6. Roehr CC, Edenharter G, Reimann S, et al. Food allergy and intolerance in children and adolescents. Clin Exp Allergy 2004;34:1534–41.
7. Schafer T, Bohler E, Ruhdorfer S, et al. Epidemiology of food allergy/food intolerance in adults: associations with other manifestations of atopy. Allergy 2001;56: 1172–9.
8. Vierk KA, Koehler KM, Fein SB, et al. Prevalence of self-reported food allergy in American adults and use of food labels. J Allergy Clin Immunol 2007;119:1504–10.
9. Rona RJ, Keil T, Summers C, et al. The prevalence of food allergy: a meta-analysis. J Allergy Clin Immunol 2007;120:638–46.
10. Liu HA, Jaramillo R, Sicherer SH, et al. National prevalence and risk factors for food allergy and relationship to asthma: results from the National Health and Nutrition Examination Survey 2005–2006. J Allergy Clin Immunol 2010;126:798–806.
11. Burney P, Summers C, Chinn S, et al. Prevalence and distribution of sensitization to foods in the European Community Respiratory Health Survey: a EuroPrevall analysis. Allergy 2010;65:1182–8.
12. Sicherer SH, Sampson HA. Peanut allergy: emerging concepts and approaches for an apparent epidemic. J Allergy Clin Immunol 2007;120:491–503.
13. Savage JH, Matsui EC, Skripak JM, et al. The natural history of egg allergy. J Allergy Clin Immunol 2007;120:1413–7.
14. Rudders SA, Banerji A, Vassallo MF, et al. Trends in pediatric emergency department visits for food-induced anaphylaxis. J Allergy Clin Immunol 2010;126:385–8.
15. Sicherer SH, Sampson HA. 9. Food allergy. J Allergy Clin Immunol 2006;117: S470–5.
16. Host A, Halken S. A prospective study of cow milk allergy in Danish infants during the first 3 years of life. Clinical course in relation to clinical and immunological type of hypersensitivity reaction. Allergy 1990;45:587–96.
17. Venter C, Pereira B, Voigt K, et al. Prevalence and cumulative incidence of food hypersensitivity in the first 3 years of life. Allergy 2008;63:354–9.
18. Skripak JM, Matsui EC, Mudd K, et al. The natural history of IgE-mediated cow's milk allergy. J Allergy Clin Immunol 2007;120:1172–7.
19. Osterballe M, Hansen TK, Mortz CG, et al. The prevalence of food hypersensitivity in an unselected population of children and adults. Pediatr Allergy Immunol 2005;16:567–73.
20. Martorell A, Plaza AM, Bone J, et al. Cow's milk protein allergy. A multi-centre study: clinical and epidemiological aspects. Allergol Immunopathol (Madr) 2006;34:46–53.
21. Hill DJ, Hosking CS, Zhie CY, et al. The frequency of food allergy in Australia and Asia. Environ Toxicol Pharmacol 1997;4:101–10.
22. Vandenplas Y, Koletzko S, Isolauri E, et al. Guidelines for the diagnosis and management of cow's milk protein allergy in infants. Arch Dis Child 2007;92:902–8.
23. Johansson SG, Bieber T, Dahl R, et al. Revised nomenclature for allergy for global use: Report of the Nomenclature Review Committee of the World Allergy Organization, October 2003. J Allergy Clin Immunol 2004;113:832–6.

24. Heine RG, Elsayed S, Hosking CS, et al. Cow's milk allergy in infancy. Curr Opin Allergy Clin Immunol 2002;2:217–25.
25. Sampson HA. Update on food allergy. J Allergy Clin Immunol 2004;113:805–19.
26. Rance F, Grandmottet X, Grandjean H. Prevalence and main characteristics of schoolchildren diagnosed with food allergies in France. Clin Exp Allergy 2005; 35:167–72.
27. Eggesbo M, Botten G, Halvorsen R, et al. The prevalence of CMA/CMPI in young children: the validity of parentally perceived reactions in a population-based study. Allergy 2001;56:393–402.
28. Venter C, Pereira B, Grundy J, et al. Prevalence of sensitization reported and objectively assessed food hypersensitivity amongst six-year-old children: a population-based study. Pediatr Allergy Immunol 2006;17:356–63.
29. Pereira B, Venter C, Grundy J, et al. Prevalence of sensitization to food allergens, reported adverse reaction to foods, food avoidance, and food hypersensitivity among teenagers. J Allergy Clin Immunol 2005;116:884–92.
30. Hu Y, Chen J, Li H. Comparison of food allergy prevalence among Chinese infants in Chongqing, 2009 versus 1999. Pediatr Int 2010;52:820–4.
31. Osterballe M, Mortz CG, Hansen TK, et al. The prevalence of food hypersensitivity in young adults. Pediatr Allergy Immunol 2009;20:686–92.
32. Zuberbier T, Edenharter G, Worm M, et al. Prevalence of adverse reactions to food in Germany—a population study. Allergy 2004;59:338–45.
33. Woods RK, Stoney RM, Raven J, et al. Reported adverse food reactions overestimate true food allergy in the community. Eur J Clin Nutr 2002;56:31–6.
34. James JM, Sampson HA. Immunologic changes associated with the development of tolerance in children with cow milk allergy. J Pediatr 1992;121: 371–7.
35. Isolauri E, Suomalainen H, Kaila M, et al. Local immune response in patients with cow milk allergy: follow-up of patients retaining allergy or becoming tolerant. J Pediatr 1992;120:9–15.
36. Vanto T, Helppila S, Juntunen-Backman K, et al. Prediction of the development of tolerance to milk in children with cow's milk hypersensitivity. J Pediatr 2004;144: 218–22.
37. Host A, Jacobsen HP, Halken S, et al. The natural history of cow's milk protein allergy/intolerance. Eur J Clin Nutr 1995;49(Suppl 1):S13–8.
38. Eggesbo M, Botten G, Halvorsen R, et al. The prevalence of allergy to egg: a population-based study in young children. Allergy 2001;56:403–11.
39. Tey D, Heine RG. Egg allergy in childhood: an update. Curr Opin Allergy Clin Immunol 2009;9:244–50.
40. Boyano-Martinez T, Garcia-Ara C, Diaz-Pena JM, et al. Prediction of tolerance on the basis of quantification of egg white-specific IgE antibodies in children with egg allergy. J Allergy Clin Immunol 2002;110:304–9.
41. Hattevig G, Kjellman B, Bjorksten B. Clinical symptoms and IgE responses to common food proteins and inhalants in the first 7 years of life. Clin Allergy 1987;17:571–8.
42. Niggemann B, Reibel S, Roehr CC, et al. Predictors of positive food challenge outcome in non-IgE-mediated reactions to food in children with atopic dermatitis. J Allergy Clin Immunol 2001;108:1053–8.
43. Hu W, Katelaris CH, Kemp AS. Recurrent egg allergy in adulthood. Allergy 2007; 62:709.
44. Young E, Stoneham MD, Petruckevitch A, et al. A population study of food intolerance. Lancet 1994;343:1127–30.

45. Kember Associates. Results of a consumer survey into attitudes towards bread, nutrition and allergy/intolerance. London: NABIM; 2009.
46. Lomer MC. The role of food hypersensitivity in gastro-intestinal disease. In: Skypala I, Venter C, editors. Food hypersensitivity: diagnosing and managing food allergies and intolerances. Oxford: Blackwells Ltd; 2008. p. 37–57.
47. McGough N, Merrikin E, Kirk E. Food hypersensitivity involving cereals: coeliac disease. In: Skypala I, Venter C, editors. Food hypersensitivity: diagnosing and managing food allergies and intolerances. Oxford: Blackwells Ltd; 2008. p. 183–202.
48. Kotaniemi-Syrjanen A, Palosuo K, Jartti T, et al. The prognosis of wheat hypersensitivity in children. Pediatr Allergy Immunol 2010;21:e421–8.
49. Keet CA, Matsui EC, Dhillon G, et al. The natural history of wheat allergy. Ann Allergy Asthma Immunol 2009;102:410–5.
50. Martin-Garcia C, Carnes J, Blanco R, et al. Selective hypersensitivity to boiled razor shell. J Investig Allergol Clin Immunol 2007;17:271–3.
51. Rodriguez V, Gracia MT, Iriarte P, et al. Allergy to dogfish. Allergy 2003;58:1315–7.
52. Koyama H, Kakami M, Kawamura M, et al. Grades of 43 fish species in Japan based on IgE-binding activity. Allergol Int 2006;55:311–6.
53. Das A, Chakraborti P, Chatterjee U, et al. Identification of allergens in Indian fishes: hilsa and pomfret exemplified by ELISA and immunoblotting. Indian J Exp Biol 2005;43:1170–5.
54. Sicherer SH, Munoz-Furlong A, Sampson HA. Prevalence of seafood allergy in the United States determined by a random telephone survey. J Allergy Clin Immunol 2004;114:159–65.
55. Ben-Shoshan M, Harrington DW, Soller L, et al. A population-based study on peanut, tree nut, fish, shellfish, and sesame allergy prevalence in Canada. J Allergy Clin Immunol 2010;125:1327–35.
56. Solensky R. Resolution of fish allergy: a case report. Ann Allergy Asthma Immunol 2003;91:411–2.
57. Dannaeus A, Inganas M. A follow-up study of children with food allergy. Clinical course in relation to serum IgE- and IgG-antibody levels to milk, egg and fish. Clin Allergy 1981;11:533–9.
58. Daul CB, Morgan JE, Lehrer SB. The natural history of shrimp hypersensitivity. J Allergy Clin Immunol 1990;86:88–93.
59. Sicherer SH, Munoz-Furlong A, Burks AW, et al. Prevalence of peanut and tree nut allergy in the US determined by a random digit dial telephone survey. J Allergy Clin Immunol 1999;103:559–62.
60. Sicherer SH, Munoz-Furlong A, Sampson HA. Prevalence of peanut and tree nut allergy in the United States determined by means of a random digit dial telephone survey: a 5-year follow-up study. J Allergy Clin Immunol 2003;112:1203–7.
61. Sicherer SH, Munoz-Furlong A, Godbold JH, et al. US prevalence of self-reported peanut, tree nut, and sesame allergy: 11-year follow-up. J Allergy Clin Immunol 2010;125:1322–6.
62. Kagan RS, Joseph L, Dufresne C, et al. Prevalence of peanut allergy in primary-school children in Montreal, Canada. J Allergy Clin Immunol 2003;112:1223–8.
63. Marklund B, Ahlstedt S, Nordstrom G, et al. Health-related quality of life among adolescents with allergy-like conditions - with emphasis on food hypersensitivity. Health Qual Life Outcomes 2004;2:65.
64. Tariq SM, Stevens M, Matthews S, et al. Cohort study of peanut and tree nut sensitisation by age of 4 years. BMJ 1996;313:514–7.

65. Grundy J, Matthews S, Bateman B, et al. Rising prevalence of allergy to peanut in children: data from 2 sequential cohorts. J Allergy Clin Immunol 2002;110:784–9.
66. Du Toit G, Katz Y, Sasieni P, et al. Early consumption of peanuts in infancy is associated with a low prevalence of peanut allergy. J Allergy Clin Immunol 2008;122: 984–91.
67. Shek LP, Cabrera-Morales EA, Soh SE, et al. A population-based questionnaire survey on the prevalence of peanut, tree nut, and shellfish allergy in 2 Asian populations. J Allergy Clin Immunol 2010;126:324–31.
68. Savage JH, Limb SL, Brereton NH, et al. The natural history of peanut allergy: extending our knowledge beyond childhood. J Allergy Clin Immunol 2007;120: 717–9.
69. Fleischer DM. The natural history of peanut and tree nut allergy. Curr Allergy Asthma Rep 2007;7:175–81.
70. Venter C, Pereira B, Grundy J, et al. Incidence of parentally reported and clinically diagnosed food hypersensitivity in the first year of life. J Allergy Clin Immunol 2006;117:1118–24.
71. Zuidmeer L, Goldhahn K, Rona RJ, et al. The prevalence of plant food allergies: a systematic review. J Allergy Clin Immunol 2008;121:1210–8.
72. Fleischer DM, Conover-Walker MK, Matsui EC, et al. The natural history of tree nut allergy. J Allergy Clin Immunol 2005;116:1087–93.
73. Kanny G, Moneret-Vautrin DA, Flabbee J, et al. Population study of food allergy in France. J Allergy Clin Immunol 2001;108:133–40.
74. Zuidmeer L, Salentijn E, Rivas MF, et al. The role of profilin and lipid transfer protein in strawberry allergy in the Mediterranean area. Clin Exp Allergy 2006; 36:666–75.

Diagnostic Testing in the Evaluation of Food Allergy

Philippe A. Eigenmann, MD[a,*], Jae-Won Oh, MD, PhD[b], Kirsten Beyer, MD[c]

KEYWORDS

• Food allergy • Diagnostic tests • Specific IgE
• Skin tests • Food challenges

The diagnosis of food allergy follows a common diagnostic frame for allergic diseases. The history is essential and allows classifying symptoms into potentially IgE-mediated or non–IgE-mediated diseases. When IgE-mediated diseases are suspected (ie, because of suggestive symptoms), the physician performs further diagnostic tests, mostly skin prick tests (SPTs) and/or measurement of serum specific IgE antibodies to the foods suspected. These tests allow identification of an immune response to potentially incriminated foods, but do not provide the diagnosis of food allergy, which is only definitive when a clear correlation between the test result and a clinical reaction (by history or positive food challenge) is established.

The history mostly focuses on potentially involved foods and the timing of the reaction in relation to the ingestion of the food, as well as the types of symptoms. Classic IgE-mediated symptoms in children may involve the skin (urticaria and/or angioedema, flares of atopic dermatitis), the gastrointestinal tract (abdominal cramps, emesis, and/or diarrhea), the respiratory system (acute rhinitis, acute asthma, and/or laryngeal symptoms), or result in generalized symptoms, such as anaphylaxis (multisystemic, severe reactions). Non–IgE-mediated symptoms in children mostly are manifested through vomiting, diarrhea, reflux, dysphagia, or blood in the stool (eg, as found in eosinophilic diseases of the gastrointestinal tract).

In addition to the history, SPTs as well as specific serum IgE measurements are routinely used to make a diagnosis. However, the diagnosis itself can be established

---

Disclosure of potential conflicts of interest: Dr Eigenmann has received speaker's honorarium and research grants from Phadia AB.
[a] Pediatric Allergy Unit, Childrens Hospital, University Hospitals of Geneva, 6, rue Willy-Donze, CH-1211 Geneva 14, Switzerland
[b] Department of Pediatrics, Hanyang University Kuri Hospital, 249–1 Kyomun-dong, Kuri-shi Kyunggi-do, Seoul, 471–020 Korea
[c] Klinik für Pädiatrie (Pneumo/Immunol), Charité, Campus Virchow-Klinikum, Augustenburger Platz 1, D-13353 Berlin, Germany
* Corresponding author.
E-mail address: Philippe.Eigenmann@hcuge.ch

Pediatr Clin N Am 58 (2011) 351–362
doi:10.1016/j.pcl.2011.02.003 **pediatric.theclinics.com**
0031-3955/11/$ – see front matter

with certainty only if the history correlates to diagnostic testing. If doubt persists, standardized oral food challenges (OFCs) are strongly recommended and necessary to establish the diagnosis with certainty.

SKIN TESTS FOR DIAGNOSIS OF FOOD ALLERGY

Immunologic responses related to food hypersensitivity may be either IgE-mediated or non–IgE-mediated. T-cell or eosinophil-mediated food hypersensitivity is the most frequent non–IgE-mediated mechanism underlying certain food allergies. Once the physician suspects a food allergy, they initially obtain a detailed history and from there initiate further procedures to prove or disprove the existence of food allergy.

SPT is the oldest procedure used for evaluating the presence of sensitization by reexposing the individual to a minute quantity of allergen. This procedure has been used since 1865, when Charles Blackley applied pollen to abraded skin by scratching. Subsequently in 1908, Mantoux[1] proposed an intracutaneous test to investigate immediate hypersensitivity diseases. Then in 1926, Lewis and Grant[2] reported the method we now use for SPT. Skin tests are a useful tool to confirm sensitization to a specific allergen. The prime advantages of this test are its simplicity, the rapidity of obtaining results, its good performance, its low cost, and its high sensitivity. The selection and number of allergens used with SPTs should be based on the history provided. Also, to avoid interpretation pitfalls of false-positive results, skin tests need to be limited to the lowest necessary number.

SPT

In the 1970s Pepys[3] suggested the use of a modified prick test procedure, using a 25-gauge hypodermic syringe needle, which permits 0.003 mL of the antigen to be absorbed into the epidermis when performed at a 45° angle to an approximate depth of 1 mm without inducing bleeding. Although this technique is no longer used, it highlighted the need for standardization of the amount introduced into the skin. Furthermore, a proper technique necessitates the use of separate needles for each test to avoid mixing the antigen solutions. Using the same needle or lancet wiped with dry cotton wool or cotton moistened with 75% ethanol between tests produces an unacceptable number of false-positive results and presents a potential risk of exposure to blood-borne pathogens.[4]

To reduce the variability of the SPT procedure, several investigators have modified the test method. Morrow Brown introduced the vertical prick puncture method, which uses a single-point device measuring 1.25 mm long. A guard prevents penetration of the needle beyond a predetermined depth. No skin lifting is used and, in using this instrument, supposedly only a small amount of antigen is delivered into the skin when compared with the Pepys prick test. By using commercially available, nonreusable, and standardized devices, the procedure is considered standard (with the limitation of the extract used) and safe.

Among other devices used for SPT, the Multi-Test (Lincoln Diagnostics, Decatur, IL, USA) has been available for more than 20 years. This test consists of a plastic device containing 8 heads, 4 on each side. Each head has 9 prongs. This device allows for a quick and easy approach and it is possible to perform multiprick puncture testing within approximately 30 seconds. However, multiheaded devices present significant variability because of the pressure applied and are considered to be more painful than single devices.[5] In general, single-point nonreusable devices are considered the preferred (standard) procedure for SPT.

Correlation of Skin Test Results with OFCs

Various studies have investigated how SPT results correlate to the outcome of OFCs, considered the gold standard for diagnosing food allergies. When correlating the size of the wheal and/or the positivity of the tests (>3 mm mean diameter) with the outcome of double-blind, placebo-controlled food challenges, significant differences in wheal sizes were noted between individuals who were allergic to egg, milk, peanut, and wheat and those who were tolerant.[6] By contrast, reactivity to soy could not be predicted based on SPT results. Cutoff values for clinical positivity were established.[6] Other groups reported different values in their population of patients,[7] indicating that the SPT results should be interpreted according to a specific population, as well as to the antigen extract used.

Precautions Before Skin Prick Testing

Before any SPT is performed, a few precautions should be followed for the safety of the patient and the accuracy of the results.[8,9] The following list of precautions, adapted from Ref.[10] are standard:

1. No testing should be performed without a physician being immediately available to treat a patient, should a systemic reaction occur.
2. Emergency equipment has to be readily available.
3. The allergenic extracts used should be standardized whenever possible. In addition, they should be manufactured free of extraneous antigenic factors.
4. Test concentrations used must be appropriate for the degree of sensitivity of the patient as determined from the history.
5. A positive (histamine) and negative control solution should always be included.
6. The test should be performed on nonlesional skin.
7. Before the test, the patients should be evaluated for increased, and nonspecific, skin reactivity (dermographism).
8. It must be determined ahead of time whether the patient uses medications (mostly antihistamines) that might interfere with the accuracy of the skin tests.
9. An accurate record of the reactions and the proper timing must be kept, and each reaction must be accurately measured.
10. An evaluation of the patient's allergic symptoms must be completed before any tests and close observation performed during the test.

In addition, the physician or technician performing SPT needs to be trained and needs to have repeated practice of skin prick testing to provide reproducible and reliable results.

Common Errors in Skin Prick Testing

The following errors are common and should be avoided:

1. When performing SPT with multiple antigens each solution should be placed 2 cm or more apart.[11]
2. Insufficient or excess penetration of the skin by the puncture instrument may lead to false-negative results. This situation occurs more frequently with plastic devices or Morrow Brown needles used by unqualified personnel.
3. Induction of bleeding, possibly leading to false-positive results.
4. Spreading of allergen solutions during the test or when the solution is wiped away.

Prick-prick Test

This procedure is performed by using native antigens (eg, a fresh fruit), and is commonly used in food-related allergic reactions. One first pricks through the fresh food and then pricks the skin of the patient. Some studies reported that the SPTs were positive 40% of the time with commercial extracts and 81% of the time using fresh foods. The overall concordance between a positive prick test and a positive challenge test is 59% with commercial extracts and 92% when fresh foods were used.[12] When a history is positive, and a commercial food antigen prick test is negative, then a prick-prick test using fresh food should be considered.

Criteria of Positivity

The wheal or the flare has been considered to assess the positivity of skin tests. For prick puncture tests, reactions generally regarded to indicate clinical allergy are usually more than 3 mm in wheal diameter and more than 10 mm in flare diameter.[13,14] An alternative criterion is a ratio of the size of the test induced by the allergen to the size that is elicited by the positive control solution. Any degree of positive response, with appropriate positive and negative controls, indicates the presence of an allergic sensitization but not necessarily the simultaneous presence of an allergic disease related to the tested allergen. Therefore, an agreement between the skin test results and the clinical history is essential in the overall interpretation of the clinical significance of the SPT.

Patch Test

Patch testing may be helpful in cases of suspected non–IgE-mediated food allergies. Majamaa and colleagues[15] tested 143 children less than 2 years of age suspected to be allergic to cow's milk by elimination diet and an OFC. Seventy-two of the 143 children had a positive OFC, and among these 26% were found to have increased IgE to cow's milk protein, 14% had an SPT, and 44% had a positive patch test to cow's milk. Most of the patients with a positive patch test had a negative SPT to cow's milk. A positive patch test suggests a delayed-type sensitivity to the tested antigen but as with all tests for food allergy the physician must evaluate whether this immunologic reaction corresponds to a clinical condition. Although patch tests might be helpful in the diagnosis of food allergy, in particular in children with eosinophilic gastrointestinal disease of atopic dermatitis, the relevance of this test in routine diagnostic testing has been questioned and cannot be generally recommended.[16]

Scratch Test

The scratch test is characterized by a superficial epidermal abrasion, approximately 2 mm long, to which an antigen is applied. This test is simple and quick to perform, but not sufficiently sensitive or specific because of the wide interindividual variation in performing the test. The major disadvantages of scratch testing are the significant numbers of false-positive reactions, the low reproducibility, and that the test is more painful than a prick test. Therefore, the Allergy Panel of the American Medical Association (AMA) Council of Scientific Affairs recommends that scratch testing should not be performed routinely.[17]

Intradermal Tests

Although intradermal tests are used in allergy diagnosis, in particular for the diagnosis of venom or drug allergy, this procedure should not be used in common clinical practice in the diagnosis of food allergy.

IN VITRO DIAGNOSIS

In vitro tests (determining serum IgE antibodies) are commonly used in the diagnostic workup of food allergy. Especially in young children, patients with severe atopic dermatitis, or patients taking antihistamines, in vitro tests may be more suitable than skin tests. Usually, the level of food-specific serum IgE antibodies is measured. Serum IgE levels can be assessed for crude allergen extracts, individual allergens, or even allergenic peptides. The results can be a simple qualitative measurement resulting in a yes or no answer for the presence of food-specific IgE or alternatively they may determine a quantitative antibody level. Screening or panel tests are available with a fixed combination of food allergens. In vitro measurements are often performed in laboratories to which patient samples are sent. However, point-of-care devices are available. These issues are discussed in detail in the following sections. Moreover, the role of total IgE testing as well as food-specific IgG4 testing is described.

Quantitative Measurement of Food-specific IgE

Increased levels of food-specific serum IgE are an indication of sensitization; however, as with skin tests, the clinical relevance of a positive test still needs to be determined. In recent years truly quantitative measurement of specific IgE has become more common. In parallel it has been shown that the level of food-specific IgE against crude allergen extracts correlates with the likelihood of clinically relevant food allergy for many food allergens. Therefore, quantitative measurement of food-specific IgE is preferred to solely qualitative measurements.[18] Several groups have described diagnostic decision points for food allergen-specific serum IgE concentrations to reduce the requirement for OFCs.[19–26] The diagnostic decision points vary between reported studies as a result of differences in patient population. Moreover, these decision points seem to be age dependent.[20] For many allergens, the likelihood of clinically relevant food allergy increases with the level of food-specific IgE. However, for some food allergens, such as wheat and soy, the correlation between the presence of food-specific IgE and clinically relevant food allergy is poor.[20]

Component-resolved Diagnosis

There is emerging evidence that component-resolved diagnosis through measurement of specific IgE to individual, most often recombinant, food allergens may be superior to measurements of specific IgE to crude allergen extracts. For example, clinically relevant peanut allergy seems to correlate with the detection of specific IgE antibodies to Ara h 2, a seed storage protein in peanuts.[27] Homolog seed storage proteins also exist in tree nuts and seeds. In hazelnut allergies, detection of specific IgE to Cor a 9[28] suggests a food allergy that might result in a life-threatening reaction, whereas detection of specific IgE solely to Cor a 1, the homolog of the birch pollen allergen Bet v 1, suggests a pollen-associated food allergy.[29,30] Similarly, positive specific IgE to the lipid transfer protein of hazelnut, Cor a 8, suggests an increased risk of severe systemic reactions. Similar improvement of the test performance and diagnostic sensitivity has been seen when using single kiwifruit allergens compared with the extract.[31] Because the measurement of specific IgE to individual food allergens increases the costs and the volume of serum needed, allergen microarray systems have been developed that enable the simultaneous detection of many allergens with minimal blood volume.[32,33] Although these new methods have not been validated for all food allergens, nevertheless for cow's milk and hen's egg the microarray system showed performance characteristics comparable with current diagnostic tests.[34]

Measurement of Food-specific IgG4

The production of specific IgG and IgG4 to food is a physiologic process. Despite this fact, tests for food-specific IgG4 represent a growing market. However, there are no controlled studies that confirm any diagnostic value of IgG4 testing in patients with food allergies, and the European Academy of Allergy and Clinical Immunology (EAACI) has taken the position that IgG4 testing in patients with suspected or proven food allergies is not indicated.[35,36] The American Academy of Allergy, Asthma & Immunology supports the EAACI's position on IgG4.[37]

Measurement of Total IgE Serum Levels

Measuring total serum IgE levels is generally not necessary in patients with food allergies. However, it might be useful in patients with atopic dermatitis. In these patients, the total serum IgE titers are sometimes high (eg, more than 1000 or 2000 international units).[38] In addition, they may have positive specific IgE tests to nearly every aeroallergen and nutritional allergen measured, raising the possibility of positive tests only relevant to sensitization and not to true allergy. Thus, in patients with atopic dermatitis, in vitro allergy testing may not provide any important information in terms of a potentially necessary diet,[39] and a high total IgE serum level might be helpful to weight the relevance of positive specific IgE testing. In addition, it had been believed that determining the ratio of food-specific IgE/total IgE compared with measuring food-specific IgE alone in predicting symptomatic food allergy would be superior. However, in a study in children with suspected hen's egg, cow's milk, wheat, or soy allergy, no benefit had been observed.[40]

Point-of-care Devices

In contrast to skin tests, the results of which are immediately available to the physician and patient, in vitro tests, usually performed in the laboratory, require processing and therefore result in delayed results. To mitigate this situation, point-of-care devices have been developed that provide immediate results. The benefit of a short turnaround time has been shown for the management of children with suspected respiratory allergies.[41–44] However, thus far these devices offer only a qualitative measurement (giving a simple yes or no answer) with regard to the presence of specific IgE antibodies. Moreover, these devices offer only a limited range of food allergens that can be tested, using crude allergen extracts rather than individual allergens. Future developments of these devices, which are not yet available in the United States, may address some of the current limitations.

OFCs

A positive SPT and/or the presence of food-specific IgE antibodies are not per se diagnostic for the existence of food allergy, because they both may indicate only sensitization to a common food (ie, indicate that the child has an atopic predisposition to possibly react to certain food proteins). When a positive test can clearly be linked to a suggestive history (eg, an anaphylactic reaction within minutes of ingestion of a food, or repeated ingestions leading to similar symptoms), an OFC is not necessary. However, when the clinical symptoms are inconclusive, such as flares of atopic dermatitis or subjective symptoms (eg, throat itching or vague abdominal pain), one cannot assume that a positive skin test or the presence of food-specific IgE antibodies truly confirms the diagnosis. In such cases, an OFC is useful. The rationale that supports a potentially risky diagnostic test rests with the challenge that families with a food-allergic child have in avoiding certain allergens, the fear for accidental ingestion, and the perceived quality of life associated with serious food allergies. The quality of life of a child suffering from peanut allergy has been shown to be inferior to that of a child suffering from insulin-dependent diabetes mellitus.[45] Also, OFCs provide parents with a definite diagnosis, in particular in unclear cases. A survey by Nguyen and colleagues[46] showed that most parents with a child with a peanut allergy were satisfied with an oral peanut food challenge to obtain a definitive diagnosis.

A physician-supervised OFC does not provide the parents with information about a safe amount of allergen that can be ingested, in particular accidentally.[47] The OFC also fails to predict the severity of future accidental allergen ingestions, a question on many parents' minds.

When Does a Patient Need an OFC?

There is a strong indication for OFCs when dealing with an unclear diagnosis (ie, allergen-specific tests do not clearly correlate with the history), as well as for follow-up of previously diagnosed food allergies. The latter is important to assess whether an allergy continues to exist as the child patient gets older. The natural history of most food allergies is that the patients outgrow them by acquisition of tolerance. For some foods (eg, milk, egg, or wheat) tolerance occurs mostly before adulthood,[48,49] whereas allergies to tree nuts or peanuts are outgrown in only a subgroup of patients.[50] Using an OFC when there is good reason to believe that tolerance has occurred can have a major positive effect on the daily lives of patients previously restricted in their dietary intake.

Open OFC

An open OFC consists of unmasked and unblinded feeding of the food to be tested. The food is given in increasing amounts over set time intervals. The first amount given is usually lower than the dose expected to provoke a reaction. The waiting time between doses is 15 to 30 minutes. The challenge continues for a total of 5 to 7 increasing doses, up to an amount equal to that of a normal serving. In OFC with cow's milk, hen's egg, peanuts, tree nuts, wheat, and soy, amounts corresponding to 3 mg, 10 mg, 30 mg, 100 mg, 300 mg, 1000 mg, and 3000 mg protein given 20 to 30 minutes apart constitute a possible protocol (**Table 1**). In case of subjective symptoms, the investigator decides whether to discontinue the OFC, whether to administer the same dose, or if the test will progress to the next amount. The test is declared positive if an objective reaction is noted, convincing to the investigator as well as to the patient or to their parents. At the end of a negative challenge, the patient should be observed for a minimum period, corresponding to the time described in the

Table 1
An example of an egg challenge procedure[a]

Time Interval to Previous Dose (min)	Amount of Egg (g)	Corresponding Amount of Proteins (g)
0	0.240	0.03
20–30	0.8	0.1
20	2.4	0.3
20	8	1
20	24	3

[a] According to symptoms, challenges can be started with lower doses (eg, 0.003 g and 0.01 g of proteins).

patient's history with regard to development of an allergic reaction to the allergen tested. In positive challenges, the patient can be discharged when all symptoms have disappeared and the risk for reoccurrence has resolved.

Blinded OFC

When subjects experience subjective or ambiguous symptoms, or high anxiety around an OFC, the test might be blinded and performed in 2 parts. For both parts, the test uses a vehicle food (ie, a food that is well tolerated by the patient). This vehicle food is used to hide the color, taste, and smell of the test food. The test food is added to 1 of 2 preparations, whereas the other contains a placebo. The order in which both preparations are given is either blinded to the investigator and the patient and the parents (double-blind procedure), or only to the patient and the parents (single-blind procedure). The time between administration of both preparations varies from 2 hours to up to several days in patients with atopic dermatitis or allergy-induced behavioral symptoms. Regardless of the time frame, safety is paramount. Therefore blinded OFCs must be organized and supervised by staff experienced in identifying potential symptoms, and trained to provide appropriate treatment if symptoms occur. Emergency medications needed onsite include antihistamines administered in case of local skin reactions, as well as epinephrine (0.01 mg/kg intramuscular) for systemic reactions. Patients also require intravenous access before each procedure. Specific guidance with regard to standard procedures used for OFCs has been published by various societies and expert groups.[51–55]

For patients who manifest a food allergy through flares of atopic dermatitis, testing needs to be adapted to their symptoms. In particular, the timing between the 2 preparations needs to take into account that the manifestation of the allergic reaction can take days or occasionally weeks in late-phase reactions.[56,57] Also for this specific manifestation of food allergies the double-blind, placebo-controlled food challenge is the preferred manner of testing.

One major pitfall in OFC is represented by the specific food chosen for the test. In particular, one should consider that certain allergens, such as the ones found in eggs and certain fruits and vegetables, are denatured by cooking. Therefore, a negative OFC test to cooked eggs may not disclose that the patient could still react to foods such as mayonnaise or desserts containing raw eggs (in which the allergen is not denatured and therefore retains its allergenic properties). Similarly, a patient might react to specific nuts or fish, but tolerate other nuts or fish. Patients have reported food-induced reactions at home after a negative physician-supervised food challenge. This situation can be explained in certain cases because the amount used during the OFC was too low (**Table 2**), or as described earlier, when foods eaten at home were uncooked, whereas testing had used cooked foods.[58]

Table 2
Suggested minimal total amounts (g) of food given (in a negative food challenge)[a]

Food	Total Amount	Corresponding Amount of Proteins (g)
Egg	35 g	4.5
Milk	134 mL	4.5
Fish	24 g	4.5
Peanut	17 g	4.5
Hazelnut	29 g	4.5

[a] The total amount can be higher and should correspond to a normal serving.

Where Should OFCs be Performed?

Most OFCs are performed by allergists in day clinics or private practice, although the limited numbers of OFCs performed in each center limits their expertise for handling more complex patients. Therefore, high-risk tests or tests requiring a blinded procedure should be performed in tertiary referral centers, where patients have access to a team that has experience with responding to emergencies during the food challenge and are cognizant of the pitfalls associated with interpreting the results of OFCs correctly.

SUMMARY

Because of the large number of children with symptoms potentially related to food allergy, the pediatrician is often asked whether that child requires referral for food allergy diagnostic workup. The history provides guidance in determining which, if any, diagnostic procedures ought to be performed. SPTs should be performed only by a skilled physician, usually a pediatric allergist. In addition, some children benefit from determining serum immunoglobulin (IgE, IgG4) levels, when possible allergen specific. If these tests are unequivocal or do not provide clear guidance for the affected families, OFC should be performed for a definite diagnosis.

REFERENCES

1. Mantoux C. Intradermoréaction de la tuberculose. CR Acad Sci 1908;147:355.
2. Lewis T, Grant R. Vascular reactions of the skin to injury. Heart 1926;13:219–25.
3. Pepys J. Skin tests. Br J Hosp Med 1984;32:120, 122, 124.
4. Piette V, Bourret E, Bousquet J, et al. Prick tests to aeroallergens: is it possible simply to wipe the device between tests? Allergy 2002;57:940–2.
5. Carr WW, Martin B, Howard RS, et al. Comparison of test devices for skin prick testing. J Allergy Clin Immunol 2005;116:341–6.
6. Eigenmann PA, Sampson HA. Interpreting skin prick tests in the evaluation of food allergy in children. Pediatr Allergy Immunol 1998;9:186–91.
7. Hill DJ, Heine RG, Hosking CS. The diagnostic value of skin prick testing in children with food allergy. Pediatr Allergy Immunol 2004;15:435–41.
8. Valyasevi MA, Maddox DE, Li JT. Systemic reactions to allergy skin tests. Ann Allergy Asthma Immunol 1999;83:132–6.
9. Wainstein BK, Studdert J, Ziegler M, et al. Prediction of anaphylaxis during peanut food challenge: usefulness of the peanut skin prick test (SPT) and specific IgE level. Pediatr Allergy Immunol 2010;21:603–11.
10. Demoly P, Bousquet J, Romano A. In vivo methods for the study of allergy. In: Adkinson NF Jr, Bochner BS, Busse WW, et al, editors. Middleton's allergy: principles and Practice. 7th edition. St Louis (MO): Mosby; 2009. p. 1268–80.
11. Demoly P, Bousquet J, Manderscheid JC, et al. Precision of skin prick and puncture tests with nine methods. J Allergy Clin Immunol 1991;88:758–62.
12. Rance F, Juchet A, Bremont F, et al. Correlations between skin prick tests using commercial extracts and fresh foods, specific IgE, and food challenges. Allergy 1997;52:1031–5.
13. Adinoff AD, Rosloniec DM, McCall LL, et al. Immediate skin test reactivity to Food and Drug Administration-approved standardized extracts. J Allergy Clin Immunol 1990;86:766–74.

14. Ahrens B, Lopes de Oliveira LC, Schulz G, et al. The role of hen's egg-specific IgE, IgG and IgG4 in the diagnostic procedure of hen's egg allergy. Allergy 2010;65(12):1554–7.
15. Majamaa H, Moisio P, Holm K, et al. Cow's milk allergy: diagnostic accuracy of skin prick and patch tests and specific IgE. Allergy 1999;54:346–51.
16. Mehl A, Rolinck-Werninghaus C, Staden U, et al. The atopy patch test in the diagnostic workup of suspected food-related symptoms in children. J Allergy Clin Immunol 2006;118:923–9.
17. AMA Council on Scientific Affairs PoA: in vivo diagnostic testing and immunotherapy for allergy. JAMA 1987;258:1363–7.
18. Beyer K. In vitro diagnosis. In: Metcalfe DD, Sampson HA, Simon RA, editors. Food allergy. 4th edition. Malden (MA): Blackwell Publishing; 2008. p. 278–84.
19. Boyano MT, Garcia-Ara C, Díaz-Pena JM, et al. Validity of specific IgE antibodies in children with egg allergy. Clin Exp Allergy 2001;31:1464–9.
20. Celik-Bilgili S, Mehl A, Verstege A, et al. The predictive value of specific immunoglobulin E levels in serum for the outcome of oral food challenges. Clin Exp Allergy 2005;35:268–73.
21. Garcia-Ara C, Boyano-Martinez T, DIaz-Pena JM, et al. Specific IgE levels in the diagnosis of immediate hypersensitivity to cows' milk protein in the infant. J Allergy Clin Immunol 2001;107:185–90.
22. Hill DJ, Hosking CS, Reyes-Benito LV. Reducing the need for food allergen challenges in young children: a comparison of in vitro with in vivo tests. Clin Exp Allergy 2001;31:1031–5.
23. Perry TT, Matsui EC, Kay Conover-Walker M, et al. The relationship of allergen-specific IgE levels and oral food challenge outcome. J Allergy Clin Immunol 2004;114:144–9.
24. Rance F, Abbal M, Lauwers-Cances V. Improved screening for peanut allergy by the combined use of skin prick tests and specific IgE assays. J Allergy Clin Immunol 2002;109:1027–33.
25. Sampson HA. Utility of food-specific IgE concentrations in predicting symptomatic food allergy. J Allergy Clin Immunol 2001;107:891–6.
26. Sporik R, Hill DJ, Hosking CS. Specificity of allergen skin testing in predicting positive open food challenges to milk, egg and peanut in children. Clin Exp Allergy 2000;30:1541–6.
27. Nicolaou N, Poorafshar M, Murray C, et al. Allergy or tolerance in children sensitized to peanut: prevalence and differentiation using component-resolved diagnostics. J Allergy Clin Immunol 2010;125:191–7.
28. Beyer K, Grishina G, Bardina L, et al. Identification of an 11S globulin as a major hazelnut food allergen in hazelnut-induced systemic reactions. J Allergy Clin Immunol 2002;110:517–23.
29. Pastorello EA, Vieths S, Pravettoni V, et al. Identification of hazelnut major allergens in sensitive patients with positive double-blind, placebo-controlled food challenge results. J Allergy Clin Immunol 2002;109:563–70.
30. Schocker F, Luttkopf D, Scheurer S, et al. Recombinant lipid transfer protein Cor a 8 from hazelnut: a new tool for in vitro diagnosis of potentially severe hazelnut allergy. J Allergy Clin Immunol 2004;113:141–7.
31. Bublin M, Pfister M, Radauer C, et al. Component-resolved diagnosis of kiwifruit allergy with purified natural and recombinant kiwifruit allergens. J Allergy Clin Immunol 2010;125:687–94, 694.e1.
32. Hiller R, Laffer S, Harwanegg C, et al. Microarrayed allergen molecules: diagnostic gatekeepers for allergy treatment. FASEB J 2002;16:414–6.

33. Schweitzer B, Kingsmore SF. Measuring proteins on microarrays. Curr Opin Biotechnol 2002;13:14–9.
34. Ott H, Baron J, Heise R, et al. Clinical usefulness of microarray-based IgE detection in children with suspected food allergy. Allergy 2008;63:1521–8.
35. Stapel SO, Asero R, Ballmer-Weber BK, et al. Testing for IgG4 against foods is not recommended as a diagnostic tool: EAACI task force report. Allergy 2008;63:793–6.
36. Taylor SL, Hefle SL, Bindslev-Jensen C, et al. A consensus protocol for the determination of the threshold doses for allergenic foods: how much is too much? Clin Exp Allergy 2004;34:689–95.
37. Bock SA. AAAAI support of the EAACI Position Paper on IgG4. J Allergy Clin Immunol 2010;125:1410.
38. Laske N, Bunikowski R, Niggemann B. Extraordinarily high serum IgE levels and consequences for atopic phenotypes. Ann Allergy Asthma Immunol 2003;91:202–4.
39. Niggemann B, Beyer K. Diagnostic pitfalls in food allergy in children. Allergy 2005;60:104–7.
40. Mehl A, Verstege A, Staden U, et al. Utility of the ratio of food-specific IgE/total IgE in predicting symptomatic food allergy in children. Allergy 2005;60:1034–9.
41. Diaz-Vazquez C, Torregrosa-Bertet MJ, Carvajal-Uruena I, et al. Accuracy of ImmunoCAP Rapid in the diagnosis of allergic sensitization in children between 1 and 14 years with recurrent wheezing: the IReNE study. Pediatr Allergy Immunol 2009;20:601–9.
42. Eigenmann PA. Are specific immunoglobulin E titres reliable for prediction of food allergy? Clin Exp Allergy 2005;35:247–9.
43. Eigenmann PA, Kuenzli M, D'Apuzzo V, et al. The ImmunoCAP Rapid Wheeze/Rhinitis child test is useful in the initial allergy diagnosis of children with respiratory symptoms. Pediatr Allergy Immunol 2009;20:772–9.
44. Sarratud T, Donnanno S, Terracciano L, et al. Accuracy of a point-of-care testing device in children with suspected respiratory allergy. Allergy Asthma Proc 2010;31:e11–7.
45. Avery NJ, King RM, Knight S, et al. Assessment of quality of life in children with peanut allergy. Pediatr Allergy Immunol 2003;14:378–82.
46. Nguyen M, Wainstein BK, Hu W, et al. Parental satisfaction with oral peanut food challenges; perception of outcomes and impact on management of peanut allergy. Pediatr Allergy Immunol 2010;21(8):1119–26.
47. Hourihane JO, Grimshaw KE, Lewis SA, et al. Does severity of low-dose, double-blind, placebo-controlled food challenges reflect severity of allergic reactions to peanut in the community? Clin Exp Allergy 2005;35:1227–33.
48. Savage JH, Matsui EC, Skripak JM, et al. The natural history of egg allergy. J Allergy Clin Immunol 2007;120:1413–7.
49. Skripak JM, Matsui EC, Mudd K, et al. The natural history of IgE-mediated cow's milk allergy. J Allergy Clin Immunol 2007;120:1172–7.
50. Bock SA, Atkins FM. The natural history of peanut allergy. J Allergy Clin Immunol 1989;83:900–4.
51. Bindslev-Jensen C, Ballmer-Weber BK, Bengtsson U, et al. Standardization of food challenges in patients with immediate reactions to foods–position paper from the European Academy of Allergology and Clinical Immunology. Allergy 2004;59:690–7.
52. Niggemann B, Beyer K. Diagnosis of food allergy in children: toward a standardization of food challenge. J Pediatr Gastroenterol Nutr 2007;45:399–404.

53. Niggemann B, Beyer K. Pitfalls in double-blind, placebo-controlled oral food challenges. Allergy 2007;62:729–32.
54. Nowak-Wegrzyn A, Assa'ad AH, Bahna SL, et al. Work Group report: oral food challenge testing. J Allergy Clin Immunol 2009;123:S365–83.
55. Rance F, Deschildre A, Villard-Truc F, et al. Oral food challenge in children: an expert review. Eur Ann Allergy Clin Immunol 2009;41:35–49.
56. Niggemann B. Role of oral food challenges in the diagnostic work-up of food allergy in atopic eczema dermatitis syndrome. Allergy 2004;59(Suppl 78):32–4.
57. Werfel T, Ballmer-Weber B, Eigenmann PA, et al. Eczematous reactions to food in atopic eczema: position paper of the EAACI and GA2LEN. Allergy 2007;62:723–8.
58. Eigenmann PA, Caubet JC, Zamora SA. Continuing food-avoidance diets after negative food challenges. Pediatr Allergy Immunol 2006;17:601–5.

Pathophysiology of Food Allergy

Brian P. Vickery, MD*, Stacy Chin, MD, A. Wesley Burks, MD

KEYWORDS

• Food allergy • IgE • Allergic sensitization • Dendritic cells
• Pathophysiology

Food allergy, which is hypothesized to result from a defect in oral tolerance, is a common, serious, and growing problem in developed countries. Whereas the immune system of all individuals recognize food antigens as foreign, patients with food allergy develop pathologic immune responses to these antigens and can rapidly experience harmful adverse symptoms upon reexposure. Although a recent meta-analysis identified variation in prevalence rates,[1] recent survey data from the Centers for Disease Control and Prevention indicate that the current prevalence of food allergy in US children is approximately 4%, an increase of almost 20% in the past decade.[2] Increases in food allergy prevalence have also been observed in methodologically rigorous birth cohort studies that use precise sampling techniques and well-defined outcome measures, suggesting that rising prevalence is not simply a result of self-diagnosis or increased recognition of the disorder.[3] Similar trends in the prevalence of asthma, allergic rhinitis, and atopic dermatitis support the general concept that atopic diseases are increasingly common.[4]

Spontaneous clinical tolerance does develop in some food-allergic individuals and tends to occur in allergen-specific patterns. For example, resolution of allergy to egg, milk, wheat, and soy can generally be expected, although this may take longer than previously appreciated. In contrast, most patients allergic to peanut, tree nuts, and seafood will not outgrow their disease and must maintain strict elimination diets. The natural history of allergy to other important proteins such as sesame and mustard is largely unknown. Furthermore, it is a common clinical scenario for a given individual

Funding Source: Food Allergy & Anaphylaxis Network; Food Allergy Project; Gerber Foundation; NIH Grant 1 R01-AI06874-01A1, NIH T32 Training Grant, and NIH Grant 1 UL1 RR024128-01 from the National Center for Research Resources (NCRR), a component of the National Institutes of Health (NIH) and NIH Roadmap for Medical Research (contents are solely the responsibility of the authors and do not necessarily represent the official view of NCRR or NIH); and the National Peanut Board.
Division of Pediatric Allergy and Immunology, Department of Pediatrics, Duke University School of Medicine, Box 2644, Durham, NC 27710, USA
* Corresponding author.
E-mail address: brian.vickery@duke.edu

Pediatr Clin N Am 58 (2011) 363–376
doi:10.1016/j.pcl.2011.02.012 **pediatric.theclinics.com**
0031-3955/11/$ – see front matter

to outgrow an early milk or egg allergy but not a peanut allergy.[5] Therefore it appears that the pathophysiology of food allergy may differ in significant antigen-specific ways even within the same patient. The overrepresentation of peanut and tree nut allergy among cases of fatal food anaphylaxis further supports the concept that certain foods tend to be more allergenic than others.[6]

However, even though there is significant heterogeneity among patients with food allergy, in practice all individuals are considered to be equally sensitive to all foods, and strict avoidance is the standard of care. This is largely because of the inability of standard diagnostic testing to predict a patient's risk for anaphylaxis, or to determine an individual's threshold dose to trigger symptoms. Therefore, affected individuals and families maintain a constant state of vigilance to avoid inadvertent exposure to even trace amounts of food allergens; however, even in the most cautious patients, accidental ingestions frequently occur.[5] Although fatalities caused by accidental ingestions are rare, parents routinely cite a fear of this outcome.[7] The inability to completely eliminate the possibility of anaphylaxis and the associated limitations in everyday activities are great sources of uncertainty and stress on affected families. Over time, health-related quality of life is seriously eroded, to a greater degree than seen in other serious chronic diseases of childhood.[8]

The gastrointestinal (GI) tract, which is the largest immunologic organ in the body, is constantly exposed to an enormous array of exogenous antigens including commensal bacteria and ingested proteins.[9] A single epithelial layer separates this antigenic load from the lymphocytes, antigen-presenting cells (APCs), stromal cells, and other immune cells in the lamina propria, which together comprise the mucosal-associated lymphoid tissue (MALT). Within the MALT, unique populations of dendritic cells (DCs) interact with dietary antigens, and determine the fate of the resulting adaptive response, ie, immunity versus tolerance.[10] In this context, immune tolerance is defined as the antigen-specific suppression of cellular or humoral immune responses. When the initial antigen exposure is mediated through the GI tract, a robust T-cell–mediated suppression develops called oral tolerance.[11] However, in the 4% to 6% of children and 2% of adults with food allergies, this mechanism appears to fail, and the ensuing immune response proceeds through 2 phases: *allergic sensitization* and *elicitation*. Allergic sensitization involves T-cell priming after DC activation, and the resultant T-helper-2 (T_H2) response is characterized by the production of interleukin-4 (IL-4), IL-5, and IL-13 from CD4+ T cells. This T_H2 response leads to B-cell immunoglobulin E (IgE) production, and this IgE binds to its high-affinity receptor on the surface of mast cells in the skin, gut, respiratory, and cardiovascular systems, arming them for reactivity upon reexposure to allergen. The elicitation of classic allergic symptoms occurs within minutes after allergen exposure, when IgE-bound mast cells recognize the allergen and become activated.[12–14]

This article covers the pathophysiology of IgE-mediated food allergy, proceeding through the steps of allergic sensitization and then elicitation. Because most of the mechanistic evidence for the pathophysiology of food allergy and tolerance is derived from experimental animals, we primarily discuss these model systems. Where possible, we review the evidence for similar phenomena in human biology and the relevant applications for clinical medicine.

THE INTRINSIC PHYSICAL PROPERTIES OF FOOD ALLERGENS

The average daily intake of protein in the US diet is approximately 1 g per kilogram of body weight, and is derived from a great variety of mammals, birds, fish, fungi, and plants. Yet amidst this wide range, only a relatively small number of foods cause the vast majority of food allergies.[5] This fact provides an important clue to the underlying pathophysiology of the disease and suggests that these main food allergens—milk, egg, wheat, soy, peanut, tree nuts, fish, and crustacea—though diverse in origin, share common characteristics that confer allergenicity. These characteristics include (1) a relatively small molecular weight, generally less than 70 kD; (2) an abundant source of the relevant allergen (eg, the seed storage proteins in nuts that are required to sustain plant growth); (3) glycosylation residues; (4) water solubility; and (5) resistance to heat and digestion. This combination of characteristics is likely unique to food allergens, which unlike inhaled or contact allergens, must pass through the harsh environment of the digestive system, beginning immediately upon entry into the oropharynx. Following ingestion, dietary proteins undergo digestion by enzymes in the saliva and stomach as well as by gastric acid. This processing results in reduced protein immunogenicity, likely by the destruction of conformational epitopes, ie, antigenic regions formed when noncontiguous amino acids are brought together by the tertiary folded structure of the protein. However, proteins that display these physicochemical properties resist this processing and thus have allergenic potential upon reaching the small intestine. Additional factors that disrupt normal digestion, such as coadministration of antacids, have been shown in animal models to result in a breakdown in oral tolerance induction.[11]

Because food antigens are nonself proteins, they are recognized as such by the MALT, and as a result all normal individuals mount immune responses to ingested food proteins.[12–14] However, once putative allergens survive the digestion process relatively intact, they must initiate a T_H2 response to result in IgE production and disease expression. There has been a great deal of recent research interest in understanding the cellular and molecular basis of allergenicity, and what intrinsic signals derived from the proteins themselves lead to allergic priming. Whereas the operative allergenic motif has long been considered to be the protein or peptide epitope owing to its central importance in T-cell stimulation, recent studies have highlighted the emerging importance of the carbohydrate residues that decorate proteins and influence T_H2 polarization.[15] Studies of inhalant allergens have also identified the intrinsic protease activity of the proteins as well as their molecular resemblance to Toll-like receptor (TLR) ligands,[16] but glycosylation appears to play a key role in allergenicity of dietary protein. This is not entirely surprising, given that the mucosal IgE system evolved to defend the host from intestinal metazoan parasites, organisms that are themselves heavily glycosylated.

Shreffler and colleagues[17] demonstrated that the cell-surface receptor Dendritic Cell–Specific Intercellular adhesion molecule-3-Grabbing Non-integrin (DC-SIGN), also known as CD209 DC-SIGN, mediates recognition of the major peanut allergen Ara h 1 by human DCs in vitro. DC-SIGN is a c-type lectin expressed on APCs that identifies conserved carbohydrate residues on pathogens and is generally considered to be a component of the innate immune system. Thus, the recognition of Ara h 1 by DC-SIGN is dependent on the carbohydrates in the peanut allergens, and furthermore this interaction is sufficient for DC activation and T_H2 skewing of naïve human T cells. This may be one example of a broader effect, because other lectins besides DC-SIGN, such as the mannose receptor and Dectin-1 and Dectin-2, appear to play important roles in recognition of allergens and activation of APCs in murine systems.[18] Interestingly, peanut allergens subjected to high-heat preparation (ie, dry roasting) undergo a nonenzymatic glycosylation reaction called the Maillard reaction. This increases the binding of IgE from peanut-allergic subjects and has been hypothesized to partially account for the disproportionate increase in peanut allergy in Westernized societies that consume roasted peanuts, as compared with other cultures with different preparation methods.[19] Other major allergens, including those from egg, shrimp, milk, and red meats (as well as dust mite and other inhalant allergens), are also known to be heavily glycosylated.

THE IMPORTANCE OF TIMING AND DOSE

Mucosal responses to soluble protein antigens early in life tend to be T_H2 biased, which has led to the general idea that this occurs by default in both animals and humans.[20] Genetics plays a clear role in mouse models, in which certain strains have exaggerated T_H2 bias, whereas others tend to be resistant to sensitization,[21] and although family studies suggest a strong genetic component in human food allergy, efforts have largely failed to identify risk alleles.[22] More recent evidence supports that impairment in T-reg induction and innate immunity may also contribute to T_H2 polarization in early life.[23] Although these findings might be expected in atopic infants, prospective birth cohort studies have shown that IgE production to egg, milk, and peanut commonly occur, even in healthy infants.[24] Importantly, although there remains some controversy, the inability of recent studies to identify a committed allergen-specific memory T_H2 response early in life suggests that allergic responses develop postnatally.[25] Several studies claimed to present evidence that allergic priming could occur in humans in utero, but these studies have largely been irreproducible, and methodologic flaws in their approach have been identified.[26]

In nonallergic individuals, the T_H2 bias appears to be transient, and IgE levels fall, possibly through a counterbalancing induction of antigen-specific T_H1 responses (ie, interferon [IFN]-γ); in contrast, these T_H2 responses consolidate and strengthen in allergic children, perhaps through induction of IL-4 signaling.[26] IL-4 is known to be a key cytokine that acts as a critical step in the allergic cascade, signaling B cells to undergo class-switch recombination and begin producing IgE. A number of cell types produce IL-4, including T_H2 cells, natural killer T (NKT) cells, and basophils; recent mouse studies have implicated basophils as a likely contributor of early IL-4 after allergen exposure.[27] Interestingly, in a large cohort of children at high risk for allergy, CD25+ cells expressed significant amounts of IL-4 after stimulation with food allergens, but did not express significant amounts of the T_H2-specific transcription factor GATA-3.[28] This indirectly suggests that in humans, a CD25+ non–T cell (ie, a basophil) may play a role in early allergic sensitization. Identifying the source of IL-4 early in human allergen priming is a key research question.

In mouse models, high-dose exposure to antigen in early life, even a single isolated dose, can produce lymphocyte anergy, whereas low-dose exposure, especially when repeated, induces tolerance through T-reg development.[29] Interestingly though, the differences in the actual dosing in these studies is quite small. Emerging evidence in human disease suggests that exposure to the proper dose of antigen during this critical period in early life is important for the shaping of the appropriate immune response to foods. Several epidemiologic studies have implicated delayed weaning patterns in the increased prevalence of peanut allergy.[30,31] Similarly, there is evidence that delayed introduction of cereals is associated with a higher risk of wheat allergy,[32] although methodologic limitations in retrospective studies make definitive conclusions difficult. Recently, European and American guidelines for the introduction of potentially allergenic solid foods were revised to reflect the position that insufficient high-quality evidence exists to support delayed weaning as a preventive (ie, tolerogenic) strategy.[33,34] However, early introduction is not automatically better, because mature immune regulation may require time. In a set of classic experiments, Strobel and Ferguson[35] showed that immunologic priming and allergic sensitization are enhanced in neonatal mouse pups fed the common experimental egg allergen ovalbumin in the first few days of life, whereas tolerance develops only after waiting 7 to 10 days to introduce antigen; if and how this "window" of priming versus tolerance translates to humans is unknown. Cow's milk is typically the first potentially allergenic exposure, often occurring early in life, and yet cow's milk is by far the most common food to which children are allergic.[5] Although oral tolerance has been shown to occur across a range of doses, frequent or continuous exposure to relatively low doses typically results in robust oral tolerance induction. Defining the most appropriate time and dose for tolerance induction in humans is a great research need. Interventional studies are under way to investigate the importance of early life oral exposure in tolerance development.

ELUDING THE DEFENSES

As we have seen, specific characteristics intrinsic to food proteins and the details of their exposure are important in determining the potential for inducing a deleterious allergic immune response. However, robust mechanisms exist within the host intestine to prevent would-be allergens from causing harm. The "first-line" features of mucosal defense serve to prevent luminal antigens from interacting with the MALT entirely. These include a hydrophobic layer of mucin oligosaccharides, which trap antigen, and both constitutive and inducible antimicrobial peptides. Secretory IgA has generally been considered to provide important tolerogenic function by binding to luminal antigens and preventing absorption (ie, "immune exclusion"), although its specific importance has been controversial.[36] A recent study showed that mice deficient in the receptor that secretes IgA and IgM into the intestinal lumen are hypersensitive to IgG-mediated anaphylaxis; nonetheless, they can be tolerized by an oral feed before systemic priming. In this model, tolerance was transferrable by CD4+CD25+ splenocytes, suggesting that cellular mechanisms can compensate for an impaired immune exclusion mechanism.[37] However, a recent case-control study from a larger placebo-controlled trial examining probiotics for allergy prevention in high-risk infants showed that the risk of atopy was inversely correlated with fecal IgA levels.[38] These data serve as one example of the complex and complementary forces that act to suppress immunity in the gut.

If a potential allergen penetrates these first few physical factors, the intestinal epithelium itself acts as a barrier to sequester luminal antigens from the MALT, and leakiness of this barrier has been postulated to result in allergic sensitization. Structural integrity of the intestinal epithelium is conferred by epithelial junction complexes, also called adherens junctions, and tight junctions. However, it may take years for complete developmental maturation of the gut barrier in healthy children.[39] In mice, the permeability of this barrier is further influenced by exposures to microbial pathogens such as viruses, alcohol, nonsteroidal anti-inflammatory drugs (NSAIDs), and other toxins, as well as cytokines such as IL-9, immune cells, and apoptotic pathways. These environmental exposures ultimately result in changes in gene expression and phosphorylation of tight junction proteins such as occludins, claudins, and JAM-ZO1 proteins, which in turn are associated with changes in intestinal mast cells and allergic sensitization.[40,41]

Interestingly, intestinal permeability was assessed in food-allergic infants by examining the lactulose/mannitol ratio in urine, and these infants were noted to have increased intestinal permeability when compared with healthy young children.[42] Investigators examined this ratio in children who had been on an allergen-free diet for at least 6 months and determined that intestinal permeability remained increased in food-allergic children, despite the absence of food allergen stimulation. Further evidence linking intestinal epithelial barrier dysfunction and food allergy comes from studies in immunosuppressed humans, who, after solid-organ transplantation, developed food allergy while on calcineurin inhibitors. Initially, investigators assumed this allergy was the result of transfer of sensitized donor lymphocytes. However, it is now theorized that medication-induced decreases in cellular adenosine triphosphate (ATP) levels altered the integrity of junctional complexes, resulting in increased intestinal permeability.[43] Mutations in the gene encoding filaggrin also lead to profound epidermal barrier dysfunction and are highly prevalent in patients with atopic dermatitis, which is in turn associated with an increased prevalence of food allergy. Acquired barrier defects associated with decreased filaggrin expression have been observed in the esophagus of patients with eosinophilic esophagitis, and are thought to be downregulated secondary to IL-13.[44] However, no studies to date have examined the mechanistic relationship of filaggrin mutations to IgE priming in the gut or clinical food allergy.[45]

Increasing evidence suggests that the mucosal epithelium is likely to play an active role in determining the host response to food allergens, which goes far beyond simply acting as an inert physical barrier. Epithelial cells are known to express major histocompatibility complex (MHC) class II molecules on their basolateral membranes and thus may act as nonprofessional APCs that do not express conventional costimulatory molecules, favoring anergy or tolerance.[46] In addition, factors derived from the gut epithelium are generally believed to condition the DCs in the stroma, dampening immune responses and promoting gut homeostasis.[47] One such factor, constitutively expressed by the gut epithelium, is thymic stromal lymphopoetin (TSLP). TSLP is an IL-7–like cytokine that has been shown to activate expression of OX40L on dendritic cells and drive T_H2 differentiation. Thus, TSLP is a critical mediator of allergic inflammation in the lung and skin. By contrast, in the gut, TSLP appears to play a regulatory role, limiting deleterious T_H1 and T_H17 inflammation in models of helminth infection and colitis.[48] Although incompletely understood, this regulation may occur at the level of the DC, which expresses the TSLP receptor and has been shown to develop tolerogenic properties after TSLP exposure. Interestingly, regulatory responses to dietary allergens are evidently normal in TSLP receptor-deficient animals.[49] These findings suggest that although allergic sensitization in the gut may be mediated or regulated via TSLP, it is not required for oral tolerance. Little is known about the role of TSLP in food sensitization in humans; however, a recent study identified TSLP gene expression in the esophagus of patients with eosinophilic esophagitis and showed that genetic variants in TSLP and the TSLP receptor are associated with the disease.[50]

THE MICROBIOME: FRIEND OR FOE?

Another critical influence on the gastrointestinal mucosal immune response is the microbial stimulation provided by the enteric flora, which by adulthood number approximately 100 trillion in the large intestine, providing essential nutritional and immunologic benefits.[51] These bacteria colonize the neonatal GI tract and begin interacting with the MALT within hours of birth. This interaction probably represents the primary stimulus for proper postnatal immune development, as germ-free mice, which are not colonized with bacteria at birth, have disorganized and poorly developed mucosal and secondary lymphoid structures. In the absence of a microbial flora, these animals have impaired antibody responses and do not develop oral tolerance.[52] In humans, specific differences have been identified in the flora of allergic and nonallergic children.[53] This suggests that although intestinal microbial colonization is required for proper immune development, certain microbes may play a significant role in skewing the immune response toward allergic sensitization. Exactly how this may occur is almost completely unknown.

The critical information provided by the microbiome is interpreted through signals from innate immune receptors, such as TLRs, which play an important role in intestinal homeostasis,[54] in the genesis of T-regs,[55] and on the outcome of allergic disease.[56] Most food allergy studies in mice use the C3H/HeJ strain, which cannot signal through TLR4, implicating the importance of its signal in promoting tolerance. Investigators have identified specific microbial products (ie, polysaccharide A from *Bacteroides fragilis*) that interact with TLRs and promote downstream induction of T-regs, which subsequently modulate intestinal inflammation in mouse models of experimental colitis.[55] However, determining the specific microbial signal(s) that is/are most critical in determining whether a response to a food protein will be allergic or toleragenic in humans has proven challenging, as evidenced by the overall disappointing results of probiotic trials on prevention and treatment of allergic disease.[57] This difficulty may be largely technical, because historically most studies have relied on culture-based methods to attempt to identify an incredibly diverse ecosystem, of which many members are fastidious or simply unculturable. New deep-sequencing technologies that focus on the unique 16s ribosomal subunit of bacterial RNA allow investigators to identify previously unknown organisms and promise to revolutionize our understanding of these critical microbes.[58] Coupling 16s rRNA sequencing techniques with high-throughput approaches allows profiling of entire bacterial communities, forming the basis of the Human Microbiome Project (HMP) to characterize the entire flora (http://nihroadmap.nih.gov/hmp/). Traditional culture-based techniques have already succeeded at identifying differences in the flora of allergic versus healthy children, and the HMP will undoubtedly shed important new light on this critical influence. If so, this will uncover new therapeutic targets to prevent or treat allergic sensitization, possibly with clinically available antimicrobial and/or pro- or pre-biotic approaches.

ANTIGEN-PRESENTING CELLS SET THE STAGE

Should allergenic food proteins survive oral and gastric digestion and evade luminal defenses, they will be detected by APCs in the MALT, likely in the context of signals provided by the commensal flora. In this way, a complex interplay of all aforementioned factors (ie, antigen character, dose, timing, and innate immune stimulation) will determine the immune response to an ingested food protein through the same final common pathway: by directly or indirectly influencing the APC. Much recent research has begun to demonstrate that mucosal DCs are probably the most critical determinant of allergic sensitization versus tolerance in naïve individuals, largely because of their location and their capacity to receive and interpret environmental signals, which lead to a specific immune response. These DCs can encounter ingested antigen in 1 of 3 ways: by extending dendrites through the paracellular space between epithelial cells to sample luminal contents, by directly interacting with the epithelial cells, and by taking up antigen in the Peyer patch, specialized lymphoid tissue that is immediately adjacent to microfold cells.[59] The properties of the antigen itself—particulate versus soluble—to a certain extent determine the route of exposure, and it is likely that each route will involve distinct DC populations.

The traditional paradigm for initiation of an immune response involves an APC encountering an antigen in the periphery and then migrating to the local lymph node to interact with T cells. Although macrophages, B cells, and others can act as

APCs, DCs are generally considered to be "professional" APCs that excel at the required functions. In their immature state, DCs sample their local environment and become activated when they encounter antigen in the context of microbial stimulation. This typically results in antigen processing, loading of the processed peptide antigen onto MHC class II molecules on the cell surface, upregulation of the costimulatory molecules necessary for T-cell stimulation, and chemotaxis to the draining lymph node. There, activated DCs interact with many T cells, and when they encounter a T cell that expresses a T-cell receptor (TCR) with the same specificity as the peptide antigen in the DC's class II molecule, an immune response ensues. When this DC–T-cell interaction occurs in the appropriate milieu (ie, significant amounts of IL-4, IL-5, and IL-13), the responding T cell is programmed to be a T_H2 cell, which can then signal B cells to generate IgE antibody. In this way, the allergic response is perpetuated. How this proallergic initial milieu is developed (a.k.a. the "original sin") in a naïve individual remains a fundamental question. There is some evidence in animals that basophils may contribute an early supply of IL-4, along with proallergic TSLP.[60] As described previously, recognition of carbohydrates by lectins may also provide key signals to DCs that drive T_H2 polarization.

Many features combine to make the intestine a unique immunologic situation, and the traditional paradigm described previously may not hold. For example, there is now evidence that IgE may be produced locally at the mucosal surface of the intestine, as it is in other mucosal sites like the respiratory tract.[12–14,61] The physical address of the DC–T-cell interaction described previously appears to be critical in determining the type of immune response that ensues. The lamina propria, which is full of lymphocytes, and the Peyer patches function as lymphoid structures, and are sufficient for induction of local immune responses. Several specialized APC populations reside within this loosely organized network and receive important signals from the epithelium and other adjacent structures. In this way, the local microenvironment provides key information to a specialized APC and influences an appropriate immune response; this likely represents a robust evolutionary adaptation to the rich antigenic environment in the gut. The health of the host depends on intestinal homeostasis, and careful recent studies in mice have highlighted the critical importance of the mesenteric lymph node (MLN) in preserving a state of nonresponsiveness. Whereas immunity can be generated locally, tolerance appears to depend on the migration, guided by the chemokine receptor CCR7, of pro-toleragenic DCs to the MLN. A key distinguishing feature of these pro-toleragenic DCs is the expression of the marker CD103.[62] By contrast, CD103-negative lamina propria DCs are strongly proinflammatory. These data suggest that tolerogenic DCs may receive site-specific signals from the intestinal epithelium through interactions with E-cadherin, a ligand of CD103; it is likely that local signals generated by the epithelium provide a unique microenvironment that licenses antigen presentation toward appropriate inflammatory versus tolerogenic outcomes.[63] Other local factors that play important roles in this complex interaction include the vitamin A analog retinoic acid and the immunosuppressive cytokine transforming growth factor-beta (TGF-β), both of which tend to induce tolerance.[64] The importance of CD103 expression and retinoic acid in regulating intestinal immune responses have also been shown in humans, implicating them as potential therapeutic targets to minimize adverse immune responses such as food allergy.

T CELLS PROMOTE ALLERGIC INFLAMMATION

At this point, the putative allergen has survived the passage into the intestine, been processed into a peptide and presented on the cell surface of an APC in the binding groove of the MHC II molecule, and then recognized by a TCR. This TCR-MHC interaction provides the first of 3 signals required for T-cell activation. The second is provided by the interaction of the costimulatory molecules CD80 and CD86 on the surface of the APC with CD28 on the surface of the T cell. The third is the signal provided by cytokines, which in the case of allergic immune responses are IL-4, IL-5, and IL-13. These 3 signals activate the T cell and cause upregulation of the transcription factor GATA-3, which is necessary and sufficient for T_H2 differentiation. This T_H2 T cell can then amplify the T_H2 cytokine response and proliferate, which results in growth and division of cells with identical specificity (ie, clonal expansion). Whereas many of these expanded T_H2 cells will eventually undergo apoptosis, some will further differentiate into memory T cells, which maintain strong T_H2 bias and serve to perpetuate allergic responses.[65] This is a critical step in the development of long-term immune memory, which can occur in patients with chronic allergy. An example is peanut allergy, which in contrast to egg or milk allergy, is not commonly outgrown.[66] It is not well understood why some allergies naturally resolve and others persist, but it is generally believed to be under the control of specialized T cells (ie, regulatory T cells) that can shut off the T_H2 response.

Newly differentiated T_H2 cells also serve one other important purpose: providing T-cell help to B cells.

B CELLS: IGE FACTORIES

In contrast to the T cell, which expresses the TCR, the antigen receptor expressed on the surface of a B cell is an immunoglobulin. B cells can thus bind allergen and interact with a CD4+ T cell that has specificity for the same allergen. When this occurs, the helper T cell signals the B cell to undergo antibody production. In the context of allergen presentation, IL-4 produced by the T_H2 cell, as well as the interaction of CD40 ligand on the T-cell surface with CD40 on the B-cell surface, causes the B cells to undergo class switch recombination and to begin making IgE. All of the previously described events culminate here in *allergic sensitization*, defined as the production of allergen-specific IgE antibodies.[67] Sensitization is a critical step in the pathophysiology of food allergy, because classical food reactions are IgE-mediated and involve symptoms characteristic of type 1 hypersensitivity, such as urticaria, angioedema, and anaphylaxis. However, it is extremely important to note that sensitization is necessary but not sufficient for the expression of clinical allergy. In other words, many healthy individuals will produce IgE antibodies to foods that they clinically tolerate; therefore, the presence of IgE can only be interpreted as a likely allergy in the context of a history that supports a pathologic role for that antibody.[68] This can be thought of as analogous to a positive purified protein derivative (PPD) test, which only confirms exposure to *Mycobacteria*. The diagnosis of tuberculosis depends on a fitting clinical history (hemoptysis, weight loss, night sweats, cavitary lung lesions, and so forth). Although the gold standard diagnostic test for food allergy is an oral food challenge, in patients with a suggestive history, high titers of food-specific IgE have been shown to be associated with a high enough probability of food allergy that challenge is not necessary.[69]

The IgE secreted by the B cell has the same specificity as the immunoglobulin expressed on the surface of the B cell (ie, it is clonal). Although IgE is by far the least prevalent antibody isotype in the circulation, allergen-specific IgE is readily detectable by both standard allergy skin-prick tests as well as in vitro immunoassays. In standard allergy tests, the IgE is detected using whole allergen, and the exact epitope specificity of the IgE is unknown. However, because food allergens are large macromolecules, they will typically activate multiple B cells in vivo and thus generate polyclonal IgE responses that have diverse specificities. Several recent studies of patients allergic to egg, peanut, shrimp, and milk have shown that the binding patterns of IgE, and in some cases the recognition of specific amino acid sequences within the allergen, are correlated with both the persistence and the severity of the allergy.[70] The IgE repertoire has been shown to be stable over the course of years in patients with peanut allergy,[71] suggesting that they are being produced by either memory B cells or perhaps long-lived plasma cells that have differentiated from B cells. It remains poorly understood how and why patients with persistent food allergy continue to make high titers of highly pathogenic antibodies in the absence of any exposure to antigen. Conversely, in children who do "outgrow" food allergy, a sustained reduction in IgE levels typically heralds the development of spontaneous clinical tolerance. Identifying the mechanisms that regulate IgE production in allergic humans is thus a critical research goal.

ELICITATION: MAST CELLS

The soluble IgE that is produced by B cells circulates and binds to the surface of mast cells and basophils, arming them for reactivity and completing a key step in the pathophysiology of allergic reactions. Mast cells are unique, highly granulated, tissue-resident cells that are increasingly recognized for a diversity of immune functions. They are found in the skin, gut, and respiratory tract, and are situated adjacent to nerves and blood vessels. Among the most important of their immune functions is the propensity to bind IgE using the high-affinity IgE receptor FcϵR1. When allergen is reencountered and recognized by cell-bound IgE, adjacent FcϵR1-IgE complexes move closer together and bring their signaling machinery into close proximity, which sets off a cascade of phosphorylation, ultimately resulting in calcium influx. When calcium enters the cell, the activated mast cell undergoes degranulation, and the contents of these granules are released into the extracellular space. The immediate liberation of preformed powerful vasoactive compounds such as histamine, platelet-activating factor, tryptase, carboxypeptidase, chymase, and heparin elicit the acute symptoms of type 1 hypersensitivity reactions in the skin, gut, respiratory, and cardiovascular systems.[72] These symptoms include urticaria, angioedema, flushing, nausea, vomiting, abdominal pain, diarrhea, wheezing, coughing/bronchospasm, rhinorrhea, and hypotension/syncope, which can occur alone or in combination, and typically begin within minutes of food ingestion. Tryptase is not uniformly elevated in food anaphylaxis, leading some to question whether basophils play a larger role than do mast cells in human food anaphylaxis; however, there is little direct evidence of their involvement. Mast cells also synthesize other mediators such as cysteinyl leukotrienes and prostaglandins upon activation, which require several hours to achieve their inflammatory effects, including recruitment and activation of secondary immune cells such as eosinophils.

SUMMARY

Although food allergy affects 12 million Americans, it is remarkable that it is not more common considering the complexities of the mucosal immune system. Robust immunologic mechanisms involving both humoral and cell-mediated responses have evolved to maintain a homeostatic environment amidst the literally billions of antigens within the intestine. To incite the allergic cascade, an ingested protein must circumvent this tolerogenic system. The sensitization phase begins when certain physicochemical characteristics increase the allergenicity of dietary proteins. Their capture by inflammatory dendritic cells in the gut results in an active immune response, which occurs under the influence of the local microenvironment. Certain key signals, such as IL-4, lead to T_H2 differentiation and propagation of the allergic T-cell response as well as isotype switching and IgE production. This allergen-specific IgE binds to the surface of mast cells and elicits mediator release within minutes to an hour after reexposure to the allergen. Bioactive mediators released by mast cells act on endothelium, smooth muscle, and epithelium to produce the symptoms characteristic of allergic reactions.

REFERENCES

1. Chafen JJ, Newberry SJ, Riedl MA, et al. Diagnosing and managing common food allergies: a systematic review. JAMA 2010;303(18):1848–56.
2. Branum AM, Lukacs SL. Food allergy among children in the United States. Pediatrics 2009;124(6):1549–55.
3. Venter C, Arshad SH, Grundy J, et al. Time trends in the prevalence of peanut allergy: three cohorts of children from the same geographical location in the UK. Allergy 2010;65(1):103–8.
4. Gupta R, Sheikh A, Strachan DP, et al. Time trends in allergic disorders in the UK. Thorax 2007;62(1):91–6.
5. Sicherer SH, Sampson HA. Food allergy. J Allergy Clin Immunol 2010; 125(2 Suppl 2):S116–25.
6. Bock SA, Munoz-Furlong A, Sampson HA. Further fatalities caused by anaphylactic reactions to food, 2001–2006. J Allergy Clin Immunol 2007;119:1016–8.
7. Gupta RS, Springston EE, Smith B, et al. Food allergy knowledge, attitudes, and beliefs of parents with food-allergic children in the United States. Pediatr Allergy Immunol 2010;21(6):927–34.
8. Cummings AJ, Knibb RC, King RM, et al. The psychosocial impact of food allergy and food hypersensitivity in children, adolescents and their families: a review. Allergy 2010;65(8):933–45.
9. Chehade M, Mayer L. Oral tolerance and its relation to food hypersensitivities. J Allergy Clin Immunol 2005;115(1):3–12.
10. Coombes JL, Powrie F. Dendritic cells in intestinal immune regulation. Nat Rev Immunol 2008;8(6):435–46.
11. Faria AM, Weiner HL. Oral tolerance. Immunol Rev 2005;206(1):232–59.
12. Gould HJ, Sutton BJ. IgE in allergy and asthma today. Nat Rev Immunol 2008; 8(3):205–17.
13. Untersmayr E, Jensen-Jarolim E. The role of protein digestibility and antacids on food allergy outcomes. J Allergy Clin Immunol 2008;121(6):1301–8.
14. Husby S, Oxelius VA, Teisner B, et al. Humoral immunity to dietary antigens in healthy adults. Occurrence, isotype and IgG subclass distribution of serum antibodies to protein antigens. Int Arch Allergy Appl Immunol 1985;77(4):416–22.
15. Berin MC, Shreffler WG. T(H)2 adjuvants: implications for food allergy. J Allergy Clin Immunol 2008;121(6):1311–20.
16. Karp CL. Guilt by intimate association: what makes an allergen an allergen? J Allergy Clin Immunol 2010;125(5):955–60.
17. Shreffler WG, Castro RR, Kucuk ZY, et al. The major glycoprotein allergen from *Arachis hypogaea*, Ara h 1, is a ligand of dendritic cell-specific ICAM-grabbing nonintegrin and acts as a Th2 adjuvant in vitro. J Immunol 2006;177(6):3677–85.
18. Wills-Karp M, Nathan A, Page K, et al. New insights into innate immune mechanisms underlying allergenicity. Mucosal Immunol 2010;3(2):104–10.

19. Nowak-Wegrzyn A, Fiocchi A. Rare, medium, or well done? The effect of heating and food matrix on food protein allergenicity. Curr Opin Allergy Clin Immunol 2009;9(3):234–7.
20. Weiner HL, Friedman A, Miller A, et al. Oral tolerance: immunologic mechanisms and treatment of animal and human organ-specific autoimmune diseases by oral administration of autoantigens. Annu Rev Immunol 1994;12(1):809–37.
21. Berin MC, Zheng Y, Domaradzki M, et al. Role of TLR4 in allergic sensitization to food proteins in mice. Allergy 2006;61(1):64–71.
22. Hong X, Tsai HJ, Wang X. Genetics of food allergy. Curr Opin Pediatr 2009;21(6):770–6.
23. Prescott SL. Allergic disease: understanding how in utero events set the scene. Proc Nutr Soc 2010;69(3):366–72.
24. Sigurs N, Hattevig G, Kjellman B, et al. Appearance of atopic disease in relation to serum IgE antibodies in children followed up from birth for 4 to 15 years. J Allergy Clin Immunol 1994;94(4):757–63.
25. Rowe J, Kusel M, Holt BJ, et al. Prenatal versus postnatal sensitization to environmental allergens in a high-risk birth cohort. J Allergy Clin Immunol 2007;119(5):1164–73.
26. Holt PG. Prenatal versus postnatal priming of allergen specific immunologic memory: the debate continues. J Allergy Clin Immunol 2008;122(4):717–8.
27. Paul WE, Zhu J. How are T(H)2-type immune responses initiated and amplified? Nat Rev Immunol 2010;10(4):225–35.
28. Sicherer SH, Wood RA, Stablein D, et al. Immunologic features of infants with milk or egg allergy enrolled in an observational study (Consortium of Food Allergy Research) of food allergy. J Allergy Clin Immunol 2010;125(5):1077–83.e8.
29. Burks AW, Laubach S, Jones SM. Oral tolerance, food allergy, and immunotherapy: implications for future treatment. J Allergy Clin Immunol 2008;121(6):1344–50.
30. Du Toit G, Katz Y, Sasieni P, et al. Early consumption of peanuts in infancy is associated with a low prevalence of peanut allergy. J Allergy Clin Immunol 2008;122(5):984–91.
31. Fox AT, Sasieni P, du Toit G, et al. Household peanut consumption as a risk factor for the development of peanut allergy. J Allergy Clin Immunol 2009;123(2):417–23.
32. Poole JA, Barriga K, Leung DY, et al. Timing of initial exposure to cereal grains and the risk of wheat allergy. Pediatrics 2006;117(6):2175–82.
33. Greer FR, Sicherer SH, Burks A. Effects of early nutritional interventions on the development of atopic disease in infants and children: the role of maternal dietary restriction, breastfeeding, timing of introduction of complementary foods, and hydrolyzed formulas. Pediatrics 2008;121(1):183–91.
34. Høst A, Halken S, Muraro A, et al. Dietary prevention of allergic diseases in infants and small children. Pediatr Allergy Immunol 2008;19(1):1–4.
35. Strobel S, Ferguson A. Immune responses to fed protein antigens in mice. 3. Systemic tolerance or priming is related to age at which antigen is first encountered. Pediatr Res 1984;18(7):588–94.
36. Brandtzaeg P. Update on mucosal immunoglobulin A in gastrointestinal disease. 9000; Publish Ahead of Print. Available at: http://journals.lww.com/co-gastroenterology/Fulltext/publishahead/Update_on_mucosal_immunoglobulin_A_in.99878.aspx. Accessed June 22, 2010.
37. Karlsson MR, Johansen F, Kahu H, et al. Hypersensitivity and oral tolerance in the absence of a secretory immune system. Allergy 2010;65(5):561–70.

38. Kukkonen K, Kuitunen M, Haahtela T, et al. High intestinal IgA associates with reduced risk of IgE-associated allergic diseases. Pediatr Allergy Immunol 2010;21(1 pt I):67–73.
39. Dahan S, Roth-Walter F, Arnaboldi P, et al. Epithelia: lymphocyte interactions in the gut. Immunol Rev 2007;215(1):243–53.
40. Forbes EE, Groschwitz K, Abonia JP, et al. IL-9– and mast cell–mediated intestinal permeability predisposes to oral antigen hypersensitivity. J Exp Med 2008; 205(4):897–913.
41. Groschwitz KR, Hogan SP. Intestinal barrier function: molecular regulation and disease pathogenesis. J Allergy Clin Immunol 2009;124(1):3–20.
42. Ventura M, Polimeno L, Amoruso A, et al. Intestinal permeability in patients with adverse reactions to food. Dig Liver Dis 2006;38(10):732–6.
43. Levy Y, Davidovits M, Cleper R, et al. New-onset post-transplantation food allergy in children—Is it attributable only to the immunosuppressive protocol? Pediatr Transplant 2009;13(1):63–9.
44. Blanchard C, Stucke EM, Burwinkel K, et al. Coordinate interaction between IL-13 and epithelial differentiation cluster genes in eosinophilic esophagitis. J Immunol 2010;184(7):4033–41.
45. van den Oord R, Sheikh A. Filaggrin gene defects and risk of developing allergic sensitisation and allergic disorders: systematic review and meta-analysis. BMJ 2009;339:b2433.
46. Hershberg RM, Cho DH, Youakim A, et al. Highly polarized HLA class II antigen processing and presentation by human intestinal epithelial cells. J Clin Invest 1998;102(4):792–803.
47. Iliev ID, Matteoli G, Rescigno M. The yin and yang of intestinal epithelial cells in controlling dendritic cell function. J Exp Med 2007;204(10):2253–7.
48. Ziegler SF, Artis D. Sensing the outside world: TSLP regulates barrier immunity. Nat Immunol 2010;11(4):289–93.
49. Blazquez AB, Berin MC. Gastrointestinal dendritic cells promote Th2 skewing via OX40L. J Immunol 2008;180(7):4441–50.
50. Sherrill JD, Gao P, Stucke EM, et al. Variants of thymic stromal lymphopoietin and its receptor associate with eosinophilic esophagitis. J Allergy Clin Immunol 2010; 126(1):160–5.e3.
51. Round JL, Mazmanian SK. The gut microbiota shapes intestinal immune responses during health and disease. Nat Rev Immunol 2009;9(5):313–23.
52. Mowat A, Parker L, Beacock-Sharp H, et al. Oral tolerance: overview and historical perspectives. Ann N Y Acad Sci 2004;1029:1–8 (1 Oral tolerance: new insights and prospects for clinical application).
53. Bjorksten B, Sepp E, Julge K, et al. Allergy development and the intestinal microflora during the first year of life. J Allergy Clin Immunol 2001;108(4):516–20.
54. Rakoff-Nahoum S, Paglino J, Eslami-Varzaneh F, et al. Recognition of commensal microflora by Toll-like receptors is required for intestinal homeostasis. Cell 2004; 118:229–41.
55. Round JL, Mazmanian SK. Inducible Foxp3+ regulatory T-cell development by a commensal bacterium of the intestinal microbiota. Proc Natl Acad Sci U S A 2010;107(27):12204–9.
56. Holt PG, Strickland DH. Soothing signals: transplacental transmission of resistance to asthma and allergy. J Exp Med 2009;206(13):2861–4.
57. Yao T, Chang C, Hsu Y, et al. Review article: probiotics for allergic diseases: realities and myths. Pediatr Allergy Immunol 2010;21(6):900–19.

58. Medini D, Serruto D, Parkhill J, et al. Microbiology in the post-genomic era. Nat Rev Microbiol 2008;6(6):419–30.
59. Mowat AM. Anatomical basis of tolerance and immunity to intestinal antigens. Nat Rev Immunol 2003;3(4):331–41.
60. Sokol CL, Medzhitov R. Emerging functions of basophils in protective and allergic immune responses. Mucosal Immunol 2010;3(2):129–37.
61. Coëffier M, Lorentz A, Manns MP, et al. Epsilon germ-line and IL-4 transcripts are expressed in human intestinal mucosa and enhanced in patients with food allergy. Allergy 2005;60(6):822–7.
62. Worbs T, Bode U, Yan S, et al. Oral tolerance originates in the intestinal immune system and relies on antigen carriage by dendritic cells. J Exp Med 2006;203(3): 519–27.
63. Belkaid Y, Oldenhove G. Tuning microenvironments: induction of regulatory T cells by dendritic cells. Immunity 2008;29(3):362–71.
64. Mucida D, Park Y, Cheroutre H. From the diet to the nucleus: vitamin A and TGF-ß join efforts at the mucosal interface of the intestine. Semin Immunol 2009;21: 14–21.
65. Galli SJ, Tsai M, Piliponsky AM. The development of allergic inflammation. Nature 2008;454(7203):445–54.
66. Flinterman AE, Pasmans SG, den Hartog Jager CF, et al. T cell responses to major peanut allergens in children with and without peanut allergy. Clin Exp Allergy 2010;40(4):590–7.
67. Geha RS, Jabara HH, Brodeur SR. The regulation of immunoglobulin E class-switch recombination. Nat Rev Immunol 2003;3(9):721–32.
68. Du Toit G, Santos A, Roberts G, et al. The diagnosis of IgE-mediated food allergy in childhood. Pediatr Allergy Immunol 2009;20(4):309–19.
69. Sampson HA. Utility of food-specific IgE concentrations in predicting symptomatic food allergy. J Allergy Clin Immunol 2001;107(5):891–6.
70. Lin J, Sampson HA. The role of immunoglobulin E-binding epitopes in the characterization of food allergy. Curr Opin Allergy Clin Immunol 2009;9(4):357–63.
71. Shreffler WG, Beyer K, Chu TH, et al. Microarray immunoassay: association of clinical history, in vitro IgE function, and heterogeneity of allergenic peanut epitopes. J Allergy Clin Immunol 2004;113(4):776–82.
72. Galli SJ, Tsai M. Mast cells in allergy and infection: versatile effector and regulatory cells in innate and adaptive immunity. Eur J Immunol 2010;40(7):1843–51.

Recognition and Management of Food-Induced Anaphylaxis

Corinne Keet, MD

KEYWORDS

• Anaphylaxis • Food allergy • Epinephrine

Food allergy is a major cause of anaphylaxis in children, and it seems that the rates of both food allergy and anaphylaxis are increasing in developed countries. Extrapolating the most conservative estimates of anaphylaxis incidence to the overall US population leads to a minimum of 25,000 cases each year.[1] Food allergy accounts for 15% to 57% of those cases.[2–7] Widespread deficiencies of concern include significant underrecognition of anaphylaxis and inadequate treatment.[8,9] One recent report estimated that at least half of likely cases of anaphylaxis are miscoded,[10] and other surveys have found even higher rates of misclassification.[11,12] Epinephrine, the primary lifesaving drug in anaphylaxis treatment, is used infrequently in emergency settings and is underprescribed as a discharge medication.[8,13] Recognizing food-induced anaphylaxis, adequately treating the episode, identifying the causative agent, and providing effective recommendations to prevent and/or live with food allergies are important aspects of care that need to be improved.

DEFINITION OF ANAPHYLAXIS

Anaphylaxis is a multisystem reaction to allergen exposure. Although the term was coined in 1902,[14] pervasive inconsistencies in its application have made interpretation of the literature difficult. In an effort to standardize research and treatment of anaphylaxis, a joint panel from the American Academy of Allergy Asthma and Immunology;

This publication was made possible in part by grant number 1KL2RR025006-01 from the National Center for Research Resources (NCRR), a component of the National Institutes of Health (NIH), and NIH Roadmap for Medical Research. Its contents are solely the responsibility of the author and do not necessarily represent the official view of NCRR or NIH. Information on NCRR is available at http://www.ncrr.nih.gov/. Information on Re-engineering the Clinical Research Enterprise can be obtained from http://nihroadmap.nih.gov/clinicalresearch/overview-translational.asp.

Division of Pediatric Allergy and Immunology, Department of Pediatrics, Johns Hopkins School of Medicine, CMSC 1102, 600 North Wolfe Street, Baltimore, MD 21287, USA
E-mail address: ckeet1@jhmi.edu

Pediatr Clin N Am 58 (2011) 377–388
doi:10.1016/j.pcl.2011.02.006 **pediatric.theclinics.com**
0031-3955/11/$ – see front matter

the American College of Allergy, Asthma and Immunology; and the Joint Council of Allergy, Asthma and Immunology agreed on a consensus definition of anaphylaxis in 2006 and recently revised it.[15,16] They define anaphylaxis as one of the following:

1. The acute onset of a reaction (minutes to hours), with involvement of the skin, mucosal tissue, or both, and at least one of the following:
   Respiratory compromise
   Reduced blood pressure or symptoms of end-organ dysfunction
2. Two or more of the following that occur rapidly after exposure to a likely allergen for that patient
   Involvement of the skin/mucosal tissue
   Respiratory compromise
   Reduced blood pressure or associated symptoms
   Persistent gastrointestinal (GI) symptoms
3. Reduced blood pressure after exposure to a known allergen.[16]

Although this definition is cumbersome, it highlights the fact that anaphylaxis is not always characterized by severe respiratory and cardiovascular compromise; persistent abdominal pain and urticaria after ingestion of a likely allergen (for that patient) also meet the definition of anaphylaxis. Generally, anaphylaxis has been understood as an IgE-mediated reaction, although the World Allergy Organization has recommended that non-IgE–mediated anaphylaxis-type reactions be included under the term. So far, US consensus panels have rejected that suggestion,[16] and in this review, anaphylaxis refers to an IgE-mediated syndrome.

PATHOPHYSIOLOGY OF ANAPHYLAXIS

The initiating event in an anaphylactic episode is the association between the allergen and membrane-bound IgE on mast cells and basophils. This association leads to aggregation of the high-affinity IgE receptor, triggering an intracellular signaling cascade that ultimately leads to calcium influx and degranulation of the cell. Activation of mast cells and basophils causes release of preformed mediators of inflammation (histamine, tryptase, carboxypeptidase A, proteoglycans, and some cytokines) and newly generated mediators (leukotrienes, cytokines including tumor necrosis factor [TNF]-α, and platelet-activating factor [PAF]). Ultimately, these mediators cause the characteristic clinical features of anaphylaxis, including vasodilation, angioedema, bronchoconstriction, and increased mucus production.[17–19]

Histamine, one of the preformed mediators released by mast cells and basophils, can recapitulate most of the signs and symptoms of anaphylaxis when administered intravenously to humans and laboratory animals.[17] Histamine acts through H1 and H2 receptors on multiple organ systems. Its effects on the vascular bed include release of nitric oxide by endothelial cells (H1 receptors) and direct relaxation of smooth muscle (H2 receptors). In the lung, bronchoconstriction is mediated by H1 receptors, whereas stimulation of both H1 and H2 receptors causes increased production of mucus. Histamine increases cardiac oxygen demand indirectly by peripheral vasodilation and via direct effects on the heart, including increased contractility, shortened depolarization, and increased heart rate. Histamine can also cause coronary artery vasospasm through the H1 receptor.[13,16,20]

Other mediators of anaphylaxis include leukotrienes and other products of arachidonic acid metabolism, including prostaglandins; PAF (discussed in more detail later); the neutral proteases such as tryptase and chymase; the proteoglycans, including heparin; and various chemokines. These mediators recruit inflammatory cells and activate complement cascades, among other mechanisms.[17]

Over the past 5 years, several studies have highlighted the role of PAF in the propagation of anaphylaxis. PAF is a preformed mediator of anaphylaxis released by mast cells, monocytes, and tissue macrophages. It is degraded by PAF-acetylhydrolase. In a seminal article published in 2008, Vadas and colleagues[21] measured PAF and PAF-acetylhydrolase in patients with varying gradations of anaphylaxis severity. They found significant correlation between PAF levels and the severity of anaphylaxis; all subjects with severe anaphylaxis had elevated PAF levels. In addition, levels of PAF-acetylhydrolase were inversely correlated with the severity of anaphylaxis.[21] Subsequently, Arias and colleagues[22] showed that blocking PAF prevents severe anaphylactic reactions, and, when combined with antihistamines, abolishes nearly all signs of anaphylaxis. Further, Kajiwara and colleagues[23] demonstrated that PAF, by itself, was capable of activating mast cells in the lung and peripheral blood but not in the skin. The role of PAF-acetylhydrolase deficiency as a risk factor for severe allergic reactions is an area of active exploration.

DIAGNOSIS OF ANAPHYLAXIS

There are 2 components to the diagnosis of food-induced anaphylaxis. The first is the recognition of an anaphylactic event, and the second is the identification of the etiologic agent.

Clinical Syndrome

As described earlier, anaphylaxis involves a combination of cutaneous, respiratory, cardiovascular, and GI symptoms. A recent review that collated information on 1865 patients with anaphylaxis found that skin symptoms are the most common manifestation of anaphylaxis, present in up to 90% of episodes.[16] In this same series, symptoms of both upper and lower respiratory compromise were common, occurring in up to 60% and 50% of published cases, respectively.[16] Perhaps because the GI mucosa is the location of exposure in food-induced anaphylaxis, GI symptoms are much more common in food-induced than in non–food-induced anaphylaxis. One series of patients referred to an allergist for anaphylaxis found that only 3.7% of cases of non–food-induced anaphylaxis had GI symptoms compared with another series in which 41% of those caused by foods had GI symptoms.[16,24] Hypotension, dizziness, and syncope are associated with up to 35% of cases of anaphylaxis in general but are much less common in food-induced anaphylaxis, in which they are rarely found in isolation from respiratory arrest. In severe food-induced reactions, respiratory symptoms predominate and are responsible for the overwhelming majority of fatalities.[25–29]

The time from ingestion of the food to onset of symptoms is usually on the order of minutes. In published reports, the median time from ingestion to symptom onset ranges from less than 5 minutes to 2 hours.[24] More severe cases tend to present earlier.[25,28,29] Usually, symptoms resolve quickly with appropriate treatment. One area of considerable controversy in the literature is the true frequency of biphasic reactions during anaphylaxis. In a biphasic reaction, symptoms of the initial reaction resolve but are followed by recurrent or new symptoms hours later. Published reports suggest that this reaction occurs in 5% to 28% of anaphylaxis cases,[30–33] and some have suggested that biphasic reactions are more common with ingested allergens, which are absorbed slowly.[34] There is also conflicting evidence about whether administration of corticosteroids or time to epinephrine delivery affects the risk for biphasic reactions.[30–33] In general, the second reaction tends to be less severe than the original reaction.

ATYPICAL FOOD-INDUCED ANAPHYLAXIS

Two unusual types of food-induced anaphylaxis, food-dependent exercise-induced anaphylaxis and carbohydrate-induced anaphylaxis, merit special comment. Food-dependent exercise-induced anaphylaxis is a rare cause of anaphylaxis.[35] In this syndrome, patients tolerate both the causative food and exercise in isolation, but not together. Typically, this syndrome presents in adolescence or in individuals in the 20s, but it can occur at any age.[36] The time between consumption of the food and onset of symptoms is frequently longer than in other kinds of food-induced anaphylaxis, as reactions have been reported hours after eating the food. Usually, symptoms begin within 30 minutes of the start of exercise, but can occur at any time during the workout and with any intensity of exercise. The initial stage usually consists of cutaneous signs and fatigue, followed by more generalized symptoms.[16]

The most common food to trigger food-dependent exercise-induced anaphylaxis is wheat, followed by other grains, nuts, and seafood.[16] Skin prick testing and food-specific IgE can help confirm the diagnosis, although the size of the skin test or level of food-specific IgE is usually lower than that found in other types of food allergy. The mechanism of exercise-induced anaphylaxis is thought to be increased permeability of the gut to undigested allergens, although this is only speculative. Exercise-induced anaphylaxis can be confused with cholinergic urticaria, in which hives occur with heating. Cholinergic urticaria is not typically accompanied by the systemic symptoms that are characteristic of exercise-induced anaphylaxis, and symptoms can be reproduced by passive heating.[16] The current recommendation for prevention of food-dependent exercise-induced anaphylaxis is to either completely avoid the food or to wait at least 6 hours between food ingestion and exercise.[16] Additional important measures are for patients to carry self-injectable epinephrine and exercise with a partner who is aware of the condition and able to assist.

Another unusual type of anaphylaxis to food has been called delayed anaphylaxis to red meat or carbohydrate-induced anaphylaxis. This condition has recently been reported in patients living in the southeastern United States and Australia who presented with anaphylaxis 3 to 6 hours after ingesting red meat.[37] Commins and colleagues[38] found that these patients had IgE to a carbohydrate found on mammalian serum albumin called galactose-α-1,3-galactose (α-gal). The condition usually begins in adulthood and seems to have a particular geographic specificity. An intriguing hypothesis to explain the age and geographic distribution of α-gal sensitization is that the bite of a tick endemic to this geographic region sensitizes people to the α-gal. Indeed, a history of tick bite is more common in patients with sensitivity to α-gal. General practitioners should be aware of this unusual type of anaphylaxis and refer patients to allergists for evaluation if it is suspected.

SEVERE AND FATAL ANAPHYLAXIS

Food-allergy–induced fatalities remain rare, although fear of fatal reactions contributes to the anxiety that exists in families with a food-allergic child.[39] Since Yunginger and colleagues[40] first described a series of deaths from food-induced anaphylaxis in 1998, the most important risk factor for a severe reaction remains a history of asthma. In the series published thus far, the prevalence of a positive history for asthma in fatal reactions has approached 100%.[25–29,40] In addition to asthma, several other features of a food allergen exposure seem to convey particular risk. Adolescence is the age at greatest risk for a fatal reaction, from increased reactivity or, more likely, because of increased risk-taking behavior. Peanuts are the most common cause of fatal reactions, causing 50% to 60% of fatal reactions. Tree nuts account for another 15% to 30% of fatal reactions.[25–29,40] In 2 reports from the United States and Great Britain attempting to account for as many food-related fatalities as possible between 2001 and 2006 (United States) and 1999 and 2006 (Great Britain), milk emerged as the next most common cause, accounting for 13% of deaths in each series.[27,29] Shellfish, fish, eggs, sesame, and selected fruits and vegetables account for most of the remaining causes.

Attempts to find other markers that prospectively identify patients at risk for severe reactions have been largely unsuccessful. Although some have found correlations between food-specific IgE titers and/or skin prick test size and the magnitude of clinical reactivity, most have found them to be poorly predictive of reaction severity with food challenge or accidental exposure.[41–47] This is, perhaps, not surprising, given that the correlation between reaction severity in the clinic and in the community is itself weak ($r^2 = 0.37$), likely because of variable exposure doses.[43] Recent studies of immunotherapy for food allergy offer an interesting opportunity to explore risk factors for reaction at a given dose. Exercise, concurrent illness, and menstrual status were identified as risk factors for unexpected or more severe reactions to a given dose.[48–50] These findings may not extend to community-based reactions, but it is likely that incident-specific factors, such as those mentioned earlier, and concurrent intake of alcohol[40] are the most important predictors of severe reactions.

DIFFERENTIAL DIAGNOSIS OF ANAPHYLAXIS

The differential diagnosis of anaphylaxis includes other illnesses that cause acute respiratory distress, syncope, rash, and/or GI distress. In children, vocal cord dysfunction, panic attacks, and vasovagal reactions (also known as vasodepressor reactions) deserve particular note. Vocal cord dysfunction is caused by abnormal adduction of the vocal cords during inspiration. It can coexist with asthma, and the wheezing and coughing can mimic anaphylaxis. Treatment is speech therapy.[51] Signs and symptoms found in vasovagal reactions, including hypotension, nausea, vomiting, and diaphoresis can mimic anaphylaxis, but these reactions lack the typical skin manifestations found in anaphylaxis. In contrast to anaphylaxis, vasovagal reactions are characterized by bradycardia, whereas anaphylaxis is usually, but not always, accompanied by tachycardia.[16] Other causes of flushing, including the red man syndrome from vancomycin, should be considered in the differential.

Miscellaneous food-related conditions that can be confused with anaphylaxis include scombroid poisoning, which mimics anaphylaxis closely, as it is caused by consumption of histamine itself, and monosodium glutamate-related flushing, which is not an IgE-mediated condition. Food protein–induced enterocolitis syndrome (FPIES) is a non-IgE–mediated disease presenting in infancy. Acute reactions usually include profound vomiting, leading to dehydration, lethargy, and hypotension, starting hours after the food is ingested. Awareness of this condition is important, as is the understanding that a negative skin prick test result or food-specific IgE does not rule it out.[52]

LABORATORY STUDIES TO CONFIRM ANAPHYLAXIS

Laboratory studies are less helpful in confirming food-induced anaphylaxis than other types of anaphylaxis. Because serum histamine levels are elevated only for 30 to 60 minutes after the onset of reaction, they are not usually measured in any type of anaphylaxis. The most commonly assessed mediator in clinical practice is tryptase. Tryptase levels in the blood peak 1.5 hours after the onset of symptoms and are measurable for up to 5 hours. However, in reports of severe and fatal anaphylactic reactions to foods, tryptase is less commonly elevated than in other types of anaphylaxis.[25,40,53–55] Because basophils have lower levels of tryptase than mast cells, some have speculated that this is a sign of the central importance of basophils in food-induced anaphylaxis, although this hypothesis has not been confirmed.

In a recent series of 76 cases of anaphylaxis from all causes, including nonfood causes, presenting to the emergency room (ER), 2 distinctive types of severe reactions were identified: those with predominantly hypotensive symptoms and those with predominant hypoxia.[18] The investigators of this series identified a consistent cytokine pattern, including the presence of interleukin (IL)-6, IL-10, TNF receptor 1, mast cell tryptase, and histamine, in hypotensive episodes but not in hypoxemic episodes, suggesting either different pathways leading to hypoxemia or a predominantly local response not reflected in the peripheral blood. Both are plausible explanations for the unique presentation of food-induced reactions. At present, there is no laboratory test that reliably confirms cases of food-induced anaphylaxis.

IDENTIFICATION OF UNDERLYING FOOD ALLERGY

Clinical history remains the most important tool to identify the cause of an acute episode of anaphylaxis. In contrast to other types of anaphylaxis, many, if not most, cases of reactions to foods occur in patients with a known history of allergy. However, the allergen is frequently hidden in other foods. Common sources of accidental peanut and tree nut exposure are baked goods, candies, and Asian foods, whereas milk can be found hidden in chocolate, bread, and baked goods.[25,29,56] Knowledge of the epidemiology and natural history of food allergy is helpful in suggesting possible triggers if the diagnosis is not yet established. The most common food allergies in childhood are caused by milk, egg, and peanut. Milk and egg allergy are typically outgrown by adulthood, although a significant and perhaps growing minority persist to at least adolescence.[57,58] In adulthood, peanut allergy remains a common cause of anaphylaxis, and tree nut and shellfish allergies emerge as important causes. Both the epidemiology and diagnosis of food allergy are reviewed in depth elsewhere in this issue.

Referral to an allergist is helpful to identify the cause of anaphylaxis and help prevent future episodes. At the time of referral, the general practitioner should ensure that the patient has been provided with a prescription for self-injectable epinephrine, given the chance for repeat episodes of anaphylaxis, especially if the cause remains elusive. For confirmation or exploration of potential allergies, the allergist either performs a specific skin prick test or tests the blood for food-specific IgE. All allergy testing needs to be interpreted in the context of a careful clinical history, as false-positive results are common. Failure to take into account dietary history and understand the predictive value of these tests frequently leads to overly restrictive elimination diets.

MANAGEMENT OF ANAPHYLAXIS

Epinephrine and Other Lifesaving Treatments

Epinephrine remains the mainstay of treatment for anaphylactic reactions. Antihistamines, glucocorticoids, and β-agonists either alone or in combination do not substitute for epinephrine's life-saving role in the treatment of anaphylaxis. Although, for obvious ethical reasons, prospective controlled studies of its use in human anaphylaxis have not been conducted, the evidence for its utility is persuasive. Epinephrine is an α-1 agonist, causing vasoconstriction leading to increased blood pressure and decreased mucosal edema; a β-1 agonist, causing increased cardiac contractility; and a β-2 agonist, reversing bronchoconstriction and inflammatory mediator release.[13,59] In controlled animal models and in human clinical experience, injected epinephrine rapidly reverses anaphylaxis. In humans, retrospective studies have shown that lack of prompt treatment with epinephrine is one of the major risk factors for death from anaphylaxis.[25–29,40,54]

The optimal method of administration of epinephrine is by intramuscular (IM) injection. Subcutaneous injection is not preferred, as administration via this method can lead to local vasoconstriction, delayed absorption, and decreased peak levels of epinephrine.[60] Injection into the vastus lateralis muscle (lateral thigh) leads to a faster peak blood level compared with deltoid injection,[60] although the clinical relevance has not been established.[16] IM administration is considerably less complicated than intravenous (IV) dosing, which lacks an established dosing regimen and is prone to dosing errors.[16,59] Moreover, IV epinephrine can lead to lethal arrhythmias.[16] The most recent practice parameter recommends restricting the use of IV epinephrine to patients with profound hypotension or failure to respond to IM epinephrine. In addition, patients who receive IV epinephrine should have continuous cardiac monitoring in place.[16]

The recommended dose for IM injection is from 0.01 mg/kg to a maximum of 0.3 mg in children, given as a 1:1000 solution (1 mg/mL). In adults, the dose is 0.2 to 0.5 mg.[16] Commercially available prefilled syringes for autoinjection (EpiPen [Dey Pharma, Basking Ridge, NJ, USA], Twinject, and Adrenaclick [Shionogi, Pharma, Atlanta, GA, USA]) are available in strengths of 0.15 and 0.3 mg. They should be administered in the lateral thigh. The package inserts for both commercially available autoinjectors suggest the 0.15-mg dose for those who weigh 15 to 30 kg and the 0.3-mg dose for those weighing more than 30 kg, but the most recent guidelines from the National Institutes of Health recommend switching to the 0.3-mg dose at approximately 25 kg because of the risk of underdosing above this weight if the smaller dosage is used.[61] Because the risks of overdose with the autoinjector use must be weighed against the demonstrated difficulty that nonprofessionals have with correctly and promptly drawing up epinephrine into a syringe,[59] the same guidelines recommend the use of the 0.15-mg autoinjector for patients down to 10 kg. In practice, self-injected epinephrine is prescribed even to smaller infants.[62] The dose may be repeated at intervals of at least 5 minutes if necessary. Ideally, epinephrine autoinjectors are prescribed on discharge from the ER after management of anaphylaxis or following consultation with a pediatric allergist for suspected food allergy.

Despite universal recommendations for the use of epinephrine in anaphylaxis, it is actually uncommonly used in home or ER treatment of food-induced anaphylaxis,[11] perhaps because patients perceive epinephrine as a dangerous medication or patients and practitioners do not think their symptoms are severe enough to merit epinephrine.[9] One review of patients presenting with food allergy to 21 ERs in North America found that, although 33% were treated for respiratory symptoms with albuterol or other inhaled treatments, only 16% received epinephrine in the ER and only 16% were prescribed epinephrine at discharge.[8] How to improve translation of practice parameters into the actual emergency treatment of anaphylaxis is an area ripe for examination. Individual action plans, which are reviewed elsewhere in this issue, are one method to improve community treatment of anaphylaxis. In general, it is recommended that epinephrine be given to food-allergic children at the first signs of a systemic reaction, before full-blown respiratory systems or hypotension develop.

β-Blockers are infrequently used in children but are associated with anaphylaxis that is difficult to treat in adults. If the patient is taking β-blockers, glucagon can be useful. Additional potentially lifesaving supportive measures include placing the patient in a supine position to maximize cardiac return, administering oxygen if needed, and giving IV fluids if hypotension develops.[16]

H1 Antihistamines

H1 antihistamines are the most commonly used medications in the treatment of anaphylactic episodes. In one multicenter sample, these medications were used in 72% of emergency visits for food allergy,[8] and others have reported rates of use consistently exceeding 50% for anaphylaxis.[13] H1 antihistamines are inverse agonists at the H1 histamine receptor in that that they bind the receptor in its inactive state, preventing signaling through the receptor. First-generation H1 antihistamines are lipophilic and can readily cross the blood-brain barrier, resulting in sedation. Second-generation antihistamines are modified so that they cannot enter the central nervous system, effectively eliminating sedation and other neurologic effects. In addition, they lack the cholinergic, α-adrenergic, and serotoninergic effects of the first-generation antihistamines, ameliorating some of the most troublesome adverse effects, including dry mouth, urinary retention, prolonged QT interval, and increased appetite.[63] Although H1 antihistamines decrease skin symptoms (itch, flush, urticaria) and nasal symptoms (rhinorrhea, congestion), they do not prevent or treat airway obstruction, wheeze, or hypotension. Suppression of the wheal and flare response to allergen takes 0.7 to 2.6 hours after oral administration.[13] Because they do not prevent the serious manifestations of anaphylaxis, they are considered secondary medications for the treatment of anaphylaxis. The most recent practice parameter suggests that they may have utility for "control of cutaneous and cardiovascular manifestations" of anaphylaxis,[16] although others recommend against their use because of their potential for both delaying lifesaving therapy and causing dangerous side effects.[64] Complications of H1 antihistamines include sedation (as mentioned earlier), other neurotoxicities such as seizure, and potentially fatal QT prolongation.

If antihistamines are to be used, they can be given by mouth, IV, or IM. For children, the dose should be 1 mg/kg up to 50 mg, whereas for adults, the dose is 25 to 50 mg, whether given IM, IV, or by mouth.[16]

H2 Antihistamines

As outlined earlier, the H2 receptor participates in the anaphylactic response, and theoretically, blockade of this receptor may interfere with cardiac, vascular, and dermal symptoms in ways distinct from that of the H1 receptor. Like H1 antihistamines, H2 antihistamines are inverse agonists that preferentially bind to the inactive state of the receptor. They are generally safe, although infusion of cimetidine should be done slowly to prevent hypotension.[16] Two randomized controlled trials of H2 antihistamines added to H1 antihistamines for the treatment of acute allergic events showed improved efficacy with both agents compared with H1 antihistamines alone for treatment of urticaria but not for itching, angioedema, or erythema.[65,66] One of the studies also showed less tachycardia after treatment with the H2 blocker than placebo. Of note, although the difference was not statistically significant, almost twice as many subjects in the H2 antihistamine group received epinephrine.[65] Several additional single case reports suggest utility for H2 antihistamines in the treatment of anaphylaxis refractory to other therapies, but their utility in anaphylaxis has not been carefully examined.[13] The most recent US practice parameter for anaphylaxis states "an H2 antagonist added to the H1 antagonist may be helpful in the management of anaphylaxis." If used, ranitidine can be given IV or IM at 1 mg/kg in adults and 12.5 to 50 mg in children.[16]

Glucocorticoids

Like H1 antihistamines, glucocorticoids have not been subjected to randomized controlled trials for anaphylaxis but are widely used in the ER setting. The onset of action of glucocorticoids is even slower than oral H1 blockers, occurring hours after administration.[13] Steroids are lipophilic, crossing the cell membrane to bind the glucocorticoid receptor, causing heat shock proteins to dissociate and the receptor to be phosphorylated and then transported to the nucleus. There they bind to glucocorticoid receptor elements and cause altered expression of a wide range of genes. Although pretreatment for 48 hours with glucocorticoids prevents the late phase response to allergen challenge, it does not affect the acute phase response.[63] Glucocorticoids can cause significant adverse events, including effects on bone and glucose metabolisms, muscle wasting, cataracts, hypertension, and skin thinning, although short-term administration is generally much safer. Mood changes and effects on glucose metabolism can occur with even very short-term use.[67] Glucocorticoids are commonly used in acute anaphylaxis to prevent biphasic reactions, although their utility for this purpose has not been conclusively demonstrated.

β-Agonists

β-Agonists may be used as an adjunct to epinephrine for the treatment of wheeze but should not replace epinephrine because they lack the widespread effects of epinephrine and do not effectively treat angioedema.[16]

SUMMARY

Even though anaphylaxis was first described centuries ago, ensuring high-quality emergency treatment of food-allergen–induced anaphylaxis and appropriate follow-up still remain a challenge in many instances. Although commonly used instead of epinephrine, antihistamines, β-agonists, and glucocorticoids do not reverse the life-threatening symptoms that are characteristic of anaphylaxis. Because almost all food-induced anaphylactic events occur in the community, provision of self-injectable epinephrine to patients at risk is essential. Patients should be referred to allergists to ensure that diagnosis of the underlying food allergy is correct and the patients and their families receive appropriate education. Although new discoveries relating to the pathophysiology and causes of anaphylaxis may ultimately alter how it is treated and prevented, the tools to prevent deaths from anaphylaxis are already available. We just need to use them.

KEY POINTS

1. Epinephrine is the treatment of choice for anaphylaxis.
2. Epinephrine is underutilized in the acute treatment of anaphylaxis.
3. Epinephrine is underprescribed for as-needed use.

ACKNOWLEDGMENTS

The author would like to acknowledge Jessica Savage, MD, for helpful comments on a draft of this manuscript.

REFERENCES

1. Keet CA, Wood RA. Food allergy and anaphylaxis. Immunol Allergy Clin North Am 2007;27(2):193–212, vi.
2. Peng MM, Jick H. A population-based study of the incidence, cause, and severity of anaphylaxis in the United Kingdom. Arch Intern Med 2004;164(3):317–9.

3. Yocum MW, Khan DA. Assessment of patients who have experienced anaphylaxis: a 3-year survey. Mayo Clin Proc 1994;69(1):16–23.
4. Brown AF, McKinnon D, Chu K. Emergency department anaphylaxis: a review of 142 patients in a single year. J Allergy Clin Immunol 2001;108(5):861–6.
5. Mehl A, Wahn U, Niggemann B. Anaphylactic reactions in children – a questionnaire-based survey in Germany. Allergy 2005;60(11):1440–5.
6. Pastorello EA, Rivolta F, Bianchi M, et al. Incidence of anaphylaxis in the emergency department of a general hospital in Milan. J Chromatogr B Biomed Sci Appl 2001;756(1–2):11–7.
7. Thong BY, Cheng YK, Leong KP, et al. Anaphylaxis in adults referred to a clinical immunology/allergy centre in Singapore. Singapore Med J 2005;46(10):529–34.
8. Clark S, Bock SA, Gaeta TJ, et al. Multicenter study of emergency department visits for food allergies. J Allergy Clin Immunol 2004;113(2):347–52.
9. Kastner M, Harada L, Waserman S. Gaps in anaphylaxis management at the level of physicians, patients, and the community: a systematic review of the literature. Allergy 2010;65(4):435–44.
10. Ross MP, Ferguson M, Street D, et al. Analysis of food-allergic and anaphylactic events in the National Electronic Injury Surveillance System. J Allergy Clin Immunol 2008;121(1):166–71.
11. Gaeta TJ, Clark S, Pelletier AJ, et al. National study of US emergency department visits for acute allergic reactions, 1993 to 2004. Ann Allergy Asthma Immunol 2007;98(4):360–5.
12. Clark S, Gaeta TJ, Kamarthi GS, et al. ICD-9-CM coding of emergency department visits for food and insect sting allergy. Ann Epidemiol 2006;16(9):696–700.
13. Simons FE. Pharmacologic treatment of anaphylaxis: can the evidence base be strengthened? Curr Opin Allergy Clin Immunol 2010;10(4):384–93.
14. Cohen SG, Mazzullo JC. Discovering anaphylaxis: elucidation of a shocking phenomenon. J Allergy Clin Immunol 2009;124(4):866–9 e861.
15. Sampson HA, Munoz-Furlong A, Campbell RL, et al. Second symposium on the definition and management of anaphylaxis: summary report—Second National Institute of Allergy and Infectious Disease/Food Allergy and Anaphylaxis Network symposium. J Allergy Clin Immunol 2006;117(2):391–7.
16. Lieberman P, Nicklas RA, Oppenheimer J, et al. The diagnosis and management of anaphylaxis practice parameter: 2010 update. J Allergy Clin Immunol 2010; 126(3):477–80, e1–42.
17. Lieberman P. Anaphylaxis. Med Clin North Am 2006;90(1):77–95, viii.
18. Stone SF, Cotterell C, Isbister GK, et al. Elevated serum cytokines during human anaphylaxis: identification of potential mediators of acute allergic reactions. J Allergy Clin Immunol 2009;124(4):786–92, e784.
19. Simons FE. Anaphylaxis. J Allergy Clin Immunol 2010;125(2 Suppl 2):S161–81.
20. Sheikh A, Ten Broek V, Brown SG, et al. H1-antihistamines for the treatment of anaphylaxis: Cochrane systematic review. Allergy 2007;62(8):830–7.
21. Vadas P, Gold M, Perelman B, et al. Platelet-activating factor, PAF acetylhydrolase, and severe anaphylaxis. N Engl J Med 2008;358(1):28–35.
22. Arias K, Baig M, Colangelo M, et al. Concurrent blockade of platelet-activating factor and histamine prevents life-threatening peanut-induced anaphylactic reactions. J Allergy Clin Immunol 2009;124(2):307–14, 314, e1–2.
23. Kajiwara N, Sasaki T, Bradding P, et al. Activation of human mast cells through the platelet-activating factor receptor. J Allergy Clin Immunol 2010;125(5):1137–45, e1136.
24. Novembre E, Cianferoni A, Bernardini R, et al. Anaphylaxis in children: clinical and allergologic features. Pediatrics 1998;101(4):E8.

25. Sampson HA, Mendelson L, Rosen JP. Fatal and near-fatal anaphylactic reactions to food in children and adolescents. N Engl J Med 1992;327(6):380–4.
26. Pumphrey RS. Lessons for management of anaphylaxis from a study of fatal reactions. Clin Exp Allergy 2000;30(8):1144–50.
27. Pumphrey RS, Gowland MH. Further fatal allergic reactions to food in the United Kingdom, 1999–2006. J Allergy Clin Immunol 2007;119(4):1018–9.
28. Bock SA, Munoz-Furlong A, Sampson HA. Fatalities due to anaphylactic reactions to foods. J Allergy Clin Immunol 2001;107(1):191–3.
29. Bock SA, Munoz-Furlong A, Sampson HA. Further fatalities caused by anaphylactic reactions to food, 2001–2006. J Allergy Clin Immunol 2007;119(4):1016–8.
30. Scranton SE, Gonzalez EG, Waibel KH. Incidence and characteristics of biphasic reactions after allergen immunotherapy. J Allergy Clin Immunol 2009;123(2):493–8.
31. Douglas DM, Sukenick E, Andrade WP, et al. Biphasic systemic anaphylaxis: an inpatient and outpatient study. J Allergy Clin Immunol 1994;93(6):977–85.
32. Mehr S, Liew WK, Tey D, et al. Clinical predictors for biphasic reactions in children presenting with anaphylaxis. Clin Exp Allergy 2009;39(9):1390–6.
33. Stark BJ, Sullivan TJ. Biphasic and protracted anaphylaxis. J Allergy Clin Immunol 1986;78(1 Pt 1):76–83.
34. Lieberman P. Biphasic anaphylactic reactions. Ann Allergy Asthma Immunol 2005;95(3):217–26 [quiz: 226, 258].
35. Barg W, Medrala W, Wolanczyk-Medrala A. Exercise-induced anaphylaxis: an update on diagnosis and treatment. Curr Allergy Asthma Rep 2011;11(1):45–51.
36. Du Toit G. Food-dependent exercise-induced anaphylaxis in childhood. Pediatr Allergy Immunol 2007;18(5):455–63.
37. Commins SP, Platts-Mills TA. Anaphylaxis syndromes related to a new mammalian cross-reactive carbohydrate determinant. J Allergy Clin Immunol 2009; 124(4):652–7.
38. Commins SP, Satinover SM, Hosen J, et al. Delayed anaphylaxis, angioedema, or urticaria after consumption of red meat in patients with IgE antibodies specific for galactose-alpha-1,3-galactose. J Allergy Clin Immunol 2009;123(2):426–33.
39. Sicherer SH, Noone SA, Munoz-Furlong A. The impact of childhood food allergy on quality of life. Ann Allergy Asthma Immunol 2001;87(6):461–4.
40. Yunginger JW, Sweeney KG, Sturner WQ, et al. Fatal food-induced anaphylaxis. JAMA 1988;260(10):1450–2.
41. Vander Leek TK, Liu AH, Stefanski K, et al. The natural history of peanut allergy in young children and its association with serum peanut-specific IgE. J Pediatr 2000;137(6):749–55.
42. Wensing M, Penninks AH, Hefle SL, et al. The distribution of individual threshold doses eliciting allergic reactions in a population with peanut allergy. J Allergy Clin Immunol 2002;110(6):915–20.
43. Hourihane JO, Grimshaw KE, Lewis SA, et al. Does severity of low-dose, double-blind, placebo-controlled food challenges reflect severity of allergic reactions to peanut in the community? Clin Exp Allergy 2005;35(9):1227–33.
44. Spergel JM, Beausoleil JL, Fiedler JM, et al. Correlation of initial food reactions to observed reactions on challenges. Ann Allergy Asthma Immunol 2004;92(2):217–24.
45. Peeters KA, Koppelman SJ, van Hoffen E, et al. Does skin prick test reactivity to purified allergens correlate with clinical severity of peanut allergy? Clin Exp Allergy 2007;37(1):108–15.
46. Benhamou AH, Zamora SA, Eigenmann PA. Correlation between specific immunoglobulin E levels and the severity of reactions in egg allergic patients. Pediatr Allergy Immunol 2008;19(2):173–9.

47. Flinterman AE, Knol EF, Lencer DA, et al. Peanut epitopes for IgE and IgG4 in peanut-sensitized children in relation to severity of peanut allergy. J Allergy Clin Immunol 2008;121(3):737–43, e710.
48. Hofmann AM, Scurlock AM, Jones SM, et al. Safety of a peanut oral immunotherapy protocol in children with peanut allergy. J Allergy Clin Immunol 2009; 124(2):286–91, 291, e1–6.
49. Varshney P, Steele PH, Vickery BP, et al. Adverse reactions during peanut oral immunotherapy home dosing. J Allergy Clin Immunol 2009;124(6):1351–2.
50. Skripak JM, Nash SD, Rowley H, et al. A randomized, double-blind, placebo-controlled study of milk oral immunotherapy for cow's milk allergy. J Allergy Clin Immunol 2008;122(6):1154–60.
51. Greenberger PA, Grammer LC. Pulmonary disorders, including vocal cord dysfunction. J Allergy Clin Immunol 2010;125(2 Suppl 2):S248–54.
52. Nowak-Wegrzyn A, Muraro A. Food protein-induced enterocolitis syndrome. Curr Opin Allergy Clin Immunol 2009;9(4):371–7.
53. Low I, Stables S. Anaphylactic deaths in Auckland, New Zealand: a review of coronial autopsies from 1985 to 2005. Pathology 2006;38(4):328–32.
54. Yunginger JW, Squillace DL, Jones RT, et al. Fatal anaphylactic reactions induced by peanuts. Allergy Proc 1989;10(4):249–53.
55. Lin RY, Schwartz LB, Curry A, et al. Histamine and tryptase levels in patients with acute allergic reactions: an emergency department-based study. J Allergy Clin Immunol 2000;106(1 Pt 1):65–71.
56. Ford LS, Taylor SL, Pacenza R, et al. Food allergen advisory labeling and product contamination with egg, milk, and peanut. J Allergy Clin Immunol 2010;126(2):384–5.
57. Skripak JM, Matsui EC, Mudd K, et al. The natural history of IgE-mediated cow's milk allergy. J Allergy Clin Immunol 2007;120(5):1172–7.
58. Savage JH, Matsui EC, Skripak JM, et al. The natural history of egg allergy. J Allergy Clin Immunol 2007;120(6):1413–7.
59. Sicherer SH, Simons FE. Self-injectable epinephrine for first-aid management of anaphylaxis. Pediatrics 2007;119(3):638–46.
60. Simons FE, Gu X, Simons KJ. Epinephrine absorption in adults: intramuscular versus subcutaneous injection. J Allergy Clin Immunol 2001;108(5):871–3.
61. Boyce JA, Assa'ad A, Burks AW, et al. Guidelines for the diagnosis and management of food allergy in the United States: report of the NIAID-sponsored expert panel. J Allergy Clin Immunol 2010;126(6 Suppl):S1–8.
62. Simons FE, Chan ES, Gu X, et al. Epinephrine for the out-of-hospital (first-aid) treatment of anaphylaxis in infants: is the ampule/syringe/needle method practical? J Allergy Clin Immunol 2001;108(6):1040–4.
63. Adkinson NF Jr, Bochner BS, Busse WW, et al, editors. Middleton's allergy. 7th edition. Philadelphia (PA): Mosby; 2009. p. 1517–89.
64. Andreae DA, Andreae MH. Should antihistamines be used to treat anaphylaxis? BMJ 2009;339:b2489.
65. Lin RY, Curry A, Pesola GR, et al. Improved outcomes in patients with acute allergic syndromes who are treated with combined H1 and H2 antagonists. Ann Emerg Med 2000;36(5):462–8.
66. Runge JW, Martinez JC, Caravati EM, et al. Histamine antagonists in the treatment of acute allergic reactions. Ann Emerg Med 1992;21(3):237–42.
67. Richards RN. Side effects of short-term oral corticosteroids. J Cutan Med Surg 2008;12(2):77–81.

Gastrointestinal Manifestations of Food Allergies

Jaime Liou Wolfe, MD[a], Seema S. Aceves, MD, PhD[b,*]

KEYWORDS

• Eosinophilic esophagitis • Eosinophilic gastroenteritis
• Food allergy • Allergy testing

INTRODUCTION

IgE-mediated food hypersensitivity affects 4% of children in the United States, with increasing incidence rates over the last 10 years. In addition, an increasing number of children with food allergy are reporting other concurrent allergic diatheses such as asthma, eczema, and allergic rhinitis. The eosinophilic gastrointestinal disorders (EGIDs), often a manifestation of food allergy, have become increasingly prevalent over the past 20 years, with eosinophilic esophagitis affecting at least 4/10,000 US children, with case reports on all continents except Africa.[1,2]

Manifestations of food allergy range from clinical anaphylaxis, mediated primarily by specific IgE and immediate hypersensitivity, to EGIDs, which are mediated through combined IgE hypersensitivity and delayed-type hypersensitivity. Subsets of EGIDs such as eosinophilic colitis seem to be largely IgE independent. Additional diseases that involve food intolerance include autoimmune processes, such as in celiac disease. Understanding the multiple mechanisms and manifestations of food allergy is of paramount importance when choosing the appropriate diagnostic modality and interpreting the test results. Immediate hypersensitivity reactions to foods are assessed by testing that evaluates the presence and/or levels of food-specific IgE. This can be achieved using skin prick testing (SPT) or serum specific IgE levels. Serum food-specific IgE levels can have prognostic usefulness in children with a history of urticaria, respiratory distress, hypotension, and other clinical symptoms of anaphylaxis. In contrast, autoantibody testing for tissue transglutaminase and endomysial IgA are used in the diagnosis of celiac disease. Food atopy patch testing is intended to evaluate a delayed hypersensitivity to foods but remains a research tool.

[a] Division of Gastroenterology, Department of Surgery, Children's National Medical Center, Washington, DC, USA
[b] Division of Allergy, Immunology, Departments of Pediatrics and Medicine, University of California, San Diego, Rady Children's Hospital, San Diego, CA, USA
* Corresponding author. Division of Allergy and Immunology, 3020 Children's Way, MC-5114, San Diego, CA 92123.
E-mail address: saceves@ucsd.edu

Pediatr Clin N Am 58 (2011) 389–405
doi:10.1016/j.pcl.2011.02.001 pediatric.theclinics.com
0031-3955/11/$ – see front matter

This article reviews the clinical manifestations, pathogenesis, testing modalities, and treatments of food allergies that involve the gastrointestinal (GI) tract.

EOSINOPHILIC ESOPHAGITIS

Clinical Features

Eosinophilic esophagitis (EoE) is a clinicopathologic condition defined by diffuse eosinophilic infiltration of the esophagus. It is becoming increasingly recognized in adults and children, and the first consensus guidelines for its diagnosis and management were published in 2007.[2] The recommended guideline diagnostic criteria were based on published literature and expert opinion, and were defined as: (1) characteristic symptoms, (2) 15 eosinophils/high power field (HPF) or greater, and (3) exclusion of other disorders, including failure of response with high-dose proton pump inhibitors (PPI) therapy, or normal pH monitoring.[2]

EoE was first described in the mid-1970s by Dobbins and colleagues[3] and Landres and colleagues,[4] who reported 2 adult men with symptoms of dysphagia, epigastric pain, esophageal spasms, and eosinophilia of the esophagus with negative pH probes. In 1993, Atwood and colleagues[5] published a retrospective review of 12 patients with increased esophageal eosinophils. In this study, 11 of 12 patients had normal pH monitoring and 7 of 12 were atopic. Most patients had dysphagia and frequent food impaction, and a mean of 56 eosinophils/HPF compared with 90 patients with pH-probe–proven gastroesophageal reflux (GER) who had mean eosinophils of 3.3 eosinophils/HPF.

Since its first description, the reports of EoE have steadily increased, with currently reported incidence rates of 1.25/10,000 and prevalence of 4.3/10,000 in children less than 19 years of age.[1] It is more common in young White males, and affected patients have high rates of concurrent atopy.[6] Greater than 70% of patients have a history of asthma, eczema, food allergies or food sensitization, environmental allergy, or chronic rhinitis, and up to 75% have a personal or family history.[2] Current reports show that a subset of patients have a genetic variant of EoE and reported disease risk genes for EoE include eotaxin-3 and thymic stromal lymphopoeitin and a single nucleotide polymorphisms at the transforming growth factor β1 (TGFβ1) promoter may have disease-modifying effects on therapeutic response. Eotaxin-3 genotype GG was statistically significant in patients with EoE versus controls and comprised 14% of the patients with EoE.[7–9]

Classic EoE symptoms include abdominal pain, vomiting, and dysphagia, although symptoms vary by age.[2] Infants and toddlers present with gagging, choking, feeding refusal, or poor growth. Whereas GER symptoms tend to improve in the second half of the first year, symptoms from EoE may not. Feeding difficulties likely arise from nausea, dysphagia, or the attempt to avoid pain with eating, which are perpetuated by continual negative reinforcement. When evaluating these children, primary swallowing dysfunction, cardiac or respiratory disease, and underlying anatomic abnormalities must also be considered and evaluated.

School-aged children tend to present with pain or vomiting. Pain can vary in location, frequency, and severity, with complaints of chest, epigastric, or periumbilical pain being most common.[2] Symptoms rarely occur in association with a particular food trigger, tend to be intermittent, and tend not to predict the severity of inflammation.[10] In some instances, parents may recall an infant in whom reflux symptoms began early in life, were associated with eczema, and worsened with the introduction of solid foods.[11]

Dysphagia and food impaction are more common in adolescents and adults. The association of dysphagia with EoE has been reported as high as 80% and is the most frequent indication for endoscopic evaluation in adults.[12–14] Endoscopic ultrasound has shown the thickening of the entire mucosa and muscular layers of the esophagus, which may affect esophageal motility.[15] Dysphagia has not been directly related to the duration of inflammation or degree of eosinophilic infiltration, but chronic inflammation with subsequent tissue remodeling has been postulated, and dysphagia complaints correlate directly with episodes of dysmotility in pediatric patients.[16] Adult patients with EoE have chronic complaints of dysphagia when treated with intermittent dilation only.[17]

Histologic Features

The esophagus, unlike other areas of the GI tract, is normally devoid of eosinophils. However, esophageal eosinophilia can occur with other diseases including GER disease, connective tissue disorders, parasitic infections, inflammatory bowel disease, and as a drug reaction. In addition, adults with allergic rhinitis can have esophageal eosinophilia during the pollen season independently of an EoE diagnosis.[18] Other causes of esophageal eosinophilia must be investigated before diagnosing primary EoE.

Histologically, EoE esophageal biopsies have several characteristic features, including eosinophil microabscesses, degranulation, and superficial layering as well as basal zone hyperplasia and vascular papillary elongation.[2] EoE is diagnosed when there are at least 15 eosinophils or more per HPF on 400× light microscopy using a hematoxylin and eosin stain (**Fig. 1**).[2] The eosinophil count of the highest density seen (peak eosinophils) is currently used in diagnosis. Unlike acid-induced esophageal eosinophilia, EoE is a patchy, diffuse disease. Procuring 5 biopsies increases the

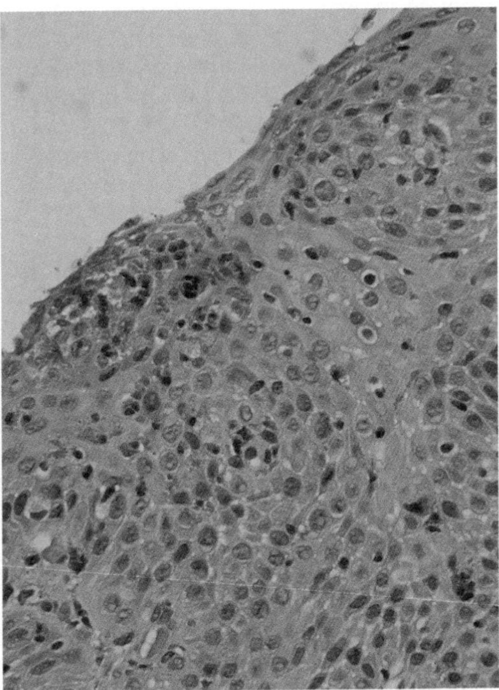

Fig. 1. Eosinophilic esophagitis. Eosinophilic abscesses and numerous eosinophils.

diagnostic yield to more than 90%. In addition, obtaining biopsies from at least 2 levels of the esophagus is recommended.[19]

Endoscopic Features

Endoscopic findings can be obvious or subtle. Up to 30% of patients with histologic EoE have an endoscopically normal mucosa.[2] However, classic EoE findings include linear furrowing, concentric rings (or felinization/trachealization), white exudates that mimic *Candida*, friability, or an attenuated subepithelial vascular pattern (**Fig. 2**).[2] Small-caliber esophagus, characterized by a uniformly narrowed esophagus, also has been described in patients with EoE with dysphagia.[20] Ongoing inflammation may lead to esophageal strictures, the most severe EoE complication reported to date.

Distinction of EoE from GER

Almost 2 decades ago, Winter and colleagues[21] reported distal and proximal esophageal eosinophilia in patients with GER. Whereas GER biopsies tend to have fewer than 7 eosinophils in the distal esophagus, EoE biopsies show significantly more severe eosinophilia.[22,23] Liacouras and colleagues[24] showed an average of 34.2 $\pm$ 9.6 eosinophils/HPF in patients with EoE compared with children with esophagitis who responded to PPI therapy (2.26 $\pm$ 1.16 eosinophils/HPF, $P<.001$). Case-control studies of patients with EoE versus GER show that EoE is more often associated with younger age, dysphagia, endoscopic findings such as rings and furrows, and eosinophil degranulation, severe basal zone hyperplasia, and lamina propria fibrosis.[25–27]

Because of the similarities in symptom complex, the clinical distinction between GER and EoE is particularly challenging. However, dysphagia and anorexia/early satiety have been reported to both correlate with inflammation, remodeling, and to distinguish GER from EoE in children.[28] Symptomatically, children with GER tend to improve with acid suppression therapy, whereas patients with EoE remain partially or completely symptomatic despite acid blockade.[2] Adult studies have shown that infusion of acid into the esophagus of patients with EoE causes significant pain.[29] However, the interplay between EoE and acid may be complex, involving an unclear relationship between eosinophilic secretory factors as well as epithelial changes

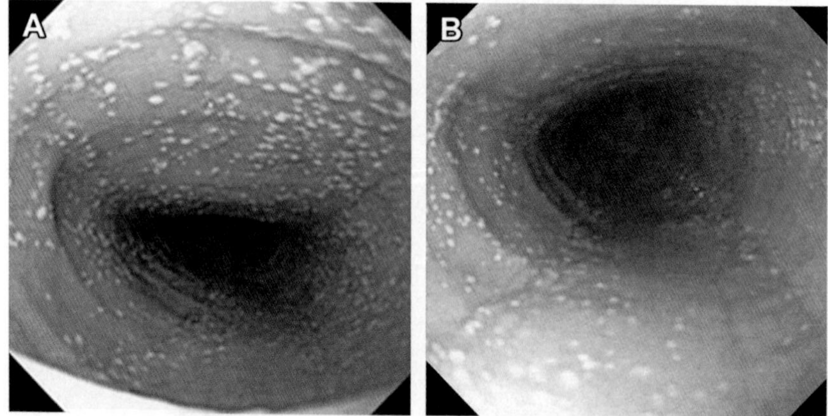

Fig. 2. Esophageal exudates in EoE (*A*). Linear furrowing and concentric rings (felinization/trachealization) in the esophagus (*B*).

secondary to acid damage.[30] Consistent with this hypothesis, Ngo and colleagues[31] described 3 patients with mean esophageal eosinophil counts of 36 (range 21–52) who responded both clinically and histologically to isolated acid suppression. For this reason, a trial of acid suppression before establishing the diagnosis of EoE is recommended.[32] In addition, this complexity underscores the importance of repeat endoscopic and biopsy evaluation after each therapeutic intervention in patients with EoE.

Disease Mechanisms

EoE combines immediate and delayed-type hypersensitive reactions to inhaled and ingested antigens. Murine EoE models have been instructive in dissecting the mechanistic pathways of esophageal inflammation. Experimental EoE is instigated by intranasal aeroallergens (*Aspergillus*, *Dermatophagoides*) and gavaged food allergens (ovalbumin).[33–35] Disease initiation depends on the presence of T cells but is independent of IgE.[36] Animals deficient in CD4+ T cells, eotaxin receptor CCR3, interleukin 15 (IL-15) receptor α, IL-13 receptor α, or IL-5 are all relatively to completely protected from experimental EoE, showing the importance of these pathways in EoE.[7,37,38]

Gene microarray studies have significantly contributed to our understanding of human EoE pathogenesis.[7] Compared with normal children or patients with GER, children with EoE have a 53-fold increase in the expression of eotaxin-3, a chemokine that functions as an eosinophil chemoattractant. Both IL-5 and IL-13 are increased and seem to function upstream of eotaxin-3. Treatment of cultured human esophageal epithelial cells from patients with EoE with IL-13 causes increased eotaxin-3 gene expression.[39] More recently, IL-15, which can function in a similar manner to IL-2, has been shown to be increased in pediatric patients with EoE, is expressed in dendritic cells in EoE, increases IL-5 and IL-13 production from T cells as well as eotaxin-3 production from epithelial cells, and is detectable in the serum of patients with EoE.[37] CD8+ cells are increased in biopsies of patients with EoE, and it is possible that IL-15 is important in their genesis and maintenance.[40,41]

IL-5 is important for both eosinophilopoesis and eosinophil trafficking into the esophagus. In addition, IL-5 in combination with eotaxins activates eosinophils. Patients with EoE show increased deposition of eosinophil granule products, including major basic protein, eosinophil derived neurotoxin, and eosinophil peroxidase.[42–44] These products can potentially affect esophageal function by increasing tissue damage and epithelial proliferation.[45]

In IgE-mediated hypersensitivity, mast cells classically mediate the downstream effects of specific IgE. EoE biopsies have shown increased numbers of mast cells as well as increased mast cell degranulation compared with non-EoE biopsies, suggesting mast cell activation.[46] In addition, there are increased numbers of tryptase-positive mast cells and IgE-positive cells as well as increased numbers of cells bearing the high-affinity IgE receptor, FcϵRI, in the esophagus of patients with EoE.[47,48] Whereas tryptase-positive mucosal mast cells are decreased after topical corticosteroid treatment,[49] the submucosal mast cell pool of tryptase-chymase double connective tissue mast cells remains static.[50] A mast cell gene profile is increased in pediatric patients with EoE.[7,51] Mast cells are increased in number in the esophageal muscularis mucosa and their products are able to affect esophageal smooth-muscle function in vitro, suggesting an important function of mast cells in EoE pathogenesis.[50] A local capacity for immunoglobulin class switch occurs in the esophagus but whether local IgE production represents a mucosal food-specific antigen response remains to be shown.[47] Increased levels of esophageal IL-13 could promote local immunoglobulin class switch to IgE production in EoE.

The role of systemic food-specific IgE remains to be further elucidated in EoE. Although most patients have sensitization to food antigens, the role of IgE in predicting foods that instigate or propagate EoE is unclear and SPT or serum IgE-based dietary eliminations are variably successful.

Pathogenesis of Complications

The most severe consequence of EoE is fixed esophageal stenosis requiring repeated dilation. Subepithelial sclerosis was first reported in adult patients with long-standing EoE.[17] Children, both with and without stricture-associated EoE, have subepithelial remodeling, an esophageal process with a pathogenesis akin to asthmatic airway remodeling.[52] Increases in TGFβ1 and its signaling pathway, phosphorylated Smad2/3, are found in the subepithelium of individuals with EoE. Increased angiogenesis, a component of esophageal remodeling, and vascular activation with vascular cell adhesion molecule 1 form adhesive conduits for inflammatory cell trafficking.[52] In addition to increased collagen deposition, increased amounts of matrix proteins such as periostin allow eosinophil accumulation.[53] Animal models have shown that IL-5 and eosinophils are necessary for tissue remodeling, whereas in vitro studies show that TGFβ1 and eotaxin-3 increase periostin expression in esophageal fibroblasts.[38]

Food Allergy Testing in EoE

Immediate hypersensitivity

Food testing that evaluates immediate hypersensitivity reactions evaluates the presence of specific IgE. SPT is performed by placing food extracts or fresh foods on the skin and pricking the skin. Cutaneous mast cells carrying food-specific IgE are stimulated to degranulate, which causes a cutaneous urticarial reaction. SPT gauges both the presence and function of specific IgE.

Serum IgE testing assesses the levels of food-specific IgE. In the context of a clinical history of anaphylaxis or immediate food hypersensitivity reaction (urticaria, vomiting, angioedema), the quantity of serum specific IgE can have predictive values for the reaction to specific foods. However, it is critical to understand that although many people generate food-specific IgE that is detectable by SPT or in vitro testing they can be clinically tolerant to the food and have no reaction on ingestion. In some cases, removal of IgE-positive foods in a clinically tolerant person can result in immediate hypersensitivity on food reintroduction, implying that continued food ingestion is important for maintaining tolerance. Although most patients with EoE have detectable levels of food-specific IgE, they do not have anaphylaxis. The reason for this remains unclear.

Serum or skin testing for foods in EoE reveals that 70% to 80% of patients with EoE have positive food testing.[2] Serum IgE testing detects more foods than SPT but the clinical implication and usefulness of low-level sensitization to foods (in the range of 1–5 IU/mL) is unclear.[54] The most commonly positive foods in patients with EoE who undergo SPT or serum IgE testing are cow's milk, hen's egg, soy, wheat, corn, rice, oat, beef, chicken, peanuts, and white potato.[54,55]

Delayed hypersensitivity

Delayed hypersensitivity testing evaluates the presence of cellular inflammation in response to foods. T-cell memory is critical to the onset of delayed-type hypersensitivity. The use of atopy patch testing has been validated, standardized, and shown to provoke a cutaneous cellular immune response in diseases such as contact dermatitis and eczema. The usual antigens in these cases are metals, occupational chemicals, and aeroallergens such as house dust mite. Food patch testing has been evaluated in EoE in order to assess foods that cause a delayed reaction. Single food extracts in Finn chambers are placed on the back for 48 hours. The reactions are read at 72 hours and graded using a scoring system that evaluates the presence and severity of erythema, induration, papules, and vesicles. The most commonly positive foods on patch testing of patients with EoE are cow's milk, hen's egg, wheat, soy, corn, barley, oat, rice, beef, and potato.[55] Positive predictive values from 1 center range from 54% (potato) to 94% (beef), whereas negative predictive values range from 59% to 97%.[55] The presence of a cutaneous cellular immune response has not yet been shown in EoE, large numbers of non-EoE control patients have not been evaluated, and the interpretation of food patch tests has not been standardized or validated yet in EoE. Food patch testing remains a research tool in EoE.

Evidence that EoE is a Food Allergic GI Disease

Murine models of esophageal eosinophilia can be promoted by food antigens, specifically ovalbumin.[35] Human data invoking foods as triggers of EoE come from the success of elimination diets as EoE therapy. Elemental formulas are the most successful dietary intervention, with histologic resolution in more than 94% of patients.[56,57] However, unpalatable taste requiring nasogastric or gastric tube insertions, lack of insurance coverage in many states, and difficulty with adherence limit the use of elemental diets.

In vitro studies looking at dendritic cells from patients with EoE and food allergic patients show increased levels of Th2 cytokine production when cultured in vitro with autologous CD4+ cells and increased serum levels of IL-5 and IL-13.[58] It is possible that, similar to patients with eosinophilic gastroenteritis (EGE), patients with EoE have increased numbers of CD4+, IL-5+, and IL-4− cells but this remains to be evaluated.[59]

Kagalwalla and colleagues[60] first described the use of an empiric 6-food elimination diet in children. Avoidance of cow's milk, hen's egg, soy, wheat, fish, shellfish, peanuts, and tree nut resulted in histologic remission in 74% of pediatric patients, again invoking immunologic food reactions in the esophagus as the basis for EoE. Consistent with atopy patch test and SPT-based diets, the most common food antigens in children were cow's milk and hen's egg. The same avoidance diet in adults leads to 70% resolution or improvement, with disease recurrence on food reintroduction. Milk and wheat were the most common adult EoE triggers (Nirmala Gonsalves, MD, personal communication, 2010).

The long-term induction of tolerance to EoE triggering foods and the potential implications for loss of tolerance and onset of IgE-mediated allergy when using diets that eliminate IgE-positive foods remain to be studied in EoE.

EoE Therapy

As a food-triggered disease, EoE can be successfully managed using elimination diets, as detailed earlier. Other mainstays of EoE management are the use of swallowed corticosteroids that deposit topically on the esophagus. By treating inflammation locally, topical corticosteroids control allergic inflammation and allow a wide diet to be consumed. Success rates vary but randomized placebo-controlled trials in children show that puff and swallowed fluticasone can be as effective as oral prednisone and significantly superior to placebo.[49,61] Oral viscous budesonide in combination with acid blockade daily is an effective EoE therapy, with response rates of 87% compared with placebo.[62] Repeat endoscopy with biopsy should be performed after changing therapy or foods, because documentation of histologic resolution is required in disease management. There are no surrogate markers, including symptoms, that obviate repeated endoscopy in patients with EoE.

Therapeutic Maneuvers in EoE

Dilation therapy and food disimpaction are required less frequently in children than in adults with EoE. However, when dilation is required, care must be taken to avoid perforation. Several case studies in the literature support a higher perforation risk in EoE, believed to be caused by mucosal remodeling and fibrosis leading to a less compliant or fragile esophageal wall.[63,64] However, recent studies have reported that perforation caused by dilation in patients with EoE may be safer than previously believed.[63,65,66] The role of antiinflammatory therapy in reducing or obviating dilations warrants further study.

EOSINOPHILIC GASTROENTERITIS

Clinical, Histologic, and Endoscopic Features

First described more than 50 years ago by Kaijser,[67] EGE is a clinicopathologic entity characterized by increased eosinophils in the stomach and small intestine, and less commonly the colon. It is rare, and the underlying pathophysiology is not clear. It is diagnosed primarily in the third to fifth decade of life, and affects both genders equally. The incidence is not clear, likely because of lack of recognition and underreporting.[68]

The definition of EGE is complicated by the baseline, normal eosinophilia of the nonesophageal regions of the GI tract. They are highest in the cecum, ascending colon, and terminal ileum.[69,70] There is no consensus guideline regarding the number of eosinophils required for diagnosis, but rather the combination of eosinophil location, depth, other histologic findings or lack thereof, the clinical context, and lack of signs of other diseases with eosinophilia help to direct diagnosis.[71]

Primary EGE can be atopic or nonatopic but is often believed be a food allergic disorder, potentially with a genetic susceptibility.[72] The most common cause of secondary EGE is parasitic infection but inflammatory bowel disease, celiac disease, and connective tissue diseases such as scleroderma can also be associated with EGE. Peripheral eosinophilia may be seen in more than 50%, but not consistently, and its significance in terms of diagnostic criteria has not been established.[73]

The stomach has been reported to be involved in 26% to 81% of cases, and the small intestine in 28% to 100% of cases.[74,75] The most frequently described symptoms are abdominal pain, diarrhea, nausea, vomiting, and weight loss.[74–77] Symptoms may wax and wane, and it is not uncommon for diagnosis to be delayed because of lack of consistency in symptoms. The most commonly accepted classification system was developed by Klein and colleagues[78] in 1970, in which the disorder was divided into 3 subtypes: mucosal, muscularis, and serosal.

Mucosal disease is the most frequently encountered, which is likely in part because of the technical limitation in obtaining deep-layer biopsies via standard endoscopy. Individuals with mucosal-type disease tend to have IgE-mediated food allergy or other atopy.[79] Other presentations of mucosal disease include anemia caused by GI bleeding, gastric and duodenal ulcers, or protein-losing enteropathy caused by malabsorption.[71,73,80–83]

Muscular disease tends to present with obstructive symptoms, and several unique presentations have been reported. Infants may present with gastric outlet obstruction, mimicking hypertrophic pyloric stenosis. Thickening of the intestinal wall, strictures, pancreatitis, intussusception, and obstruction by a cecal mass have also been described.[75,77,84,85] Diagnosis of muscular and serosal types may require laparotomy and full-thickness biopsy.

Serosal disease is associated with abdominal bloating, marked increase in eosinophils, ascites, increased peripheral eosinophilia, and better response to steroids. Talley and colleagues[74] published one of the largest experiences with EGE, in which they compared symptoms, allergic history, and serum parameters among patients with EGE and control individuals and reported that abdominal bloating and peripheral eosinophil count were the only parameters found to be statistically different. However, obstructive jaundice, acute abdomen, intussusception, and bowel obstruction have also been described.[86–91]

Diagnosis

Endoscopy and histology are required for diagnosis. Endoscopic findings vary from normal to nodular with friability, erythema, polypoid lesions, or ulcerations.[72] Biopsies show increased eosinophils but the histologic finding of eosinophilia must be evaluated in the clinical context, and secondary causes such as inflammatory bowel disease and celiac disease that can also be associated with intestinal eosinophilia must be evaluated. Like EoE, EGE disease is patchy and therefore multiple biopsies should be obtained.

Diagnosis is made more difficult by the technical limitation of standard endoscopy. The distal limit of upper endoscopic biopsies is the third portion of the duodenum, whereas the proximal limit of colonic endoscopies is the terminal ileum. With newer endoscopic techniques such as balloon enteroscopy, more distal small bowel biopsies may be obtained and aid in EGE recognition.

There are no radiographic findings specific to EGE, although computed tomography of the abdomen may show nodular and irregular thickening of gastric folds.[91] Ultrasound may also be helpful in assessing antral and bowel wall thickness.[92] Barium contrast may show bowel wall thickening or strictures.

Pathogenesis

Patients with atopic EGE often have multiple food sensitizations with positive SPT. However, elimination diets based on SPT results have variable success. However, elemental formula can have significant success.[93] Together the success of these interventions speaks to the important role of food intolerance in EGE.

Because the usual response of the GI tract is tolerogenic, shifts in sensitization to foods can lead to significant intestinal disease, and the role of food antigens in EGE continues to be investigated. Most recently Prussin and colleagues[59] reported that peripheral, food-specific CD4+ T cells in allergic patients with anaphylaxis produce both IL-4 and IL-5, whereas allergic EGE was singularly associated with a Th2 population that was IL-4−/IL-5+ cells. The numbers of IL-4+,5+ cells in peanut-allergic patients directly correlated with IgE levels. However, the link between the presence of peripheral IL-4−,5+ cells and GI T cells and eosinophils remains ambiguous. In addition, earlier work showed that patients with allergic EGE had duodenal CD4+/IL-4+ cells that proliferated to milk.[94] These cells were also noted to release IL-5 and IL-13 but not IL-4 in response to antigen, again implicating the importance of these interleukins to food-related GI disease. Together, these studies provide evidence for a mechanism of eosinophil chemoattraction and activation via IL-5 in patients with a GI Th2 phenotype and EGE.

Treatment

Patients with cow's milk allergy and EGE can have IgE to casein and whey proteins. It is reasonable to perform SPT to foods and, if not limited by the numbers of positive foods, to trial an elimination diet. Amino acid-based formulas can be trialed for EGE if there are multiple positive foods on IgE testing or if no food triggers can be found on IgE testing but the patient wishes to pursue dietary management. Although proliferative responses of peripheral blood mononuclear cells have been reported for milk, peanut, and soy proteins in patients with EGE, the extension of this disease mechanism to food patch testing has not been studied rigorously.

A recent clinical trial reported that the biologic agent anti-IgE was successful in decreasing eosinophil counts and symptoms in patients with EGE, underscoring a role for IgE in EGE.[95] Although IL-5 can drive esophageal eosinophilia, its role in the pathogenesis of EGE remains less clear and trials that were geared to assess the role of anti-IL-5 therapy in EoE showed that there were no changes in the levels of T cells, eosinophils, or mast cells in the duodenal or gastric mucosa of patients with EoE treated with anti-IL-5.[96]

The treatment of EGE can be complex, requiring systemic immunomodulatory therapy with prednisone, 6-mercaptopurine, and azathioprine.[97] Because EGE is characterized by relapses and remissions, patients often require recurrent steroid courses, with serosal disease having been reported to respond to systemic corticosteroids. Long-term remission may be possible with the use of the leukotriene receptor antagonist montelukast.[98] Because EGE has been associated with infections from helminths and *Helicobacter pylori* as well as systemic processes such as lupus erythematosis and posttransplantation syndrome, it is of paramount importance to determine if the disease is primary or secondary EGE before embarking on therapy. Depending on the location of intestinal involvement, topical corticosteroids such as entocort, a formulation of budesonide that targets right-sided intestinal disease, can be instituted.

EOSINOPHILIC COLITIS/PROCTOCOLITIS

Most commonly a benign disease of infancy, milk and soy trigger proctocolitis manifests as bloody, mucus-containing stools in infancy and is easily treated by the removal of the triggering antigen. Up to 60% of cases occur in breastfed babies, with onset during the first 6 months of life, and resolution by age 2 years old, with many children tolerating regular diets by 1 year of age.[99,100] Dietary elimination leads to rapid resolution of symptoms within 72 to 96 hours.[99] Because the diagnosis is based on clinical history and improvement with elimination of cow's milk in the breastfeeding mother, or with a semihydrolyzed or extensively hydrolyzed formula, neither flexible sigmoidoscopy nor colonoscopy is routinely indicated. Gross visual findings in the rectosigmoid colon may reveal erythema or erosions, whereas histologically one may see acute inflammation and eosinophilia. Although T cells are likely the source of immunologic memory, the use of food patch testing is not warranted in these infants.

FOOD PROTEIN-INDUCED ENTEROCOLITIS SYNDROME

Food protein–induced enterocolitis syndrome (FPIES) is a non–IgE-mediated food allergic disorder characterized by severe GI or systemic reactions to a food trigger, particularly milk or soy. Symptoms resolve with elimination of exposure to the inciting food. After the first case series in 1967 of 21 infants with diarrhea and variable hemodynamic instability with exposure to milk protein,[101] the diagnostic criteria have been formalized to include: (1) onset of symptoms typically at age less than 2 months, (2) diagnosis at age younger than 9 months; and (3) resolution of symptoms when the food antigen is eliminated.[102]

FPIES typically presents with significant GI symptoms, primarily vomiting and diarrhea within 4 hours of food ingestion.[103] More than 75% of infants appear ill, and in some patients, systemic signs such as hypotension necessitate hospitalization.[103] Common presentation in infants includes a septic appearance with a metabolic acidosis, dehydration, lethargy, and bloody stools. Because of this, children are often evaluated first for sepsis, metabolic disorders, or acute abdominal processes before the recognition of the triggering food antigen. Other signs such as hypoalbuminemia, poor weight gain, hypothermia, thrombocytosis, peripheral polymorphonuclear lymphocytosis, and methemoglobinemia have also been reported.[102–105] The severity of symptoms and lack of awareness of FPIES often delay the diagnosis.

Milk and soy are the most common food triggers, with as high as a 50% cross-reactivity between milk and soy.[102,106] Solid foods have also been implicated, particularly rice.[105,107,108] Most patients have negative SPTs and serum IgE test results.[102] Patch testing may be a promising modality to aid in diagnosis.[109]

FPIES is a clinical diagnosis. The gold standard for diagnosis is a positive oral food challenge but this is often not necessary and can be dangerous if the reaction involves hypotension. When challenges are done, intravenous access and a minimum of 4 hours of observation are necessary. Endoscopy is not routine because the diagnosis can often be made clinically based on symptoms with exposure to the food trigger, and improvement with removal of the causative food. Histologic changes include increased eosinophils in the lamina propria and focal cryptitis, with overall preservation of architecture.[110–112]

SUMMARY

Food reactions can have GI manifestations that cause significant tissue disease and patient morbidity. It is essential to use the proper diagnostic testing, including endoscopy with biopsy and food allergy testing, and to interpret test results appropriately in order to choose the best therapeutic intervention. New manifestations of food allergies, especially EoE, are increasing in prevalence and constitute a new and significant health care burden.

REFERENCES

1. Noel RJ, Putnam PE, Rothenberg ME. Eosinophilic esophagitis. N Engl J Med 2004;26(351):940–1.
2. Furuta GT, Liacouras CA, Collins MH, et al. Eosinophilic esophagitis in children and adults: a systematic review and consensus recommendations for diagnosis and treatment. Gastroenterology 2007;133:1342–63.
3. Dobbins JW, Sheahan DG, Behar J. Eosinophilic gastroenteritis with esophageal involvement. Gastroenterology 1977;72(6):1312–6.
4. Landres RT, Kuster GG, Strum WB. Eosinophilic esophagitis in a patient with vigorous achalasia. Gastroenterology 1978;74(6):1298–301.
5. Attwood SE, Smyrk TC, Demeester TR, et al. Esophageal eosinophilia with dysphagia. A distinct clinicopathologic syndrome. Dig Dis Sci 1993;38(1):109–16.
6. Orenstein SR, Shalaby TM, Di Lorenzo C, et al. The spectrum of pediatric eosinophilic esophagitis beyond infancy: a clinical series of 30 children. Am J Gastroenterol 2000;95(6):1422–30.

7. Blanchard C, Wang N, Stringer KF, et al. Eotaxin-3 and a uniquely conserved gene-expression profile in eosinophilic esophagitis. J Clin Invest 2006;116: 536–47.
8. Rothenberg ME, Spergel JS, Sherrill JD, et al. Common variants at 5q22 associate with pediatric eosinophilic esophagitis. Nat Genet 2010;42:289–91.
9. Aceves SS, Newbury RO, Chen D, et al. Resolution of remodeling in eosinophilic esophagitis correlates with epithelial response to topical corticosteroids. Allergy 2010;65:109–15.
10. Pentiuk S, Putnam PE, Collins MH, et al. Dissociation between symptoms and histological severity in pediatric eosinophilic esophagitis. J Pediatr Gstroenterol Nutr 2009;48:152–60.
11. Putnam PE. Eosinophilic esophagitis in children: clinical manifestations. Gastroenterol Clin North Am 2008;37:369–81.
12. Sgouros SN, Bergele C, Mantides A. Eosinophilic esophagitis in adults: a systematic review. Eur J Gastroenterol Hepatol 2006;18:211–7.
13. Desai TK, Stecevic V, Chang CH, et al. Association of eosinophilic inflammation with esophageal food impaction in adults. Gastrointest Endosc 2005;61:795–801.
14. Kapel RC, Miller JK, Torres C, et al. Eosinophilic esophagitis: a prevalent disease in the United States that affects all age groups. Gastroenterology 2008;134:1316–21.
15. Fox VL, Nurko S, Teitelbaum JE, et al. High-resolution EUS in children with eosinophilic "allergic" esophagitis. Gastrointest Endosc 2003;57:30–6.
16. Nurko S, Rosen R, Furuta GT. Esophageal dysmotility in children with eosinophilic esophagitis: a study using prolonged manometry. Am J Gastroenterol 2009;104:3050–7.
17. Straumann A, Spichtin HP, Grize L, et al. Natural history of primary eosinophilic esophagitis: a follow-up of 30 adult patients for up to 11.5 years. Gastroenterology 2003;125:1660–9.
18. Onbasi K, Sin AZ, Doganavsargil B, et al. Eosinophil infiltration of the oesophageal mucosa in patients with pollen allergy during the season. Clin Exp Allergy 2005;35:1423–31.
19. Gonsalves N, Policarpio-Nicolas M, Zhang Q, et al. Histopathologic variability and endoscopic correlates in adults with eosinophilic esophagitis. Gastrointest Endosc 2006;64:313–9.
20. Vasilopoulos S, Murphy P, Auerbach A, et al. The small-caliber esophagus: an unappreciated cause of dysphagia for solids in patients with eosinophilic esophagitis. Gastrointest Endosc 2002;55(1):99–106.
21. Winter HS, Madara JL, Stafford RJ, et al. Intraepithelial eosinophils: a new diagnostic criterion for reflux esophagitis. Gastroenterology 1982;83:818–23.
22. Ruchelli E, Wenner W, Voytek T, et al. Severity of esophageal eosinophilia predicts response to conventional gastroesophageal reflux therapy. Pediatr Dev Pathol 1999;2(1):15–8.
23. Steiner SJ, Gupta SK, Croffie JM, et al. Correlation between number of eosinophils and reflux index on same day esophageal biopsy and 24 hour esophageal pH monitoring. Am J Gastroenterol 2004;99:801–5.
24. Liacouras C, Wenner WJ, Brown K, et al. Primary eosinophilic esophagitis in children: successful treatment with oral corticosteroids. J Ped Gastro Nutr 1998;26:380–5.
25. Dellon ES, Gibbs WB, Fritchie KJ, et al. Clinical, endoscopic, and histologic findings distinguish eosinophilic esophagitis from gastroesophageal reflux disease. Clin Gastroenterol Hepatol 2009;7:1305–13.

26. Parfitt JR, Gregor JC, Suskin NG, et al. Eosinophilic esophagitis in adults: distinguishing features from gastroesophageal reflux disease: a study of 41 patients. Mod Pathol 2006;19:90–6.
27. Aceves SS, Newbury RO, Dohil R, et al. Distinguishing eosinophilic esophagitis in pediatric patients: clinical, endoscopic, and histologic features of an emerging disorder. J Clin Gastroenterol 2007;41:252–6.
28. Aceves SS, Newbury RO, Dohil MA, et al. A symptom scoring tool for identifying pediatric patients with eosinophilic esophagitis and correlating symptoms with inflammation. Ann Allergy Asthma Immunol 2009;103:401–6.
29. Krarup AL, Villadsen GE, Mejlgaard E, et al. Acid hypersensitivity in patients with eosinophilic esophagitis. Scan J Gastroenterol 2010;45:273–81.
30. Spechler SJ, Genta RM, Souza RF. Thoughts on the complex relationship between gastroesophageal reflux disease and eosinophilic esophagitis. Am J Gastroenterol 2007;102:1301–6.
31. Ngo P, Furuta GT, Antonioli DA, et al. Eosinophils in the esophagus–peptic or allergic eosinophilic esophagitis? Case series of three patients with esophageal eosinophilia. Am J Gastroenterol 2006;101:1666–70.
32. Walsh SV, Antonioli DA, Goldman H, et al. Allergic esophagitis in children: a clinicopathological entity. Am J Surg Pathol 1999;23:390–6.
33. Mishra A, Hogan SP, Brandt EB, et al. An etiological role for aeroallergens and eosinophils in experimental esophagitis. J Clin Invest 2001;107:83–90.
34. Rayapudi M, Mavi P, Zhu X, et al. Indoor insect allergens are potent inducers of experimental eosinophilic esophagitis in mice. J Leukoc Biol 2010;88: 337–46.
35. Song DJ, Cho JY, Lee SY, et al. Anti-Siglec-F antibody inhibits oral egg allergen-induced intestinal eosinophilic inflammation in a mouse model. Clin Immunol 2009;131:157–69.
36. Mishra A, Schlotman J, Wang M, et al. Critical role for adaptive T-cell immunity in experimental eosinophilic esophagitis in mice. J Leukoc Biol 2007;81: 916–24.
37. Xiang Z, Wang M, Mavi P, et al. Interleukin-15 expression is increased in human eosinophilic esophagitis and mediates pathogenesis in mice. Gastroenterology 2010;139:182–93.
38. Mishra A, Wang M, Pemmaraju VR, et al. Esophageal remodeling develops as a consequence of tissue specific IL-5-induced eosinophilia. Gastroenterology 2008;134:204–14.
39. Blanchard C, Mingler MK, Vicario M, et al. IL-13 involvement in eosinophilic esophagitis: transcriptome analysis and reversibility with glucocorticoids. J Allergy Clin Immunol 2007;120:1292–300.
40. Lucendo AJ, Navarro M, Comas C, et al. Immunophenotypic characterization and quantification of the epithelial inflammatory infiltrate in eosinophilic esophagitis through stereology: an analysis of the cellular mechanisms of the disease and the immunologic capacity of the esophagus. Am J Surg Pathol 2007;31: 598–606.
41. Teitelbaum J, Fox V, Twarog F, et al. Eosinophilic esophagitis in children: immunopathological analysis and response to fluticasone propionate. Gastroenterology 2002;122:1216–25.
42. Mueller S, Aigner T, Neureiter D, et al. Eosinophil infiltration and degranulation in oesophageal mucosa from adult patients with eosinophilic oesophagitis: a retrospective and comparative study on pathological biopsy. J Clin Pathol 2006;59: 1175–80.

43. Kephart GM, Alexander JA, Arora AS, et al. Marked deposition of eosinophil derived neurotoxin in adult patients with eosinophilic esophagitis. Am J Gastroenterol 2010;105:298–307.
44. Protheroe C, Woodruff SA, dePetris G, et al. A novel histologic scoring system to evaluate mucosal biopsies from patients with eosinophilic esophagitis. Clin Gastroenterol Hepatol 2009;7:749–55.
45. Mulder DJ, Pacheco I, Hurlbut DJ, et al. FGF-9 induced proliferative response to eosinophilic inflammation in oesophagitis. Gut 2009;58:166–73.
46. Kirsch R, Bokhary R, Marcon MA, et al. Activated mucosal mast cells differentiate eosinophilic (allergic) esophagitis from gastroesophageal reflux disease. J Pediatr Gastroenterol Nutr 2007;44:20–6.
47. Vicario M, Blanchard C, Stringer KF, et al. Local B cells and IgE production in oesophageal mucosa in eosinophilic oesophagitis. Gut 2010;59:12–20.
48. Yen EH, Hornick JL, Dehlink E, et al. Comparative analysis of FcER1 expression patterns in patients with eosinophil and reflux esophagitis. J Pediatr Gastroenterol Nutr 2010;51(5):584–92.
49. Konikoff MR, Noel RJ, Blanchard C, et al. A randomized, double blind, placebo-controlled trial of fluticasone propionate for pediatric eosinophilic esophagitis. Gastroenterology 2006;131:1381–91.
50. Aceves SS, Chen D, Newbury RO, et al. Mast cells infiltrate the esophageal smooth muscle in patients with eosinophilic esophagitis, express TGFb1 and increase esophageal smooth muscle contraction. J Allergy Clin Immunol 2010;126:1198–204.
51. Albonia JP, Blanchard C, Butz BB, et al. Involvement of mast cells in eosinophilic esophagitis. J Allergy Clin Immunol 2010;126:140–9.
52. Aceves SS, Newbury RO, Dohil R, et al. Esophageal remodeling in pediatric eosinophilic esophagitis. J Allergy Clin Immunol 2007;119:206–12.
53. Blanchard C, Mingler MK, McBride M, et al. Periostin facilitates eosinophil tissue infiltration in allergic lung and esophageal responses. Mucosal Immunol 2008;1:289–96.
54. Erwin EA, James HR, Gutekunst HM, et al. Serum IgE measurement and detection of food allergy in pediatric patients with eosinophilic esophagitis. Ann Allergy Asthma Immunol 2010;104:496–502.
55. Spergel JM, Brown-Whitehorn T, Beausoleil JL, et al. Predictive values for skin prick test and atopy patch test for eosinophilic esophagitis. J Allergy Clin Immunol 2007;119:509–11.
56. Markowitz JE, Spergel JM, Ruchelli E, et al. Elemental diet is an effective treatment for eosinophilic esophagitis in children and adolescents. Am J Gastroenterol 2003;98:777–82.
57. Liacouras CA, Spergel JM, Ruchelli E, et al. Eosinophilic esophagitis: a 10-year experience in 381 children. Clin Gastroenterol Hepatol 2005;3:1198–206.
58. Frischmeyer-Guerrerio PA, Guerrerio AL, Chichester KL, et al. Dendritic cell and T cell responses in children with food allergy. Clin Exp Allergy 2011;41(1):61–71.
59. Prussin C, Lee J, Foster B. Eosinophilic gastrointestinal disease and peanut allergy are alternatively associated with IL-5+ and IL-5-Th2 responses. J Allergy Clin Immunol 2009;124:1326–32.
60. Kagalwalla AF, Sentongo TA, Ritz S, et al. Effect of six-food elimination diet on clinical and histologic outcomes in eosinophilic esophagitis. Clin Gastroenterol Hepatol 2006;4:1097–102.

61. Schaefer ET, Fitzgerald JF, Molleston JP, et al. Comparison of oral prednisone and topical fluticasone in treatment of eosinophilic esophagitis: a randomized trial in children. Clin Gastroenterol Hepatol 2008;6:165–73.
62. Dohil R, Newbury R, Fox L, et al. Oral viscous budesonide is effective in children with eosinophilic esophagitis in a randomized placebo controlled trial. Gastroenterology 2010;139:418–29.
63. Dellon ES, Gibbs WB, Rubinas TC, et al. Esophageal dilation in eosinophilic esophagitis: safety and predictors of clinical response and complications. Gastrointest Endosc 2010;71:706–12.
64. Straumann A, Bussmann C, Zuber M, et al. Eosinophilic esophagitis: analysis of food impaction and perforation in 251 adolescent and adult patients. Clin Gastroenterol Hepatol 2008;6:598–600.
65. Schoepfer AM, Gonsalves N, Bussmann C, et al. Esophageal dilation in eosinophilic esophagitis: effectiveness, safety, and impact on the underlying inflammation. Am J Gastroenterol 2010;105:1062–70.
66. Jacobs JW Jr, Spechler SJ. A systematic review of the risk of perforation during esophageal dilation for patients with eosinophilic esophagitis. Dig Dis Sci 2010; 55:1512–5.
67. Kaijser R. Allergic disease of the gut from the point of view of the surgeon. Arch Klin Chir 1937;188:36–64, 183:195–201.
68. Oh HE, Chetty R. Eosinophilic gastroenteritis: a review. J Gastroenterol 2008;43: 741–50.
69. Lowichik A, Weinberg AG. A quantitative evaluation of mucosal eosinophils in the pediatric gastrointestinal tract. Mod Pathol 1996;9(2):110–4.
70. DeBrosse CW, Case JW, Putnam PE, et al. Quantity and distribution of eosinophils in the gastrointestinal tract of children. Pediatr Dev Pathol 2006;9(3): 210–8.
71. Kelly KJ. Eosinophilic gastroenteritis. J Pediatr Gastroenterol Nutr 2000;30: S28–35.
72. Simon D, Wardlaw A, Rothenberg ME. Organ specific eosinophilic disorders of the skin, lung, and gastrointestinal tract. J Allergy Clin Immunol 2010;126:3–13.
73. Redondo-Cerezo E, Cabello MJ, González Y, et al. Eosinophilic gastroenteritis: our recent experience: one-year experience of atypical onset of an uncommon disease. Scand J Gastroenterol 2001;36:1358–60.
74. Talley NJ, Shorter RG, Phillips SF, et al. Eosinophilic gastroenteritis: a clinicopathological study of patients with disease of the mucosa, muscle layer, and subserosal tissues. Gut 1990;31:54–8.
75. Lee CM, Changchien CS, Chen PC, et al. Eosinophilic gastroenteritis: 10 years experience. Am J Gastroenterol 1993;88:70–4.
76. Guajardo JR, Plotnick LM, Fende JM, et al. Eosinophil-associated gastrointestinal disorders: a world-wide-web based registry. J Pediatr 2002;141(4):576–81.
77. Chen MJ, Chu CH, Lin SC, et al. Eosinophilic gastroenteritis: clinical experience with 15 patients. World J Gastroenterol 2003;9(12):2813–6.
78. Klein NC, Hargrove RL, Sleisenger MH, et al. Eosinophilic gastroenteritis. Medicine 1970;40:299–319.
79. Gonsalves N. Food allergies and eosinophilic gastrointestinal illness. Gastroenterol Clin North Am 2007;36:75–91.
80. Siaw EK, Sayed K, Jackson RJ. Eosinophilic gastroenteritis presenting as acute gastric perforation. J Pediatr Gastroenterol Nutr 2006;43:691–4.
81. Markowitz JE, Russo P, Liacouras CA. Solitary duodenal ulcer: a new presentation of eosinophilic gastroenteritis. Gastrointest Endosc 2000;52:673–6.

82. Friesen CA. Clinical efficacy and pharmacokinetics of montelukast in dyspeptic children with duodenal eosinophilia. J Pediatr Gastroenterol Nutr 2004;38: 343–51.
83. Jacobson LB. Diffuse eosinophilic gastroenteritis: an adult form of allergic gastroenteropathy. Report of a case with probable protein-losing enteropathy. Am J Gastroenterol 1970;54:580–8.
84. Tursi A, Rella G, Inchingolo CD, et al. Gastric outlet obstruction due to gastroduodenal eosinophilic gastroenteritis. Endoscopy 2007;39:E184.
85. Lyngbaek S, Adamsen S, Aru A, et al. Recurrent acute pancreatitis due to eosinophilic gastroenteritis. Case report and literature review. JOP 2006;9:211–7.
86. Whitaker IS, Gulati A, McDaid JO, et al. Eosinophilic gastroenteritis presenting as obstructive jaundice. Eur J Gastroenterol Hepatol 2004;16:407–9.
87. Tran D, Salloum L, Tshibaka C, et al. Eosinophilic gastroenteritis mimicking acute appendicitis. Am Surg 2000;66(10):990–2.
88. Shweiki E, West JC, Klena JW, et al. Eosinophilic gastroenteritis presenting as an obstructing cecal mass–a case report and review of the literature. Am J Gastroenterol 1999;94:3644–5.
89. Yun MY, Cho YU, Park IS, et al. Eosinophilic gastroenteritis presenting as small bowel obstruction: a case report and review of the literature. World J Gastroenterol 2007;13:1758–60.
90. Siahanidou T, Mandyla H, Dimitriadis D, et al. Eosinophilic gastroenteritis complicated with perforation and intussusception in a neonate. J Pediatr Gastroenterol Nutr 2001;32:335–7.
91. Vitellas KM, Bennett WF, Bova JG, et al. Radiographic manifestations of eosinophilic gastroenteritis. Abdom Imag 1995;20:406–13.
92. Maroy B. Nonmucosal eosinophilic gastroenteritis: sonographic appearance at presentation and during follow-up of response to prednisone therapy. J Clin Ultrasound 1998;26:483–6.
93. Chehade M, Magid MS, Mofidi S, et al. Allergic eosinophilic gastroenteritis with protein losing enteropathy: intestinal pathology, clinical course, and long term follow up. J Pediatr Gastroenterol Nutr 2006;42:516–21.
94. Beyer K, Castro R, Birnbaum A, et al. Human milk specific mucosal lymphocytes of the gastrointestinal tract display a Th2 cytokine profile. J Allergy Clin Immunol 2002;109:707–13.
95. Foroughi S, Foster B, Kim NY, et al. Anti-IgE treatment of eosinophil associated gastrointestinal disorders. J Allergy Clin Immunol 2007;120:594–601.
96. Conus S, Straumann A, Bettler E, et al. Mepolizumab does not alter levels of eosinophils, T cells, and mast cells in the duodenal mucosa in eosinophilic esophagitis. J Allergy Clin Immunol 2010;120:175–6.
97. Netzer P, Gschossmann JM, Staumann A, et al. Corticosteroid dependent eosinophilic oesophagitis: azathioprine and 6-mercaptopurine can induce and maintain long term remission. Eur J Gastroenterol Hepatol 2007;19:865–9.
98. Quack I, Sellin L, Buchner NJ, et al. Eosinophilic gastroenteritis in a young girl–long term remission under montelukast. BMC Gastroenterology 2005;5:24–9.
99. Garcia-Careaga M Jr, Kerner JA. Gastrointestinal manifestations of food allergies in pediatric patients. Nutr Clin Pract 2005;20:526–35.
100. Lake AM. Food-induced eosinophilic proctocolitis. J Pediatr Gastroenterol Nutr 2000;30:S58–60.
101. Gryboski J. Gastrointestinal milk allergy in infancy. Pediatrics 1967;40:354–62.
102. Sicherer SH, Eigenmann PA, Sampson HA. Clinical features of food protein-induced enterocolitis syndrome. J Pediatr 1998;133(2):214–9.

103. Nowak-Wegrzyn A, Muraro A. Food protein-induced enterocolitis syndrome. Curr Opin Allergy Clin Immunol 2009;9:371–7.
104. Hwang JB, Lee SH, Kang YN, et al. Indexes of suspicion of typical cow's milk protein-induced enterocolitis. J Korean Med Sci 2007;22:993–7.
105. Mehr S, Kakakios A, Frith K, et al. Food protein-induced enterocolitis syndrome: 16-year experience. Pediatrics 2009;123:e459–64.
106. Burks AW, Casteel HB, Fiedorek SC, et al. Prospective oral food challenge study of two soybean protein isolates in patients with possible milk or soy protein enterocolitis. Pediatr Allergy Immunol 1994;5:40–5.
107. Nowak-Wegrzyn A, Sampson HA, Wood RA, et al. Food protein-induced enterocolitis syndrome caused by solid food proteins. Pediatrics 2003;111(4):829–35.
108. Levy Y, Danon YL. Food protein-induced enterocolitis syndrome–not only due to cow's milk and soy. Pediatr Allergy Immunol 2003;14(4):325–9.
109. Fogg MI, Brown-Whitehorn TA, Pawlowski NA, et al. Atopy patch test for the diagnosis of food protein-induced entero-colitis syndrome. Pediatr Allergy Immunol 2006;17(5):351–5.
110. Goldman H, Provjanksy R. Allergic proctitis and gastroenteritis in children. Am J Surg Pathol 1986;10:75–86.
111. Machida HM, Catto Smith AG, et al. Allergic colitis in infancy: clinical and pathologic aspects. J Pediatr Gastroenterol Nutr 1994;19(1):22–6.
112. Arvola T, Ruuska T, Keränen J, et al. Rectal bleeding in infancy: clinical, allergological, and microbiological examination. Pediatrics 2006;117(4):e760–8.

Milk and Soy Allergy

Jacob D. Kattan, MD[a], Renata R. Cocco, MD[b],
Kirsi M. Järvinen, MD, PhD[a,*]

KEYWORDS

• Cow's milk • Soy • Allergy • Cross-reactivity • Diagnosis
• Management • Natural history

EPIDEMIOLOGY

General population birth cohorts report a prevalence of cow's milk allergy (CMA) of 2.2% to 2.8% at 1 year of age,[1,2] similar to the rate found in another large cohort followed for 18 to 34 months.[3] Of those with CMA, about 60% have IgE-mediated CMA.[4] A recent study from Israel by Katz and colleagues[5] reported a much lower rate of CMA in infants (0.5%) than in 3-year-old children (0.6%).[6] The investigators also reported a rate of 0.5% for non-IgE–mediated CMA in infants, equivalent to the rate of IgE-mediated CMA in infants.[5] Childhood CMA is more prevalent in boys than girls.[7] Regarding severe allergic reactions, cow's milk (CM) comprises 10% to 19% of food-induced anaphylaxis cases seen both in the field and in emergency departments in pediatric and mixed-age populations. CM is the third most common food product to cause anaphylaxis, following peanut and tree nuts.[8–11]

In general, soy allergy is not as common as CMA, even in atopic children. Bruno and colleagues[12] found a prevalence of 1.2% in a cohort of 505 children suffering from allergic diseases and 0.4% in 243 children who had been fed soy protein formula in the first 6 months of life for supposed prevention of allergic diseases. In population-based studies, 2 European cohorts pointed to rates varying from 0.0%[13] to 0.7%[14] for children in double-blind placebo-controlled food challenge. Also, up to 10% to 14% of patients with CMA also present with soy protein allergy.[15–17] In a study by Klemola and colleagues,[16] adverse reactions to soy were seen more often in milk-allergic individuals younger than 6 months. In this study, at 2-year follow-up, sensitization to soy proteins was not higher in infants fed soy formula than in those fed extensively hydrolyzed formulas (P = .082; n = 70).[18] One recent study reported

This work was supported by funding from the NIH K12 HD052890 (K.M.J.).
The authors have nothing to disclose.

[a] Division of Pediatric Allergy and Immunology, Department of Pediatrics, Jaffe Institute for Food Allergy, The Mount Sinai School of Medicine, Box 1198, One Gustave L. Levy Place, New York, NY 10029-6574, USA
[b] Division of Allergy, Clinical Immunology and Rheumatology, Department of Pediatrics, Federal University of São Paulo, Rua dos Otonis, 725, São Paulo, SP, CEP 04025-002, Brazil
* Corresponding author.
E-mail address: kirsi.jarvinen-seppo@mssm.edu

Pediatr Clin N Am 58 (2011) 407–426
doi:10.1016/j.pcl.2011.02.005 **pediatric.theclinics.com**
0031-3955/11/$ – see front matter

that of 66 infants with IgE-mediated CMA, none had a proven allergy to soy, with 64 of 66 tolerating soy in their diets.[5]

Dietary exposure to milk, soy, and products containing either or both vary in different parts of the world. Traditional Asian cuisine includes less milk sources than the Western cuisine but includes several natural soy sources. Meanwhile, the consumption of soy-containing food additives (soy isolate, soy concentrate, and soy flour) is increasing in Western diets. This interesting geographic divergence may lead to a difference in the prevalence of soy and milk allergy between different populations, but this has not been confirmed.

CLINICAL MANIFESTATIONS

Patients with CMA and soy allergy present with a wide range of IgE-mediated and non-IgE–mediated clinical syndromes (**Table 1**).[19–23] IgE-mediated reactions occur immediately or within 1 to 2 hours of ingestion, whereas non-IgE–mediated reactions generally have a delayed onset beyond 2 hours of ingestion.[24] Both humoral and/or cell-mediated mechanisms play a role in mixed manifestations, which may present with acute or chronic symptoms, making the causal relationship to foods more difficult to detect. Clinical symptoms of CMA commonly appear during the first months of life, usually within days or weeks after feeding with CM-based formulas have been started or may sometimes be seen in exclusively breast-fed infants.[25,26] With such an early age of onset, symptoms of an erythematous rash or hives shortly after intake of CM (or infrequently soy) formula are suggestive of food allergy. The role of food allergy in causing flares of atopic dermatitis is less clear, although up to one-third of moderate to severe atopic dermatitis may in fact be because of CMA.[27,28]

Table 1
Presentation of CMA and soy allergy

IgE Mediated	
Cutaneous	Urticaria Angioedema
Gastrointestinal	Oral itching and abdominal pain Nausea and vomiting Diarrhea
Respiratory	Rhinoconjunctivitis Wheeze and asthma exacerbation Laryngeal edema
Systemic	Anaphylaxis
Mixed IgE mediated and non-IgE mediated	
Cutaneous	Atopic dermatitis
Gastrointestinal	Eosinophilic esophagitis and gastroenteritis
Non-IgE mediated	
Gastrointestinal	Dietary protein enterocolitis/proctitis/proctocolitis Protein-losing enteropathy GER[a] Colic[a] Constipation[a]
Respiratory	Pulmonary hemosiderosis (ie, Heiner syndrome; mostly caused by milk allergy)

[a] Controversial.

Immediate IgE-Mediated Reactions

Immediate IgE-mediated skin reactions include hives and angioedema. Gastrointestinal manifestations include mouth and lip pruritus, abdominal pain, vomiting, and diarrhea. A variety of respiratory tract symptoms that generally involve IgE-mediated responses, including rhinorrhea and wheezing, may also be seen, although isolated asthma or rhinitis is unusual.[29] Occupational and household exposures involving inhalation of cooking or processing vapors containing milk droplets may cause respiratory symptoms, and casual contact by touching can cause localized urticaria.

Milk is also the third most common food responsible for fatal or near-fatal food-induced anaphylactic reactions (8%–15% cases).[10,30–32] Although severe soy allergy reactions have been reported, they are far less common than CMA reactions. Moreover, the small number of fatal allergic reactions to soy included some patients with concomitant severe peanut allergy and/or asthma.[33,34] Foucard and Malmheden Yman[35] described 4 deaths presumably caused by soy allergy in severely peanut-allergic asthmatic children with previous tolerance to soy. By contrast, Sicherer and colleagues[34] reported no severe allergic reactions to soy challenge in 13 years of experience with double-blind placebo-controlled food challenges. In a more recent study on allergic reactions during inpatient oral food challenges (OFCs), 7% of soy challenges were severe enough to require administration of epinephrine.[36] A report on patients with soy and birch pollen allergy describes 25% patients with more severe reactions, including throat or chest tightness during double-blind placebo-controlled food challenges with soy.[37]

Mixed Reactions

Atopic dermatitis

CMA and soy allergy play a pathogenic role in a subset of patients, primarily infants and children, with atopic dermatitis. It is recommended that patients with atopic dermatitis be treated with topical medications before considering a food allergy because most cases do not seem to be caused by food allergy. However, approximately 40% of infants and young children with moderate to severe atopic dermatitis have a food allergy, with hen's eggs, CM, soy, and wheat accounting for about 90% of allergenic foods.[6,38,39] CMA was found in 17% of children with atopic dermatitis and clinically significant IgE-mediated food hypersensitivity referred to a university-based dermatology clinic.[27] In a multicenter study performed in Brazil, 12 of 13 children (median age 5.4 years) with atopic eczema and IgE-mediated soy allergy confirmed by open challenges also had high levels of specific IgE for other foods, including milk, egg, wheat, and peanuts, as well as pollens (Cocco RR et al, unpublished data, 2007).

Eosinophilic gastroenteropathies

Milk and soy are among the major allergens in allergic eosinophilic esophagitis (AEE), a disorder characterized by eosinophilic inflammation of the esophagus. Symptoms are suggestive of gastroesophageal reflux (GER) but do not respond to conventional reflux therapies.[19] Feeding problems, vomiting, abdominal pain, dysphagia, and food impaction may also be seen. The role of food allergy in eosinophilic gastroenteritis, which is the eosinophilic gastroenteropathy of the stomach and intestines, is less clear than in eosinophilic esophagitis. Symptoms include abdominal pain, nausea, vomiting, diarrhea, and weight loss.[40]

Delayed Non-IgE–Mediated Reactions

Food protein–induced enterocolitis

Dietary protein–induced syndromes of enteropathy and enterocolitis are not IgE mediated and typically present with profuse vomiting and diarrhea within 2 to 3 hours after ingestion of the offending allergen, causing profound dehydration and lethargy.[40] Three quarters of infants with food protein–induced enterocolitis (FPIES) appear acutely ill, and about 15% have hypotension requiring hospitalization.[41] Mehr and colleagues[42] reported that a quarter of acute FPIES episodes in young infants manifested with hypothermia less than 36°C. Patients may present with diarrhea with occult blood loss, and fecal smears reveal leukocytes and eosinophils. Chronic exposure to the offending allergen results in a less acute clinical presentation of failure to thrive and hypoalbuminemia.[40,43] Sicherer and colleagues[44] reported that FPIES was elicited most often by CM and soy protein, with 7 of 16 patients having sensitivity to both. Similarly, Burks and colleagues[45] reported that 6 of 10 patients with FPIES reacted to both milk and soy. Our preliminary data on 76 patients with FPIES showed that CM was the trigger in 58% and soy in 47% of patients.[46] Among children with milk FPIES, 45% had soy FPIES, and among children with soy FPIES, 56% had milk FPIES.

Protein-induced allergic enterocolitis/proctitis/proctocolitis

Protein-induced allergic enterocolitis/proctitis/proctocolitis usually presents by 6 months of life in an otherwise well-appearing breast-fed or formula-fed infant with blood-streaked, mucous, loose stools and occasionally diarrhea.[40] CM and soy are the major causative foods. Most breast-fed infants with allergic proctocolitis respond to maternal elimination of CM proteins, although some require the additional elimination of soy[47] or conversion to extensively hydrolyzed formula. Other causes, such as viruses, may have a similar presentation.[48]

GER

Although debated, symptoms of GER may be associated with CMA. However, GER is not likely to be the sole presentation of CMA or soy allergy. Underlying causes of GER, such as eosinophilic esophagitis and dietary protein-induced gastroenteropathy, should be ruled out in patients with GER symptoms and suspected CMA.

Infantile colic

The role of milk protein in infantile colic and constipation in childhood remains controversial.[7,49–54] Improvement in colic symptoms after CM elimination or change of formula, followed by worsening of symptoms with challenge in some infants has been demonstrated.[7,50,51] Colic and fussiness are common in early infancy but are not likely to be isolated manifestations of CMA or soy allergy.

Constipation

Also a controversial topic, CM allergy/intolerance has been suggested as a cause of constipation in infants and children, especially in those with refractory chronic constipation. In up to half of the children with refractory chronic constipation, as demonstrated by one group, symptoms were shown to be related to CM in double-blind or open food challenges.[54,55] Biopsy findings demonstrate proctitis with eosinophil infiltration of the rectal mucosa and a reduced thickness of the rectal mucous layer,[54] as well as lymphonodular hyperplasia in the terminal ileum and colon.[55] A case report describes difficulty of spontaneous defecation mimicking Hirschsprung disease.[29] Other rare gastrointestinal presentations described in neonates include bilious vomiting, massive bloody stools with peripheral eosinophilia, eosinophilic infiltration in the lamina propria, and CM-specific IgE in the serum supporting the diagnosis of CMA.[56,57] However, in a recent study, no association was found between timing of introduction of CM or soy and onset of functional constipation, although history of CMA in the first year of life was significantly associated with functional constipation in childhood.[58]

Heiner syndrome

Heiner syndrome is a rare food hypersensitivity pulmonary disease that primarily affects infants. This syndrome is mostly caused by CM. The symptoms include cough, wheezing, hemoptysis, nasal congestion, dyspnea, recurrent otitis media, recurrent fever, anorexia, vomiting, colic, diarrhea, hematochezia, and failure to thrive.[59] Radiological evidence of pulmonary infiltrates and high serum titers of precipitating antibodies (IgG) to CM proteins are seen. Milk-specific IgE may be detected, and there is pulmonary hemosiderosis in some cases. Improvement of both clinical and radiological findings occurs after strict milk avoidance.[59]

PATHOGENESIS

Acute (IgE-mediated) reactions to milk are caused by various milk allergens. Caseins and whey proteins account for approximately 80% and 20% of total milk protein, respectively.[60] The caseins include α_{s1}-, α_{s2}-, β-, and κ-caseins (Bos d 8) and comprise 32%, 10%, 28%, and 10% of the total protein, respectively. The most important whey allergens are α-lactalbumin (Bos d 4) and β-lactoglobulin (BLG, Bos d 5), comprising 5% and 10% of total milk protein, respectively.[60–62] Other minor milk allergens include bovine serum albumin (BSA, Bos d 6), lactoferrin, and immunoglobulins (Bos d 7).[17,62] Sequential IgE-binding epitopes of the major milk allergens have been identified,[63–67] and several have been investigated for mutational analysis.[68–70] The pathogenesis and causative allergens in non-IgE–mediated CMA and milk allergy caused by mixed IgE-mediated and non-IgE–mediated processes are less well understood.

Cooking diminishes the allergenicity of whey proteins, particularly that of BLG, presumably by denaturation of heat-labile proteins, resulting in loss of conformational epitopes.[71,72] This diminishing of allergenicity because of cooking may explain why many CM-allergic patients tolerate extensively heated milk.[73] Similarly, yogurt cultures, which ferment and acidify milk, contain less intact whey protein,[72] and therefore, individuals with CMA exclusively sensitized to whey proteins may tolerate yogurt-based dairy products.

The specificity of soy allergens is variable and complex. As many as 28 different soy proteins were recognized as being able to bind IgE in soy-allergic patients.[74,75] However, only a few of these proteins are considered major allergens, defined as those to which more than 50% of tested population reacted.[76] In this context, only the birch pollen–related allergens, Gly m 3 (a profilin) and Gly m 4 (a PR-10 protein), in addition to soybean hull proteins, Gly m 1 and Gly m 2 (see later), have been officially accepted as soybean allergens by the International Union of Immunological Societies Allergen Sub-Committee (http://www.allergen.org?Allergen.aspx). Several other soy proteins have been characterized, including storage proteins (β-conglycinin and glycinin, named Gly m 5 and Gly m 6, respectively),[77–79] the thiol protease Gly m Bd 30 k (possibly a major soybean allergen),[80–82] the soybean Kunitz trypsin inhibitor,[83–85] and the 2S albumin soy protein.[85] The 2 soybean major storage proteins, β-conglycinin and glycinin, are 7S and 11S globulins and account for about 30% and 40% of the total seed proteins, respectively. Sensitization to both of these allergens has been shown to be a potential indicator for severe allergic reactions to soy.[86] Specific linear IgE-binding epitopes on some soy allergens have been identified,[78,81] and mutational analysis is underway.[82]

Soybeans are also aeroallergens, although the pathology and allergen reactivity profiles are different for ingestion versus inhalation, whereby soy hull antigens (Gly m 1 and Gly m 2), not present in soy protein isolates, seem to dominate.[87] The hydrophobic soybean hull proteins Gly m 1 and Gly m 2 have been described to be relevant in respiratory soy allergy, which is acquired through inhalation of soy proteins.[88]

Soy allergy may also develop secondary to initial sensitization to birch pollen and resulting cross-reactivity (see later). A retrospective analysis of specific IgE to foods and inhalants from 273 children by The German Multi-Centre Allergy Study revealed that IgE sensitization to soy in infancy is relatively uncommon and mostly primary (generated by food ingestion). On the other hand, IgE sensitization is more frequent at school age because of cross-reacting pollen antigens via inhalation.[89]

CROSS-REACTIVITY

Mammals that are phylogenetically related have quite similar milk protein expression.[90] As an example, significant amino acid sequence homology and resulting high rate of clinical cross-reactivity render sheep or goat milk inappropriate feeding alternatives for most CM-allergic individuals.[91,92] However, some patients with primary goat's or sheep's milk allergy may tolerate CM and vice versa.[93,94] Some patients with CMA may tolerate milk from other mammals, such as camels, pigs, reindeer, horses, and donkeys.[92,95–100] Clinical allergy to human milk has been shown in one case report, and sensitization to human milk with immediate-type skin reaction has been reported in another one, although confirmatory clinical data are missing and the clinical significance is largely unknown.[101,102] The authors identified IgE-reactive human epitopes that were cross-reactive with bovine milk and human milk epitopes that were non–cross-reactive using peptides representing the known IgE-binding regions of bovine milk proteins and the corresponding highly similar peptides on human milk.[103] Cross-reactivity between different mammalian milks has been reviewed in detail elsewhere.[104]

Serum albumin is thought to be involved in cosensitization to milk and beef, reported in 13% to 20% of children with CMA.[105] Clinical cross-reactivity may be more pronounced with less well-cooked meat. In another study, 7 of 8 patients with persistent CMA who were sensitized to CM, BSA, and animal dander recognized serum albumin in different raw, but not heated, meats (beef, lamb, deer, and pork) and epithelia (dog, cat, and cow).[106]

Cosensitization to soy is common in patients with CMA, but clinical coallergy due to cross-sensitization based on cross-reactive proteins between milk and soy is not.[62] In one study, cosensitization without clinical reactivity to soy milk was noted in 17% of patients with CMA.[107] Several other studies suggest that most individuals with CMA tolerate soy or soy formula, and reactions in those who do not tolerate soy are non–IgE-mediated (see "Epidemiology"). The soy protein component that cross-reacts with casein has been identified as the A5-B3 glycinin molecule, although findings have not been reproduced.[108]

Clinical cross-reactivity between peanut and soy, both legumes, is extremely rare, despite the high degree of cross-sensitization based on IgE binding and skin tests.[109,110] Green and colleagues[111] found that 7% of 140 peanut-allergic patients were allergic to soy as determined from a combination of history taking, serum food-specific IgE level tests, skin prick tests (SPTs), and OFCs. Consistent with this, Bernhisel-Broadbent and Sampson[112] performed open or double-blind placebo-controlled food challenges in 69 highly atopic children with at least 1 positive skin test result to a legume and found that 6.5% of the peanut-allergic children reacted to soy. In their study, among the 43% of patients with a positive skin test result for soy, only 11.5% were soy reactive.[112] Another study found that 6% of individuals with positive soy skin test results reacted to soy.[113]

Soy proteins can also elicit allergic oropharyngeal or systemic reactions in adult patients sensitized to major birch pollen allergen Bet v 1. This reaction results from cross-reactivity to pathogenesis-related protein (PR-10) from soy, designated as the allergen starvation-associated message 22 or, more recently, as Gly m 4.[37,114] Relevant studies in children are lacking, although the same phenomenon is seen in the clinical setting. The content of Gly m 4 in soy food products strongly depends on the degree of food processing.[37] A prevalence of 10% of soy allergy was reported among Central European patients sensitized to birch pollen, which was caused by IgE cross-reactivity between the major birch pollen allergen, Bet v 1, and its homologous protein in soy, Gly m 4.[37]

DIAGNOSIS

The diagnosis of CMA or soy allergy is based on the clinical history; allergy testing, when it is available (diagnostic tests for non–IgE-mediated manifestations are limited); and, if needed, a diagnostic trial including elimination of the suspected food, challenge, and reelimination. In breast-fed infants, CM/soy protein is restricted in the maternal diet, and in formula-fed infants, either extensively hydrolyzed or amino acid–based infant formula may be used.[115] If there is no improvement on a milk or soy avoidance diet, the food in question may not be responsible for the symptoms. Alternatively, the diet may not have been restricted enough and additional foods may be considered suspicious.

The double-blind placebo-controlled food challenge is the gold standard for the diagnosis of food allergy. Numerous efforts have been made to standardize these challenges, which are time consuming and expensive endeavors and induce severe and potential life-threatening allergic reactions. OFCs should be approached cautiously even in children with sensitization to CM without a history of clinical reactions who have undergone a long-term (median 2.3 years in one study) elimination of CM because the challenge has a potential to elicit severe immediate allergic reactions to CM.[116] The indications and conduct of controlled OFCs in children with suspected food-related symptoms have been reviewed recently.[117]

IgE-Mediated Reactions

Although SPT and specific IgE testing may reveal sensitization to a food allergen, this sensitivity may not translate to clinical symptoms in up to half of the sensitized population.[118,119] However, in the context of a convincing reaction to ingestion of milk or soy protein and the presence of milk-specific or soy-specific IgE, a diagnosis of CMA or soy allergy is likely. In the setting of a convincing history but negative tests or sensitization in the presence of an unconvincing history, an oral milk or soy challenge may be needed. In infants, skin tests may not be as useful in ruling out CMA because detectable levels of milk-specific IgE are less frequent.[120] Higher concentrations of CM-specific IgE and larger skin test wheals generally correlate with an increased likelihood of a reaction on ingestion. However, these values are not predictive of the nature or severity of reaction to milk and are based on few clinical studies in selected populations.

Several studies have investigated the relationship between the specific IgE levels and SPT wheal size and CM and the outcome of milk double-blind placebo-controlled food challenges to identify cutoff values above which there is a high likelihood of a positive OFC (**Table 2**).[121–127] Such cutoff values could eliminate the need for a challenge. A CM-specific IgE level of 15 kU_A/L using the ImmunoCAP (Phadia, Uppsala, Sweden) assay is 95% predictive of a clinical reaction to milk ingestion.[122] A level of

Table 2
Cutoff values based on 95% positive predicted values for CM-specific IgE and SPT in children with CMA

	Age (y)	95% PPV	Methods
CM-specific IgE			
Sampson,[122] 2001	—	15 kU_A/L	CAP System FEIA[a]
Garcia-Ara et al,[123] 2001	<1	5 kU_A/L	CAP System FEIA[a]
van der Gugten et al,[125] 2008	<2.5	7.5 kU_A/L	CAP System FEIA[a]
SPT			
Hill et al,[124] 2004	<2 All children	100% PPV: 6-mm wheal 100% PPV: 8-mm wheal	CM allergen extract
Verstege et al,[126] 2005	—	12.5-mm wheal or 2.7 SI[b]	Fresh CM
Calvani et al,[127] 2007	—	15-mm wheal	Fresh CM

[a] Phadia, Uppsala, Sweden.
[b] SI, ratio of allergen-induced wheal diameter to histamine-induced wheal diameter.

5 kU_A/L in children younger than 2 years is similarly predictive of a reaction.[123] Similar analyses have been performed for skin testing using a commercial CM extract; a wheal diameter of 6 mm in children who are 2 years or younger and 8 mm in children older than 2 years is 95% predictive of a clinical reaction.[124] The limiting factor is that positive predictive values (PPVs) have been obtained from highly selected pediatric populations and may not be applied to less-selected patient populations.[128] Furthermore, the predictive values for clinical reactivity associated with food-specific IgE levels determined by ImmunoCAP should not be applied to results from other laboratory assays.[129]

Regarding soy allergy, the performance of specific IgE levels for predicting clinical reactivity is poorer.[121,122,130] Several studies point out the dissociation between high levels of specific IgE to soy proteins and low rates of clinical symptoms confirmed by means of double-blind placebo-controlled food challenges.[113,131,132] A soybean IgE level of 65 kU_A/L or higher has a high specificity (99%) but only 86% PPV in predicting clinical allergy.[122]

Non-IgE–Mediated Reactions

IgE tests are not helpful if the symptoms do not suggest an IgE-mediated reaction, such as delayed gastrointestinal reactions and some cases of atopic dermatitis. Atopy patch testing (APT) may provide additional information in these cases, although there are currently no standardized reagents, application methods, or guidelines for interpretation of APT. At present, this type of testing cannot be recommended outside research settings.

The diagnosis of AEE is based on clinical presentation and biopsy with 15 or more eosinophils per high-power field after aggressive therapy with anti-GER medications and the disappearance of eosinophils after an appropriate elimination diet.[133] Some experts use SPT and APT to guide elimination diets,[134] whereas others empirically remove common foods allergens such as CM, soy, egg, wheat, peanuts, and tree nuts.[135] In one study, although the combination of SPT and APT correctly identified an appropriate diet in about 70% of the population with resolution of the symptoms and biopsies (the remaining 30% required an elemental diet), the negative predictive value (NPV) for milk APT was unacceptably low.[136]

In FPIES, IgE-based allergy testing is commonly negative, and a presumptive diagnosis is made based on a typical presentation, resolution of symptoms on elimination diets, and exclusion of other causes. In a small cohort of 19 infants with FPIES most commonly to CM and soy, APT was found to have a PPV of 75% and a NPV of 100%.[137] Another study suggested that a diagnosis for CM protein–induced enterocolitis is supported by a gastric juice analysis with more than 10 leukocytes per high-power field, when vomiting or lethargy after an OFC is not apparent or is difficult to interpret.[138]

Experimental Tools for Diagnosis

As mentioned earlier, APT has been suggested as an addition to the workup for children with suspected CMA, although results are conflicting.[134,136,137,139–147] The most recent studies found no additional value of APT when compared with specific IgE measurement in the diagnosis of CMA or soy allergy.[145,146]

Most recently, protein microarrays using purified natural CM allergen components have been introduced to the diagnostic armamentarium of milk allergy.[148] These microarrays showed performance characteristics comparable to the current diagnostic tests with the advantages of using small blood volumes (ideal for small children) and multiplex detection of responses to several proteins. Peptide microarray immunoassay is a novel method that can be used to analyze IgE and IgG4 binding to sequential epitopes on individual milk allergens and has been shown to differentiate between tolerant and milk-reactive patients.[67] Further studies are needed to validate its utility in clinical practice.

An allergenic source, such as soybeans, may contain several allergenic proteins or allergenic components. The component-resolved diagnosis (CRD) is a method that provides a detailed analysis of the sensitization profile in individual patients.[149] CRD may be especially useful to differentiate specific IgE binding that is clinically relevant or associated with more severe reactions from that caused by IgE cross-reactivity and milder or no reactions. Evaluation of patients with soy allergy from Switzerland, Denmark, and Italy identified that IgE binding to Gly m 5 or Gly m 6 was found in 86% (6/7) of individuals with anaphylaxis to soy but in only 55% (6/11) and 33% (4/12) of individuals with moderate and mild soy-related symptoms, respectively.[86]

Diagnostic Pitfalls

Digestion, various processing methods (heating, cooking), and fermentation may influence the amount of relevant allergen in a final food product. Thus, tolerance of milk or soy in processed foods may not exclude allergy in forms such as liquid CM, soy milk, or ice cream. Furthermore, CM may be initially missed as a potential allergen because of the ubiquitous nature of milk proteins or misdiagnosis as egg allergy because egg proteins are commonly present in the same foods. Milk should also be considered as a possible contaminant in infants reacting to mixed jarred baby foods and in individuals reacting to soy milk because of use of common production lines. Tolerance of soy oil and soy lecithin does not exclude the possibility of soy allergy because these soy products are tolerated by most patients with soy allergy.[150]

NATURAL HISTORY

Children with CMA should be monitored for development of tolerance because most outgrow their allergy in childhood. Non-IgE–mediated CMA has a better prognosis and tends to resolve more quickly than IgE-mediated CMA. An earlier report indicated that most children with IgE-mediated CMA became tolerant by 3 years of age.[2] However, a more recent study argued that IgE-mediated CMA is more persistent, with only 64% of children developing tolerance by 12 years of age.[151] It is unclear whether these differing results are because of population differences or a change in the natural history of milk allergy. Several prognostic indicators for the development of tolerance include lower initial level of milk-specific IgE,[151] faster rate of decline of milk-specific IgE level over time,[152] lack of specific IgE to a set of specific sequential epitopes on milk allergens,[153] and absence of concomitant allergic rhinitis or asthma.[151,154]

Regarding soy allergy, most people become tolerant over time, although as with CMA, it may take longer than previously thought. Savage and colleagues[155] retrospectively described the natural history of 133 patients allergic to soy (88% with concomitant peanut allergy) with a variety of clinical reactions and found that approximately 50% of the children outgrew their allergy by age 7 years and 69% by age 10 years. By age 6 years, peak soy-specific IgE level less than 10 kU_A/L was predictive of more than 50% chance of outgrowing allergy, but peak level more than 50 kU_A/L suggested a chance of tolerance development of more than 20%. Although soy allergy is commonly considered to have an early onset, the study identified a subset of patients with late-onset soy allergy whose symptoms started after tolerating soy on a regular basis in their diet. The investigators suggested that such late-onset soy allergy may be related to either birch pollen cross-reactivity or persistent peanut allergy, as indicated by a very high peanut-specific IgE levels at their last follow-up. The prevalence of soy sensitization progressively increased with age from 2% at 2 years to 7% at 10 years in the German Multi-Centre Allergy Study, which followed 1314 children from birth to age 13 years.[89]

FPIES responds well to dietary elimination of the offending food, with tolerance usually developing within 3 years of life,[41] although rate of tolerance development varies between studies and populations. Occasionally, FPIES may persist into the teenage years. Earlier reports suggested that within 2 years, 60% of milk and 20% of soy-induced FPIES resolves.[44] Our preliminary data on 76 individuals with FPIES show that most patients with milk FPIES become tolerant by 3 to 4 years, but the natural history was not as favorable for soy.[46] However, a recent study by Korean investigators on 23 infants with milk FPIES reported that 64% tolerated milk at 10 months and 92% tolerated soy at 10 months.[156]

MANAGEMENT

Avoidance

The mainstay of therapy for any food allergy is complete avoidance of the culprit food. Elimination of milk can pose nutritional concerns because milk is an important source of fat and protein in early childhood. Also, eliminating milk from the diet can be difficult because of the ubiquitous nature of CM protein in candy, custard, pudding, sherbet, luncheon meats, hot dogs, sausages, margarine, salad dressing, breaded foods, and more. CM protein may be found in some milk, cream, and butter substitutes, even in those labeled nondairy. CM may contaminate shrimp because some establishments store shrimp in milk to avoid the development of a fishy odor. In addition, breads and pastries may be brushed with milk. Exposure to food allergens via cross-contact (ie, inadvertent exposure to the allergenic food by contamination of "safe" foods with small amounts of the culprit food) can happen anywhere the food is served and because of shared utensils, counters contaminated with dairy product, and shared grills. Furthermore, up to 10% to 40% of products with advisory labeling, such as "may contain milk," have indeed been shown to contain milk.[157,158]

Soy lecithins are commonly used in the food industry as emulsifiers. Concerns about reactivity with soy lecithin and soy oil by soy-allergic patients exist based on the likelihood of contamination with soy proteins. However, evidence[159] and clinical experience suggest that proteins present in both soy lecithin and oil have little allergenicity.

Many individuals with CMA can tolerate extensively heated or baked forms of milk or small amounts of soy protein as an ingredient. However, the only currently available diagnostic test to determine which individuals can tolerate such products (unless it is currently in their diet) is an OFC. During oral challenge to extensively heated milk, severe reactions can occur, and extreme caution is advised. It can be argued that it is reasonable to allow individuals to continue to eat milk or soy in more processed forms (eg, in baked goods) than what triggered their reactions (eg, straight milk, ice cream, soy milk, or soybeans) if they have eaten these forms regularly and in the recent past, although it is unclear whether exposure in this form in the diet induces, prevents, or delays the development of tolerance. It is advisable that these patients avoid more intermediate forms of cooked or processed milk or soy, such as pudding, yogurt, or soy flour, and that anyone who has reacted to such intermediate forms avoid all forms of milk.

Substitutes

In children younger than 12 months, extensively hydrolyzed casein or whey protein formulas are commonly tolerated but occasionally amino acid–based formulas are indicated. For older individuals avoiding milk, calcium supplementation is recommended. Because of the small risk of allergic reactions to soy in milk-allergic individuals, soy protein–based formulas are not indicated in the management of IgE-mediated milk allergy in those younger than 6 months[160] or documented CM protein–induced enteropathy or enterocolitis. The Nutrition Committees of the European Society of Pediatric Gastroenterology, Hepatology and Nutrition (ESPGHAN) and the American Academy of Pediatrics (AAP) differ regarding the use of soy infant formula in the treatment of infants with CMA.[15,161] The guidelines published by the ESPGHAN and an Australian expert panel consider transition to soy infant formula after 6 months of age,[161] whereas the AAP recommends the use of soy infant formula before the use of an extensive hydrolysate in the treatment of CMA, regardless of age, with the consideration of extensively hydrolyzed formula.[15] Soy infant formula remains a valid option to feed term infants if breast-feeding is not possible and if CM formula is not tolerated.[162] However, because of the reported high frequency of sensitivity to both CM and soy antigens in infants with documented CM protein–induced enteropathy or enterocolitis, soy protein–based formulas are not indicated, and instead, CM hydrolyzed protein formulas should be used for these infants. The routine use of isolated soy protein–based formula has no proven value in the prevention of atopic disease in healthy or high-risk infants.[15]

Oral Immunotherapy

There is a growing evidence of the efficacy of oral immunotherapy with milk protein in the treatment of milk allergy. According to the current knowledge, such therapies induce desensitization as opposed to long-term tolerance and are currently investigational. These therapies are discussed in detail elsewhere in this issue.

SUMMARY

CMA affects 2% to 3% and soy allergy about 0.4% of young children. These allergies present with a wide range of IgE-mediated and non-IgE–mediated clinical syndromes. Diagnosis is based on a supervised OFC, but convincing clinical history taking and measurement of CM–specific IgE can aid in the diagnosis of IgE-mediated CMA and occasionally eliminate the need for OFCs. The close resemblance and resultant cross-reactivity between proteins from soy and other related plants such as peanut and the lack of predictive values for clinical reactivity often make the diagnosis of soy allergy far more challenging. Furthermore, diagnostic tests for non-IgE–mediated manifestations are lacking. Avoidance of the culprit food protein is the mainstay of therapy, although there is a growing body of evidence on the efficacy of investigational new therapies such as oral or sublingual immunotherapy. Despite concerns regarding cosensitization or allergy to soy in CM-allergic subjects, soy-based formulas continue to be a management option for CM-allergic infants with IgE-mediated reactions, especially those older than 6 months. These formulas are not suitable for prevention of milk allergy or as a treatment of milk-induced enterocolitis, for which extensively hydrolyzed CM-based formulae are recommended because of a high prevalence of concomitant soy allergy. Natural history is favorable for most milk- and soy-allergic children, although recovery may take several years in most of them.

REFERENCES

1. Schrander JJ, van den Bogart JP, Forget PP, et al. Cow's milk protein intolerance in infants under 1 year of age: a prospective epidemiological study. Eur J Pediatr 1993;152(8):640–4.
2. Host A, Halken S. A prospective study of cow milk allergy in Danish infants during the first 3 years of life. Clinical course in relation to clinical and immunological type of hypersensitivity reaction. Allergy 1990;45(8):587–96.
3. Saarinen KM, Juntunen-Backman K, Jarvenpaa AL, et al. Supplementary feeding in maternity hospitals and the risk of cow's milk allergy: a prospective study of 6209 infants. J Allergy Clin Immunol 1999;104(2 Pt 1):457–61.
4. Sampson HA. Food allergy. Part 1: immunopathogenesis and clinical disorders. J Allergy Clin Immunol 1999;103(5 Pt 1):717–28.
5. Katz Y, Rajuan N, Goldberg MR, et al. Early exposure to cow's milk protein is protective against IgE-mediated cow's milk protein allergy. J Allergy Clin Immunol 2010;126(1):77–82 e1.
6. Niggemann B, Sielaff B, Beyer K, et al. Outcome of double-blind, placebo-controlled food challenge tests in 107 children with atopic dermatitis. Clin Exp Allergy 1999;29(1):91–6.
7. Iacono G, Carroccio A, Montalto G, et al. Severe infantile colic and food intolerance: a long-term prospective study. J Pediatr Gastroenterol Nutr 1991;12(3):332–5.
8. Jarvinen KM, Sicherer SH, Sampson HA, et al. Use of multiple doses of epinephrine in food-induced anaphylaxis in children. J Allergy Clin Immunol 2008;122(1):133–8.
9. Colver AF, Nevantaus H, Macdougall CF, et al. Severe food-allergic reactions in children across the UK and Ireland, 1998–2000. Acta Paediatr 2005;94(6):689–95.
10. Bock SA, Munoz-Furlong A, Sampson HA. Further fatalities caused by anaphylactic reactions to food, 2001–2006. J Allergy Clin Immunol 2007;119(4):1016–8.
11. Uguz A, Lack G, Pumphrey R, et al. Allergic reactions in the community: a questionnaire survey of members of the anaphylaxis campaign. Clin Exp Allergy 2005;35(6):746–50.
12. Bruno G, Giampietro PG, Del Guercio MJ, et al. Soy allergy is not common in atopic children: a multicenter study. Pediatr Allergy Immunol 1997;8(4):190–3.

13. Osterballe M, Hansen TK, Mortz CG, et al. The prevalence of food hypersensitivity in an unselected population of children and adults. Pediatr Allergy Immunol 2005;16(7):567–73.
14. Roehr CC, Edenharter G, Reimann S, et al. Food allergy and non-allergic food hypersensitivity in children and adolescents. Clin Exp Allergy 2004;34(10): 1534–41.
15. Bhatia J, Greer F, American Academy of Pediatrics Committee on Nutrition. Use of soy protein-based formulas in infant feeding. Pediatrics 2008;121(5):1062–8.
16. Klemola T, Vanto T, Juntunen-Backman K, et al. Allergy to soy formula and to extensively hydrolyzed whey formula in infants with cow's milk allergy: a prospective, randomized study with a follow-up to the age of 2 years. J Pediatr 2002;140(2):219–24.
17. Zeiger RS, Sampson HA, Bock SA, et al. Soy allergy in infant and children with IgE-associated cow's milk allergy. J Pediatr 1999;134(5):614–22.
18. Klemola T, Kalimo K, Poussa T, et al. Feeding a soy formula to children with cow's milk allergy: the development of immunoglobulin E-mediated allergy to soy and peanuts. Pediatr Allergy Immunol 2005;16(8):641–6.
19. Sicherer SH, Sampson HA. Food allergy: recent advances in pathophysiology and treatment. Annu Rev Med 2009;60:261–77.
20. Host A. Cow's milk protein allergy and intolerance in infancy. Some clinical, epidemiological and immunological aspects. Pediatr Allergy Immunol 1994;5(Suppl 5): 1–36.
21. Heine RG, Elsayed S, Hosking CS, et al. Cow's milk allergy in infancy. Curr Opin Allergy Clin Immunol 2002;2(3):217–25.
22. Brill H. Approach to milk protein allergy in infants. Can Fam Physician 2008; 54(9):1258–64.
23. Salvatore S, Vandenplas Y. Gastroesophageal reflux and cow milk allergy: is there a link? Pediatrics 2002;110(5):972–84.
24. Sicherer SH, Teuber S, Adverse Reactions to Foods Committee. Current approach to the diagnosis and management of adverse reactions to foods. J Allergy Clin Immunol 2004;114(5):1146–50.
25. Jarvinen KM, Suomalainen H. Development of cow's milk allergy in breast-fed infants. Clin Exp Allergy 2001;31(7):978–87.
26. de Boissieu D, Matarazzo P, Dupont C. Allergy to extensively hydrolyzed cow milk proteins in infants: identification and treatment with an amino acid-based formula. J Pediatr 1997;131(5):744–7.
27. Eigenmann PA, Sicherer SH, Borkowski TA, et al. Prevalence of IgE-mediated food allergy among children with atopic dermatitis. Pediatrics 1998;101(3):E8.
28. Werfel T, Ballmer-Weber B, Eigenmann PA, et al. Eczematous reactions to food in atopic eczema: position paper of the EAACI and GA2LEN. Allergy 2007;62(7): 723–8.
29. James JM. Respiratory manifestations of food allergy. Pediatrics 2003;111 (6 Pt 3):1625–30.
30. Sampson HA, Mendelson L, Rosen JP. Fatal and near-fatal anaphylactic reactions to food in children and adolescents. N Engl J Med 1992;327(6):380–4.
31. Pumphrey RS. Fatal anaphylaxis in the UK, 1992–2001. Novartis Found Symp 2004;257(116):28 [discussion: 128–32, 157–60, 276–85].
32. Pumphrey RS, Gowland MH. Further fatal allergic reactions to food in the United Kingdom, 1999–2006. J Allergy Clin Immunol 2007;119(4):1018–9.
33. Yunginger JW, Nelson DR, Squillace DL, et al. Laboratory investigation of deaths due to anaphylaxis. J Forensic Sci 1991;36(3):857–65.

34. Sicherer SH, Morrow EH, Sampson HA. Dose-response in double-blind, placebo-controlled oral food challenges in children with atopic dermatitis. J Allergy Clin Immunol 2000;105(3):582–6.
35. Foucard T, Malmheden Yman I. A study on severe food reactions in Sweden—is soy protein an underestimated cause of food anaphylaxis? Allergy 1999;54(3):261–5.
36. Jarvinen KM, Amalanayagam S, Shreffler WG, et al. Epinephrine treatment is infrequent and biphasic reactions are rare in food-induced reactions during oral food challenges in children. J Allergy Clin Immunol 2009;124(6):1267–72.
37. Mittag D, Vieths S, Vogel L, et al. Soybean allergy in patients allergic to birch pollen: clinical investigation and molecular characterization of allergens. J Allergy Clin Immunol 2004;113(1):148–54.
38. Sicherer SH, Sampson HA. Food hypersensitivity and atopic dermatitis: pathophysiology, epidemiology, diagnosis, and management. J Allergy Clin Immunol 1999;104(3 Pt 2):S114–22.
39. Ellman LK, Chatchatee P, Sicherer SH, et al. Food hypersensitivity in two groups of children and young adults with atopic dermatitis evaluated a decade apart. Pediatr Allergy Immunol 2002;13(4):295–8.
40. Maloney J, Nowak-Wegrzyn A. Educational clinical case series for pediatric allergy and immunology: allergic proctocolitis, food protein-induced enterocolitis syndrome and allergic eosinophilic gastroenteritis with protein-losing gastroenteropathy as manifestations of non-IgE-mediated cow's milk allergy. Pediatr Allergy Immunol 2007;18(4):360–7.
41. Nowak-Wegrzyn A, Muraro A. Food protein-induced enterocolitis syndrome. Curr Opin Allergy Clin Immunol 2009;9(4):371–7.
42. Mehr SS, Kakakios AM, Kemp AS. Rice: a common and severe cause of food protein-induced enterocolitis syndrome. Arch Dis Child 2009;94(3):220–3.
43. Hwang JB, Lee SH, Kang YN, et al. Indexes of suspicion of typical cow's milk protein-induced enterocolitis. J Korean Med Sci 2007;22(6):993–7.
44. Sicherer SH, Eigenmann PA, Sampson HA. Clinical features of food protein-induced enterocolitis syndrome. J Pediatr 1998;133(2):214–9.
45. Burks AW, Casteel HB, Fiedorek SC, et al. Prospective oral food challenge study of two soybean protein isolates in patients with possible milk or soy protein enterocolitis. Pediatr Allergy Immunol 1994;5(1):40–5.
46. Jarvinen KM, Sickles L, Nowak-Wegrzyn A. Clinical characteristics of children with food protein-induced enterocolitis (FPIES). J Allergy Clin Immunol 2010;125(2):AB85.
47. Anveden-Hertzberg L, Finkel Y, Sandstedt B, et al. Proctocolitis in exclusively breast-fed infants. Eur J Pediatr 1996;155(6):464–7.
48. Arvola T, Ruuska T, Keranen J, et al. Rectal bleeding in infancy: clinical, allergological, and microbiological examination. Pediatrics 2006;117(4):e760–8.
49. Hill DJ, Hosking CS. Infantile colic and food hypersensitivity. J Pediatr Gastroenterol Nutr 2000;30(Suppl):S67–76.
50. Lucassen PL, Assendelft WJ, Gubbels JW, et al. Infantile colic: crying time reduction with a whey hydrolysate: a double-blind, randomized, placebo-controlled trial. Pediatrics 2000;106(6):1349–54.
51. Jakobsson I, Lothe L, Ley D, et al. Effectiveness of casein hydrolysate feedings in infants with colic. Acta Paediatr 2000;89(1):18–21.
52. Iacono G, Carroccio A, Cavataio F, et al. Chronic constipation as a symptom of cow milk allergy. J Pediatr 1995;126(1):34–9.

53. Iacono G, Cavataio F, Montalto G, et al. Intolerance of cow's milk and chronic constipation in children. N Engl J Med 1998;339(16):1100–4.
54. Carroccio A, Scalici C, Maresi E, et al. Chronic constipation and food intolerance: a model of proctitis causing constipation. Scand J Gastroenterol 2005; 40(1):33–42.
55. Turunen S, Karttunen TJ, Kokkonen J. Lymphoid nodular hyperplasia and cow's milk hypersensitivity in children with chronic constipation. J Pediatr 2004;145(5):606–11.
56. Hirose R, Yamada T, Hayashida Y. Massive bloody stools in two neonates caused by cow's milk allergy. Pediatr Surg Int 2006;22(11):935–8.
57. Kawai M, Kubota A, Ida S, et al. Cow's milk allergy presenting Hirschsprung's disease-mimicking symptoms. Pediatr Surg Int 2005;21(10):850–2.
58. Kiefte-de Jong JC, Escher JC, Arends LR, et al. Infant nutritional factors and functional constipation in childhood: the Generation R study. Am J Gastroenterol 2010;105(4):940–5.
59. Moissidis I, Chaidaroon D, Vichyanond P, et al. Milk-induced pulmonary disease in infants (Heiner syndrome). Pediatr Allergy Immunol 2005;16(6):545–52.
60. Wal JM. Bovine milk allergenicity. Ann Allergy Asthma Immunol 2004;93 (5 Suppl 3):S2–11.
61. Docena GH, Fernandez R, Chirdo FG, et al. Identification of casein as the major allergenic and antigenic protein of cow's milk. Allergy 1996;51(6): 412–6.
62. Natale M, Bisson C, Monti G, et al. Cow's milk allergens identification by two-dimensional immunoblotting and mass spectrometry. Mol Nutr Food Res 2004;48(5):363–9.
63. Busse PJ, Jarvinen KM, Vila L, et al. Identification of sequential IgE-binding epitopes on bovine alpha(s2)-casein in cow's milk allergic patients. Int Arch Allergy Immunol 2002;129(1):93–6.
64. Chatchatee P, Jarvinen KM, Bardina L, et al. Identification of IgE- and IgG-binding epitopes on alpha(s1)-casein: differences in patients with persistent and transient cow's milk allergy. J Allergy Clin Immunol 2001;107(2):379–83.
65. Chatchatee P, Jarvinen KM, Bardina L, et al. Identification of IgE and IgG binding epitopes on beta- and kappa-casein in cow's milk allergic patients. Clin Exp Allergy 2001;31(8):1256–62.
66. Jarvinen KM, Chatchatee P, Bardina L, et al. IgE and IgG binding epitopes on alpha-lactalbumin and beta-lactoglobulin in cow's milk allergy. Int Arch Allergy Immunol 2001;126(2):111–8.
67. Cerecedo I, Zamora J, Shreffler WG, et al. Mapping of the IgE and IgG4 sequential epitopes of milk allergens with a peptide microarray-based immunoassay. J Allergy Clin Immunol 2008;122(3):589–94.
68. Han N, Jarvinen KM, Cocco RR, et al. Identification of amino acids critical for IgE-binding to sequential epitopes of bovine kappa-casein and the similarity of these epitopes to the corresponding human kappa-casein sequence. Allergy 2008;63(2):198–204.
69. Cocco RR, Jarvinen KM, Sampson HA, et al. Mutational analysis of major, sequential IgE-binding epitopes in alpha s1-casein, a major cow's milk allergen. J Allergy Clin Immunol 2003;112(2):433–7.
70. Cocco RR, Jarvinen KM, Han N, et al. Mutational analysis of immunoglobulin E-binding epitopes of beta-casein and beta-lactoglobulin showed a heterogeneous pattern of critical amino acids between individual patients and pooled sera. Clin Exp Allergy 2007;37(6):831–8.

71. Chen WL, Hwang MT, Liau CY, et al. Beta-lactoglobulin is a thermal marker in processed milk as studied by electrophoresis and circular dichroic spectra. J Dairy Sci 2005;88(5):1618–30.
72. Ehn BM, Ekstrand B, Bengtsson U, et al. Modification of IgE binding during heat processing of the cow's milk allergen beta-lactoglobulin. J Agric Food Chem 2004;52(5):1398–403.
73. Nowak-Wegrzyn A, Bloom KA, Sicherer SH, et al. Tolerance to extensively heated milk in children with cow's milk allergy. J Allergy Clin Immunol 2008; 122(2):342–7.
74. Shibasaki M, Suzuki S, Tajima S, et al. Allergenicity of major component proteins of soybean. Int Arch Allergy Appl Immunol 1980;61(4):441–8.
75. Awazuhara H, Kawai H, Maruchi N. Major allergens in soybean and clinical significance of IgG4 antibodies investigated by IgE- and IgG4-immunoblotting with sera from soybean-sensitive patients. Clin Exp Allergy 1997;27(3):325–32.
76. Cinader B. Chairman's report to the WHO-IUIS Nomenclature Committee, Kyoto, 25 August 1983. Immunology 1984;52(3):585–7.
77. Ogawa T, Bando N, Tsuji H, et al. Alpha-subunit of beta-conglycinin, an allergenic protein recognized by IgE antibodies of soybean-sensitive patients with atopic dermatitis. Biosci Biotechnol Biochem 1995;59(5):831–3.
78. Beardslee TA, Zeece MG, Sarath G, et al. Soybean glycinin G1 acidic chain shares IgE epitopes with peanut allergen Ara h 3. Int Arch Allergy Immunol 2000;123(4):299–307.
79. Helm RM, Cockrell G, Connaughton C, et al. A soybean G2 glycinin allergen. 1. Identification and characterization. Int Arch Allergy Immunol 2000;123(3):205–12.
80. Ogawa T, Bando N, Tsuji H, et al. Investigation of the IgE-binding proteins in soybeans by immunoblotting with the sera of the soybean-sensitive patients with atopic dermatitis. J Nutr Sci Vitaminol (Tokyo) 1991;37(6):555–65.
81. Helm R, Cockrell G, Herman E, et al. Cellular and molecular characterization of a major soybean allergen. Int Arch Allergy Immunol 1998;117(1):29–37.
82. Helm RM, Cockrell G, Connaughton C, et al. Mutational analysis of the IgE-binding epitopes of P34/Gly m Bd 30K. J Allergy Clin Immunol 2000;105(2 Pt 1):378–84.
83. Moroz LA, Yang WH. Kunitz soybean trypsin inhibitor: a specific allergen in food anaphylaxis. N Engl J Med 1980;302(20):1126–8.
84. Burks AW, Cockrell G, Connaughton C, et al. Identification of peanut agglutinin and soybean trypsin inhibitor as minor legume allergens. Int Arch Allergy Immunol 1994;105(2):143–9.
85. Gu X, Beardslee T, Zeece M, et al. Identification of IgE-binding proteins in soy lecithin. Int Arch Allergy Immunol 2001;126(3):218–25.
86. Holzhauser T, Wackermann O, Ballmer-Weber BK, et al. Soybean (Glycine max) allergy in Europe: Gly m 5 (beta-conglycinin) and Gly m 6 (glycinin) are potential diagnostic markers for severe allergic reactions to soy. J Allergy Clin Immunol 2009;123(2):452–8.
87. Codina R, Lockey RF, Fernandez-Caldas E, et al. Purification and characterization of a soybean hull allergen responsible for the Barcelona asthma outbreaks. II. Purification and sequencing of the Gly m 2 allergen. Clin Exp Allergy 1997; 27(4):424–30.
88. Gonzalez R, Polo F, Zapatero L, et al. Purification and characterization of major inhalant allergens from soybean hulls. Clin Exp Allergy 1992;22(8):748–55.
89. Matricardi PM, Bockelbrink A, Beyer K, et al. Primary versus secondary immunoglobulin E sensitization to soy and wheat in the Multi-Centre Allergy Study cohort. Clin Exp Allergy 2008;38(3):493–500.

90. D'Auria E, Agostoni C, Giovannini M, et al. Proteomic evaluation of milk from different mammalian species as a substitute for breast milk. Acta Paediatr 2005;94(12):1708–13.
91. Bellioni-Businco B, Paganelli R, Lucenti P, et al. Allergenicity of goat's milk in children with cow's milk allergy. J Allergy Clin Immunol 1999;103(6):1191–4.
92. Vita D, Passalacqua G, Di Pasquale G, et al. Ass's milk in children with atopic dermatitis and cow's milk allergy: crossover comparison with goat's milk. Pediatr Allergy Immunol 2007;18(7):594–8.
93. Tavares B, Pereira C, Rodrigues F, et al. Goat's milk allergy. Allergol Immunopathol (Madr) 2007;35(3):113–6.
94. Ah-Leung S, Bernard H, Bidat E, et al. Allergy to goat and sheep milk without allergy to cow's milk. Allergy 2006;61(11):1358–65.
95. Katz Y, Goldberg MR, Zadik-Mnuhin G, et al. Cross-sensitization between milk proteins: reactivity to a "kosher" epitope? Isr Med Assoc J 2008;10(1): 85–8.
96. Suutari TJ, Valkonen KH, Karttunen TJ, et al. IgE cross reactivity between reindeer and bovine milk beta-lactoglobulins in cow's milk allergic patients. J Investig Allergol Clin Immunol 2006;16(5):296–302.
97. Businco L, Giampietro PG, Lucenti P, et al. Allergenicity of mare's milk in children with cow's milk allergy. J Allergy Clin Immunol 2000;105(5):1031–4.
98. Restani P, Beretta B, Fiocchi A, et al. Cross-reactivity between mammalian proteins. Ann Allergy Asthma Immunol 2002;89(6 Suppl 1):11–5.
99. Monti G, Bertino E, Muratore MC, et al. Efficacy of donkey's milk in treating highly problematic cow's milk allergic children: an in vivo and in vitro study. Pediatr Allergy Immunol 2007;18(3):258–64.
100. Alessandri C, Mari A. Efficacy of donkey's milk in treating cow's milk allergic children: major concerns. Pediatr Allergy Immunol 2007;18(7):625–6.
101. Makinen-Kiljunen S, Plosila M. A father's IgE-mediated contact urticaria from mother's milk. J Allergy Clin Immunol 2004;113(2):353–4.
102. Schulmeister U, Swoboda I, Quirce S, et al. Sensitization to human milk. Clin Exp Allergy 2008;38(1):60–8.
103. Jarvinen KM, Sampson HA. Recognition of human milk peptides by IgE antibodies from infants with cow's milk allergy. J Allergy Clin Immunol 2008; 121(2):S214.
104. Jarvinen KM, Chatchatee P. Mammalian milk allergy: clinical suspicion, cross-reactivities and diagnosis. Curr Opin Allergy Clin Immunol 2009;9(3):251–8.
105. Martelli A, De Chiara A, Corvo M, et al. Beef allergy in children with cow's milk allergy; cow's milk allergy in children with beef allergy. Ann Allergy Asthma Immunol 2002;89(6 Suppl 1):38–43.
106. Vicente-Serrano J, Caballero ML, Rodriguez-Perez R, et al. Sensitization to serum albumins in children allergic to cow's milk and epithelia. Pediatr Allergy Immunol 2007;18(6):503–7.
107. Osterballe M, Mortz CG, Hansen TK, et al. The prevalence of food hypersensitivity in young adults. Pediatr Allergy Immunol 2009;20(7):686–92.
108. Rozenfeld P, Docena GH, Anon MC, et al. Detection and identification of a soy protein component that cross-reacts with caseins from cow's milk. Clin Exp Immunol 2002;130(1):49–58.
109. Sicherer SH. Clinical implications of cross-reactive food allergens. J Allergy Clin Immunol 2001;108(6):881–90.
110. Bock SA, Atkins FM. The natural history of peanut allergy. J Allergy Clin Immunol 1989;83(5):900–4.

111. Green TD, LaBelle VS, Steele PH, et al. Clinical characteristics of peanut-allergic children: recent changes. Pediatrics 2007;120(6):1304–10.
112. Bernhisel-Broadbent J, Sampson HA. Cross-allergenicity in the legume botanical family in children with food hypersensitivity. J Allergy Clin Immunol 1989; 83(2 Pt 1):435–40.
113. Magnolfi CF, Zani G, Lacava L, et al. Soy allergy in atopic children. Ann Allergy Asthma Immunol 1996;77(3):197–201.
114. Kleine-Tebbe J, Vogel L, Crowell DN, et al. Severe oral allergy syndrome and anaphylactic reactions caused by a Bet v 1-related PR-10 protein in soybean, SAM22. J Allergy Clin Immunol 2002;110(5):797–804.
115. Vandenplas Y, Koletzko S, Isolauri E, et al. Guidelines for the diagnosis and management of cow's milk protein allergy in infants. Arch Dis Child 2007; 92(10):902–8.
116. Flinterman AE, Knulst AC, Meijer Y, et al. Acute allergic reactions in children with AEDS after prolonged cow's milk elimination diets. Allergy 2006;61(3): 370–4.
117. Niggemann B, Beyer K. Diagnosis of food allergy in children: toward a standardization of food challenge. J Pediatr Gastroenterol Nutr 2007;45(4): 399–404.
118. Niggemann B, Rolinck-Werninghaus C, Mehl A, et al. Controlled oral food challenges in children—when indicated, when superfluous? Allergy 2005;60(7): 865–70.
119. Sampson HA. Food allergy. Part 2: diagnosis and management. J Allergy Clin Immunol 1999;103(6):981–9.
120. Bock SA, Sampson HA. Food allergy in infancy. Pediatr Clin North Am 1994; 41(5):1047–67.
121. Sampson HA, Ho DG. Relationship between food-specific IgE concentrations and the risk of positive food challenges in children and adolescents. J Allergy Clin Immunol 1997;100(4):444–51.
122. Sampson HA. Utility of food-specific IgE concentrations in predicting symptomatic food allergy. J Allergy Clin Immunol 2001;107(5):891–6.
123. Garcia-Ara C, Boyano-Martinez T, Diaz-Pena JM, et al. Specific IgE levels in the diagnosis of immediate hypersensitivity to cows' milk protein in the infant. J Allergy Clin Immunol 2001;107(1):185–90.
124. Hill DJ, Heine RG, Hosking CS. The diagnostic value of skin prick testing in children with food allergy. Pediatr Allergy Immunol 2004;15(5):435–41.
125. van der Gugten AC, den Otter M, Meijer Y, et al. Usefulness of specific IgE levels in predicting cow's milk allergy. J Allergy Clin Immunol 2008;121(2): 531–3.
126. Verstege A, Mehl A, Rolinck-Werninghaus C, et al. The predictive value of the skin prick test weal size for the outcome of oral food challenges. Clin Exp Allergy 2005;35(9):1220–6.
127. Calvani M, Alessandri C, Frediani T, et al. Correlation between skin prick test using commercial extract of cow's milk protein and fresh milk and food challenges. Pediatr Allergy Immunol 2007;18(7):583–8.
128. Miceli Sopo S, Radzik D, Calvani M. The predictive value of specific immunoglobulin E levels for the first diagnosis of cow's milk allergy. A critical analysis of pediatric literature. Pediatr Allergy Immunol 2007;18(7):575–82.
129. Wang J, Godbold JH, Sampson HA. Correlation of serum allergy (IgE) tests performed by different assay systems. J Allergy Clin Immunol 2008;121(5): 1219–24.

130. Ballmer-Weber BK, Holzhauser T, Scibilia J, et al. Clinical characteristics of soybean allergy in Europe: a double-blind, placebo-controlled food challenge study. J Allergy Clin Immunol 2007;119(6):1489–96.
131. Giampietro PG, Ragno V, Daniele S, et al. Soy hypersensitivity in children with food allergy. Ann Allergy 1992;69(2):143–6.
132. Burks AW, James JM, Hiegel A, et al. Atopic dermatitis and food hypersensitivity reactions. J Pediatr 1998;132(1):132–6.
133. Furuta GT, Liacouras CA, Collins MH, et al. Eosinophilic esophagitis in children and adults: a systematic review and consensus recommendations for diagnosis and treatment. Gastroenterology 2007;133(4):1342–63.
134. Spergel JM, Andrews T, Brown-Whitehorn TF, et al. Treatment of eosinophilic esophagitis with specific food elimination diet directed by a combination of skin prick and patch tests. Ann Allergy Asthma Immunol 2005;95(4): 336–43.
135. Kagalwalla AF, Sentongo TA, Ritz S, et al. Effect of six-food elimination diet on clinical and histologic outcomes in eosinophilic esophagitis. Clin Gastroenterol Hepatol 2006;4(9):1097–102.
136. Spergel JM, Brown-Whitehorn T, Beausoleil JL, et al. Predictive values for skin prick test and atopy patch test for eosinophilic esophagitis. J Allergy Clin Immunol 2007;119(2):509–11.
137. Fogg MI, Brown-Whitehorn TA, Pawlowski NA, et al. Atopy patch test for the diagnosis of food protein-induced enterocolitis syndrome. Pediatr Allergy Immunol 2006;17(5):351–5.
138. Hwang JB, Song JY, Kang YN, et al. The significance of gastric juice analysis for a positive challenge by a standard oral challenge test in typical cow's milk protein-induced enterocolitis. J Korean Med Sci 2008;23(2):251–5.
139. Isolauri E, Turjanmaa K. Combined skin prick and patch testing enhances identification of food allergy in infants with atopic dermatitis. J Allergy Clin Immunol 1996;97(1 Pt 1):9–15.
140. Majamaa H, Moisio P, Holm K, et al. Cow's milk allergy: diagnostic accuracy of skin prick and patch tests and specific IgE. Allergy 1999;54(4):346–51.
141. Vanto T, Juntunen-Backman K, Kalimo K, et al. The patch test, skin prick test, and serum milk-specific IgE as diagnostic tools in cow's milk allergy in infants. Allergy 1999;54(8):837–42.
142. Roehr CC, Reibel S, Ziegert M, et al. Atopy patch tests, together with determination of specific IgE levels, reduce the need for oral food challenges in children with atopic dermatitis. J Allergy Clin Immunol 2001;107(3):548–53.
143. Stromberg L. Diagnostic accuracy of the atopy patch test and the skin-prick test for the diagnosis of food allergy in young children with atopic eczema/dermatitis syndrome. Acta Paediatr 2002;91(10):1044–9.
144. Breuer K, Heratizadeh A, Wulf A, et al. Late eczematous reactions to food in children with atopic dermatitis. Clin Exp Allergy 2004;34(5):817–24.
145. Mehl A, Rolinck-Werninghaus C, Staden U, et al. The atopy patch test in the diagnostic workup of suspected food-related symptoms in children. J Allergy Clin Immunol 2006;118(4):923–9.
146. Devillers AC, de Waard-van der Spek FB, Mulder PG, et al. Delayed- and immediate-type reactions in the atopy patch test with food allergens in young children with atopic dermatitis. Pediatr Allergy Immunol 2009;20(1):53–8.
147. Canani RB, Ruotolo S, Auricchio L, et al. Diagnostic accuracy of the atopy patch test in children with food allergy-related gastrointestinal symptoms. Allergy 2007;62(7):738–43.

148. Ott H, Baron JM, Heise R, et al. Clinical usefulness of microarray-based IgE detection in children with suspected food allergy. Allergy 2008;63(11):1521–8.
149. Lidholm J, Ballmer-Weber BK, Mari A, et al. Component-resolved diagnostics in food allergy. Curr Opin Allergy Clin Immunol 2006;6(3):234–40.
150. Bush RK, Taylor SL, Nordlee JA, et al. Soybean oil is not allergenic to soybean-sensitive individuals. J Allergy Clin Immunol 1985;76(2 Pt 1):242–5.
151. Skripak JM, Matsui EC, Mudd K, et al. The natural history of IgE-mediated cow's milk allergy. J Allergy Clin Immunol 2007;120(5):1172–7.
152. Shek LP, Soderstrom L, Ahlstedt S, et al. Determination of food specific IgE levels over time can predict the development of tolerance in cow's milk and hen's egg allergy. J Allergy Clin Immunol 2004;114(2):387–91.
153. Jarvinen KM, Beyer K, Vila L, et al. B-cell epitopes as a screening instrument for persistent cow's milk allergy. J Allergy Clin Immunol 2002;110(2):293–7.
154. Levy Y, Segal N, Garty B, et al. Lessons from the clinical course of IgE-mediated cow milk allergy in Israel. Pediatr Allergy Immunol 2007;18(7):589–93.
155. Savage JH, Kaeding AJ, Matsui EC, et al. The natural history of soy allergy. J Allergy Clin Immunol 2010;125(3):683–6.
156. Hwang JB, Sohn SM, Kim AS. Prospective follow-up oral food challenge in food protein-induced enterocolitis syndrome. Arch Dis Child 2009;94(6):425–8.
157. Crotty MP, Taylor SL. Risks associated with foods having advisory milk labeling. J Allergy Clin Immunol 2010;125(4):935–7.
158. Ford LS, Taylor SL, Pacenza R, et al. Food allergen advisory labeling and product contamination with egg, milk, and peanut. J Allergy Clin Immunol 2010;126(2):384–5.
159. Awazuhara H, Kawai H, Baba M, et al. Antigenicity of the proteins in soy lecithin and soy oil in soybean allergy. Clin Exp Allergy 1998;28(12):1559–64.
160. Allen KJ, Davidson GP, Day AS, et al. Management of cow's milk protein allergy in infants and young children: an expert panel perspective. J Paediatr Child Health 2009;45(9):481–6.
161. ESPGHAN Committee on Nutrition, Agostoni C, Axelsson I, et al. Soy protein infant formulae and follow-on formulae: a commentary by the ESPGHAN Committee on Nutrition. J Pediatr Gastroenterol Nutr 2006;42(4):352–61.
162. Vandenplas Y, De Greef E, Devreker T, et al. Soy infant formula: is it that bad? Acta Paediatr 2011;100(2):162–6.

Current Understanding of Egg Allergy

Jean-Christoph Caubet, MD[a,b], Julie Wang, MD[a,*]

KEYWORDS

• Egg • Allergy • Food • Children • Hypersensitivity • IgE
• Ovomucoid • Ovalbumin

After cow's milk, hen's egg allergy is the second most common food allergy in infants and young children.[1–5] The estimated prevalence of egg allergy varies depending on method of data collection or definition. A recent meta-analysis of the prevalence of food allergy estimated that egg allergy affects 0.5% to 2.5% of young children.[6] The major limitation of this meta-analysis was significant variability in study design that made direct comparisons difficult. Most studies included in the meta-analysis were based on self-reports of food allergy, which tend to overestimate the prevalence. Some studies used skin prick test and food-specific IgE levels to confirm sensitization to the allergen; however, only 3 studies used double-blind, placebo-controlled food challenges, the gold standard, to confirm the diagnosis of food allergy.[7–9] In these 3 studies of unselected populations, the prevalence of egg allergy ranged from 0.0004% in a cohort of German children aged up to 17 years,[7] to 0.6% in nursery school children in Mexico,[8] to 1.6% in 3-year-old Danish children.[9] From Norway, Eggesbo and colleagues[2] reported an estimated point prevalence of allergy to egg in children aged 2.5 years of 1.6% (confidence interval [CI] 1.3%–2.0%), with an upper estimate of the cumulative incidence by this age calculated roughly at 2.6% (CI 1.6%–3.6). A similar prevalence of 1.3% was reported from the United States.[1] Although prevalence depends primarily on nutritional habits in different population, the heterogeneity in egg allergy prevalence may not reflect genuine difference between populations but may be related only to difference in the design and conduct of the primary studies. Egg allergy is closely associated with atopic dermatitis and was found to be present in about two-thirds of children with positive oral food challenges (OFC)

Potential conflicts of interest – none.

[a] Division of Pediatric Allergy and Immunology, Pediatrics Mount Sinai School of Medicine, One Gustave L. Levy Place, Box 1198, New York City, NY 10029, USA
[b] Department of Child and Adolescent, University Hospitals of Geneva and Medical School of the University of Geneva, Geneva, Switzerland
* Corresponding author.
E-mail address: julie.wang@mssm.edu

Pediatr Clin N Am 58 (2011) 427–443
doi:10.1016/j.pcl.2011.02.014 **pediatric.theclinics.com**
0031-3955/11/$ – see front matter

performed for allergy evaluation of atopic dermatitis.[10] The risks of sensitization to aeroallergens[11] and asthma[12] are also increased in children with egg allergy.

PATHOGENESIS

Egg allergy may be defined as an adverse reaction of immunologic nature induced by egg proteins,[13] and includes IgE antibody–mediated allergy as well as other allergic syndromes such as atopic dermatitis and eosinophilic esophagitis, which are mixed IgE-mediated and cell-mediated disorders. IgE-mediated food allergy, also known as type I food allergy, accounts for most of the food-induced responses and is characterized by the presence of allergen-specific IgE antibodies. Five major allergenic proteins from the egg of the domestic chicken (*Gallus domesticus*) have been identified; these are designated Gal d 1 to Gal d 5.[14] Most of the allergenic egg proteins are found in egg white (**Table 1**), including ovomucoid (Gal d 1, 11%), ovalbumin (Gal d 2, 54%), ovotransferrin (Gal d 3, 12%), and lysozyme (Gal d 4, 3.4%).[15] Although ovalbumin (OVA) is the most abundant protein in hen's egg white, ovomucoid (OVM) has been shown to be the dominant allergen in egg.[16–18]

The allergenicity of proteins depends mostly, but not exclusively, on their resistance to heat and digestive enzymes,[19] reflecting their capacity to stimulate a specific immune response.[14] To elicit a sustained immune response, the immunogen should ideally stimulate both T and B cells. The portion of the immunogen that binds specifically with membrane receptors on T or B cells is called an epitope, which can be sequential or conformational. Sequential epitopes are determined by contiguous amino acids, whereas conformational epitopes contain amino acids from different regions of the protein that are in close proximity because of the folding of the protein. Conformational epitopes can be destroyed with heating or partial hydrolysis, which alters the tertiary structure of the protein. Egg-specific IgE molecules that identify sequential or conformational epitopes of OVM and OVA can distinguish different clinical phenotypes of egg allergy. It has been shown that patients with egg allergy with IgE antibodies reacting against sequential epitopes tend to have persistent allergy, whereas those with IgE antibodies primarily to conformational epitopes tend to have transient allergy.[20]

Egg proteins differ in their physical properties and can be related to different clinical patterns of egg allergy. The importance of OVM may be because of its unique characteristics such as relative stability against heat[21] and digestion with proteinases,[22] and its strong allergenicity,[15] compared with other egg white components. These characteristics are possibly related to the presence of strong disulfide bonds that stabilize this highly glycosylated protein.[18] In 2 different studies, children with persistent egg allergy had significantly higher specific IgE levels to OVM than children who outgrew their egg allergy.[15,20] In the report by Jarvinen and colleagues,[20] 7 patients with persistent egg allergy had IgE that recognized 4 sequential epitopes of OVM. In contrast, none of the 11 children with transient egg allergy had specific IgE to these epitopes. Gastric digestion has been shown to reduce the allergenicity of OVM,[23] which can explain why some patients have skin contact reactions to egg, but not ingestion reactions.[24]

In contrast, OVA epitopes are heat labile,[25] suggesting that children who have specific IgE primarily to OVA are likely to tolerate heat-denatured forms of egg. However, using the sera from patients with egg allergy, reports have shown that the antigenicity of OVA could resist heat treatment in certain conditions.[26] By using OVA, a recent study[27] investigated the T-cell immunogenicity of chemically glycated proteins termed advanced glycation end products (AGEs), produced by the Maillard reaction that occurs between reducing sugars and proteins during thermal processing of foods. The glycation structures of AGEs are suggested to function as pathogenesis-

Table 1
Major egg white allergens

Allergen	Common Name	Content (%)	Mw (kDa)	Carbohydrate (%)	IgE Binding Activity — Digestive — Heat Treated	IgE Binding Activity — Digestive — Enzyme Treated	Allergenic Activity	Test Code (In Vitro Tests)
Gal d 1	Ovomucoid	11	28	25	Stable	Stable	+++	f233
Gal d 2	Ovalbumin	54	45	3	Unstable	Unstable	++	f232
Gal d 3	Ovotransferrin/ conalbumin	12	76.6	2.6	Unstable	Unstable	+	f323
Gal d 4	Lysozyme	3.4	14.3	0	Unstable	Unstable	++	k208

Data from Benhamou AH. State of the art for egg allergy. Allergy 2010;65:283–9.

related immune epitopes in food allergy. They showed that T-cell immunogenicity of OVA can be enhanced by the Maillard reaction, indicating a critical role for thermal processing in the allergenicity of OVA.

In egg yolk, α-livetin (Gal d 5) is the major allergen and is involved in the bird-egg syndrome, which is described later.[28,29] Several other allergens have been identified in egg yolk, including vitellenin (apovitellenin I) and apoprotein B (apovitellenin VI), although their roles in food allergy remain unclear. Manufactured food products often contain trace amounts of egg lecithin as emulsifiers, but ingestion of trace amounts of egg lecithin is probably insufficient to elicit allergic reactions.[14]

Regarding non–IgE-mediated as well as mixed IgE-mediated and non–IgE-mediated egg allergy, the pathogenesis is less clear. Egg allergy has been implicated as a trigger for atopic dermatitis and allergic eosinophilic esophagitis. Only few cases of enteropathy induced by egg are reported in the literature.

CLINICAL FEATURES

Allergy to hen's egg usually presents in the second half of the first year of life, with a median age of presentation of 10 months.[30] This reflects the typical age of the first dietary exposure to egg. It has been shown that most reactions occur on first known exposure to egg, particularly in sensitized children with atopic dermatitis.[31,32] The development of sensitization in these patients may be caused by exposure in utero [33] or via exposure to egg proteins through maternal breast milk.[34,35] Mouse models suggest that sensitization may also occur via epicutaneous exposure (before gut mucosa exposure) and may play a role in the development of atopic dermatitis and asthma.[36,37]

IgE-mediated Reactions

IgE-mediated reactions are the most common type of allergic reactions to egg. Children typically present with rapid onset of urticaria or angioedema, usually within minutes to 2 hours after ingestion. Although cutaneous symptoms are most common, immediate reactions involving the gastrointestinal or respiratory tracts are reported as well. The severity of reactions can be unpredictable, potentially life threatening, and can vary from episode to episode. Anaphylaxis can occur with exposure to egg, and asthmatics, in particular, are at high risk for severe allergic reactions.[38–40] Egg accounted for 7% of severe anaphylactic reactions in infants and children in a German survey.[41] Fatal reactions to egg are rare, but have been reported.[42] Ingestion of raw or undercooked egg may trigger more severe clinical reactions than well-cooked egg.[43]

Egg allergy is also associated with other types of IgE-mediated allergies, mostly in the adult population. Occupational asthma has been reported in bakery workers who are frequently exposed to aerosolized egg and in people who work in factories that process eggs.[44] In bird-egg syndrome, the primary sensitization is to airborne bird allergens and there is secondary sensitization or cross-reactivity with albumin in egg yolk (Gal d 5). These patients experience respiratory symptoms such as rhinitis and/or asthma with bird exposure and allergic symptoms when egg is ingested.[29,45] Food-dependent, exercise-induced anaphylaxis with egg as the trigger has also been reported.[46]

Mixed and Non–IgE-mediated Reactions

Egg proteins not only trigger IgE-mediated allergy, but can also be involved in non–IgE-mediated and mixed IgE-mediated and non–IgE-mediated reactions. These disorders include atopic dermatitis and the eosinophilic gastroenteropathies.

Atopic dermatitis

Egg allergy can manifest as atopic dermatitis, especially in infants and young children. In an international multicenter study of children with atopic dermatitis, egg sensitization was found to be closely associated with early-onset, moderate-to-severe atopic dermatitis.[13] A small randomized trial of egg avoidance in children with egg sensitization and atopic dermatitis found that egg elimination decreases the extent and severity of the skin symptoms, showing the clinical relevance of egg sensitization in these patients.[47] Isolated delayed reactions (ie, flares of atopic dermatitis usually after 6 to 48 hours) are suggestive of non–IgE-mediated reactions and are likely caused by T-cell–mediated mechanisms. Late reactions are more difficult to identify. A combination of immediate allergy symptoms and delayed skin reactions is also described in a significant proportion of children.[48] More than 10% of the children who reacted to an OFC developed isolated atopic dermatitis flares after 16 hours or later.[49]

The combination of egg allergy and atopic dermatitis is a risk factor for asthma. In a small cohort of children with both these allergic conditions, 80% also suffered from asthma.[50] Children with asthma are at increased risk for more severe allergic reactions to foods.

Gastroenteropathies

A small number of children with egg allergy present with gastrointestinal symptoms, including allergic eosinophilic esophagitis (EoE). This inflammatory disorder is characterized by high numbers of intraepithelial eosinophils in the esophagus and is mediated by mixed IgE-mediated and non–IgE-mediated processes.[51–53] Egg was found to be the second most common allergen triggering symptoms in a series of more than 500 patients with EoE. This was confirmed on endoscopy after allergy evaluation with skin prick testing and patch testing.[54] Elimination of food triggers has been found to be an effective treatment of EoE.

Food protein–induced enteropathy caused by egg has been reported.[55] A 5-month-old boy developed protein-losing enteropathy and hypogammaglobulinemia, which was triggered by egg exposure in maternal breast milk. After maternal elimination of egg, resolution of symptoms occurred. Furthermore, reintroduction of egg into the maternal diet caused recurrence of symptoms. Recently, food protein–induced enterocolitis syndrome to egg has also been reported.[56]

DIAGNOSIS

The diagnostic workup of suspected food allergy should start with a detailed history and physical examination of the patients. The next step may include in vitro and/or in vivo allergy tests that are used to support the diagnosis of egg allergy. These tests may include measurement of food-specific IgE antibodies, skin prick tests, atopy patch test, diagnostic elimination diet, and/or OFC. These different diagnostic tools are discussed later, with a focus on the diagnosis of egg allergy.

IgE-mediated Reactions

The history of an immediate reaction consistent with typical allergic symptoms, supported by evidence of specific IgE antibodies, establishes the diagnosis. Either skin prick tests or in vitro tests for IgE are usually performed initially.

Skin prick testing is a quick, useful test for determining the presence of specific IgE antibodies to egg. Traditionally, taken with a good clinical history, cutoff levels for skin prick test wheal size of 3 mm or greater than the negative saline control[31] have been used to support a clinical diagnosis. Higher cutoff levels have been proposed, which are associated with higher specificity and positive predictive values, although in younger children (<2 years) smaller skin prick test wheals are more likely to be predictive of egg allergy than in older children.[57] Specifically, a wheal size of 5 mm or greater has been reported to provide a 100% positive predictive value (PPV) for children less than 2 years of age, whereas for older children, a wheal size of 7 mm has a reported 100% PPV[58,59] (**Table 2**). Children with test results greater than these cutoffs are presumed to be clinically reactive, and OFC are avoided in these cases. Because of a high negative predictive value (91% for skin prick test <3 mm[60]), a negative prick test can be helpful to rule out an allergy to egg. Skin prick testing has low specificity, therefore isolated positive tests in the absence of clinical suspicion may not indicate clinical allergy.

Egg white–specific IgE can be measured using standardized, in vitro IgE assays providing a quantitative measurement. There is a positive correlation between increasing levels of egg white–specific IgE and the likelihood of clinical reactivity to egg. A range of predictive cutoff values for the diagnosis of egg allergy have been proposed. Studies using the ImmunoCAP (Phadia, Uppsala, Sweden) have shown that an IgE level of 7 kUA/L to egg has a 95% PPV for clinical reactivity to egg for children more than 2 years of age; for children 2 years of age or less, a level of 2 kUA/L has a 95% PPV.[30,60–63] Although there is a demonstrable relationship between serum IgE levels and challenge outcome, there is poor agreement between cutoff levels identified by different centers (**Table 3**).[30,64–68] This may be because of differences in inclusion criteria, significance level, challenge method and outcome criteria, subject age, and prevalence of egg allergy and eczema between studies. These variables should be taken into account when interpreting cutoff levels for any given patient population. Similar to skin prick testing, the measurement of specific IgE to egg in the absence of a history of egg ingestion is discouraged because the test has poor sensitivity and low negative predictive value. The presence of undetectable IgE levels to egg (<0.35 kUA/L) does not exclude clinical reactivity to egg.[60–62]

It has been suggested that quantification of OVM antibodies could be useful in guiding the physician in deciding whether to perform an OFC. Recently published data suggest that a concentration of IgE antibodies to OVM higher than approximately 11 kUA/L (positive decision point) indicates a high risk of reacting to heated (as well as

Table 2
Diagnostic decision points for skin prick test wheal diameter to egg (Pharmacia ImmunoCAP)

References	Year	Age Group (y)	Number of Patients	PPV	SPT Wheal Diameter (mm)
Sampson and Ho[64]	1997	Children and adolescents	100	85	≥3
Sporik et al[59]	2000	<2 >2	39 82	100	≥5 ≥7
Boyano-Martinez et al[30]	2001	<2	81	93	≥3
Hill et al[58]	2004	<2 >2	90 555	100	≥5 ≥7
Verstege et al[57]	2005	All children (range 0.3–14.5) <1 >1	160 26 134	95	≥13 ≥11.2 ≥13.3

Data from Tey D. Egg allergy in childhood: an update. Current Opinion in Allergy and Clinical Immunology 2009;9:244–50.

Table 3
Diagnostic decision points for egg-specific serum IgE levels (Pharmacia ImmunoCAP)

References	Year	Age Group (y)	Challenge	PPV	Egg-Specific IgE (kUA/L)
Sampson and Ho[64]	1997	Children and adolescents	126	95	6.0
Boyano-Martinez et al[30]	2001	0–2	94	94	>0.35
Roehr et al[63]	2001	2 mo–11.2	42	100	17.5
Osterballe and Bindslev-Jensen[66]	2003	0.5–4.9	56	95	1.5
Celik-Bilgili et al[65]	2005	All children (range 0.1–16.1) ≤1 >1	227 41 186	95	12.6 10.9 13.2
Komata et al[67]	2007	All children (range 0.2–14.6) ≤1 1–2 >2	764 N/A N/A N/A	95	25.5 13.0 23.0 30.0
Benhamou et al[68]	2008	Median 47 mo	51	100	7

Data from Tey D. Egg allergy in childhood: an update. Current Opinion in Allergy and Clinical Immunology 2009;9:244–50.

less-heated or undercooked) egg.[69] A concentration lower than approximately 1 kUA/L (negative decision point) suggests that there is a low risk of reaction to heated egg, even if the patients might well react to less-heated or undercooked egg. Further studies are required to confirm these data in other populations, and this test is not currently used in practice.

Although these tests provide an indication of likelihood of clinical reactivity to egg, neither is able to predict the severity of allergic reactions that may occur with each individual, nor the natural history of the allergy. However, the rate of decline of specific IgE levels with time is a prognostic indicator for the development of tolerance.[70]

Standardized, double-blind, placebo-controlled OFCs remain the gold standard for the diagnosis of food allergy. A physician-supervised OFC is required if the history and/or IgE test results do not clearly indicate an allergy. OFC should always be performed by well-trained physicians and health personnel, and emergency equipment must be readily available. The food is gradually administered with increasing doses because it may cause immediate, potentially severe, symptoms.

Asthma

The diagnosis of suspected occupational asthma caused by egg allergy, which is also IgE mediated, involves skin prick testing, pulmonary function testing, and possible bronchoprovocation challenge.

Mixed IgE-mediated and Non–IgE-mediated Disorders

Skin prick test and specific IgE test are useful for detecting an IgE-mediated sensitization, but do not provide information regarding non–IgE-mediated mechanisms of allergy. For mixed IgE-mediated disorders, including atopic dermatitis or allergic gastrointestinal disorders, the results need to be correlated with the clinical picture and, when necessary, confirmed with a positive challenge. Atopy patch tests with egg white may provide additional information in these cases.[52]

Differential Diagnosis

Gastrointestinal symptoms, such as vomiting and diarrhea, occurring after ingestion of undercooked egg can be caused by food poisoning, such as salmonella or campylobacter infection, rather than allergy. Unlike food allergy reactions, symptoms are generally delayed and occur 8 to 72 hours after exposure. Allergies to foods other than egg should also be considered in the differential diagnosis, especially if the reactions occurred to foods that contained multiple ingredients.

Cross-reactivity

Serologic and clinical cross-reactivity with other bird eggs (turkey, duck, goose, seagull, and quail) have been reported.[71,72] A minority of patients with allergy to egg are reactive to chicken meat as well. Chicken serum albumin (Gal d 5) is responsible for this cross-reactivity.[28]

MANAGEMENT

The management of egg allergy is similar to that of other food allergies. It requires education on avoidance and management of allergic reactions in the event of accidental exposure. Hen's egg is a versatile ingredient used in food from many cultures, including a wide range of manufactured food products (**Table 4**). The dietary avoidance of egg can thus be challenging[73] and can pose significant quality-of-life concerns. To ensure that elimination of egg does not result in nutritional deficiency, and in particular for those who have additional dietary limitations (eg, vegetarian diet or multiple food allergies), a dietician should be involved in the care of the patient.

Patients must be counseled about the potential for accidental exposure to food allergens via cross-contamination. This exposure can occur wherever food is being prepared or served, including restaurants and bakeries. In addition, egg whites and shells are used as clarifying agents and can be found in soup stocks, consommés, wine, alcohol-based beverages, and coffee drinks. Egg white is also used as a wash for bread products. Counseling should also include a discussion about egg

Table 4
How to read a label for an egg-free diet

Avoid Foods that Contain Eggs or Any of these Ingredients:	Egg Protein is Sometimes Found in the Following:
Albumin (also spelled as albumen)	Baked goods
Egg (dried, powdered, solids, white, yolk)	Egg substitutes
Eggnog	Lecithin
Globulin	Macaroni
Lysozyme	Marzipan
Mayonnaise	Marshmallows
Meringue (meringue powder)	Nougat
Ovalbumin	Pasta
Ovovitellin	
Surimi	

Data from The Food Allergy and Anaphylaxis Network.

Box 1
Substitutions for egg in recipes

Two tablespoons of fruit puree (binding only)

One tablespoon of ground flax seeds, 3 tablespoons water (binding only)

One and one-half tablespoons water, 1.5 tablespoons oil, 1 teaspoon baking powder (leavening and blinding)

One teaspoon baking powder, 1 tablespoon liquid, 1 tablespoons vinegar (leavening and binding)

Potato-based commercial egg substitute from Ener-G foods (leavening and binding)

One packet of gelatin, 2 tablespoons warm water; mix when ready to use (leavening and binding)

One teaspoon yeast dissolved in one-quarter cup water (leavening and binding)

Data from The Food Allergy and Anaphylaxis Network.

alternatives and substitutes because commercial products marketed as egg substitutes may have egg ingredients (**Box 1**).

Careful reading of ingredient labels is essential and legislation has been enacted in the United States mandating clear labeling of food packages to identify the presence of the 8 major food allergens, including egg (as well as milk, tree nuts, peanuts, wheat, soybeans, fish, and crustacean shellfish).[74] Some products in the United States may have advisory labeling, such as "may contain egg." This type of labeling is not currently regulated. Based on a recent study,[75] avoidance of advisory-labeled products should be recommended because they present a small, but real, risk of allergic reactions, especially products from small companies. Other countries are addressing issues of food labeling as well. Since November 2005, prepackaged food sold within the European Union have been required by law to list egg in the ingredient panel if it is a deliberately added component of the product, however little the amount.

Several studies have found that most individuals with egg allergy can tolerate extensively heated or baked egg.[76–79] However, identification of these patients remains difficult and the only currently available diagnostic test to determine which patients can tolerate extensively heated egg (unless it is currently in their diet) is an OFC. Patients may be allowed to continue to eat egg in more processed forms than what triggered their reaction(s) if they have eaten egg in these forms regularly and in the recent past (similar to passing an oral food challenge). In most cases, this involves patients who reacted to lightly cooked egg (eg, scrambled egg, French toast), but have a history of tolerating extensively heated egg (eg, muffins, waffles). However, patients should avoid more intermediate forms of cooked egg, such as meatballs/meatloaf, breaded foods, casseroles, custard, mayonnaise, and hardboiled egg.

There are several caveats that should be discussed with patients when considering inclusion of certain heated forms of egg in the diet. It is possible that a patient may have a reaction caused by ingestion of a larger amount of egg or more lightly cooked egg than usual (eg, undercooked muffins or cookies). Furthermore, the effect of including heated egg in the diet on the natural history of egg allergy is unknown. However, patients who have reacted to intermediately cooked or extensively heated egg should avoid all forms of egg. An OFC to extensively heated egg may be considered by an allergy specialist if a patient is not currently eating egg in this form but the patient (or parents of the patient) wishes to introduce it into the diet. Caution is needed, because severe reactions can occur from this type of oral food challenge.[79]

In addition, the effect of ingesting heated egg on the course of the allergy is not yet understood. However, it has been recently shown that ingestion of extensively heated egg in children with egg allergy is associated with favorable immunologic changes.[79] Continued ingestion of extensively heated egg for tolerant children showed a decrease in OVA-IgE/IgG4 and OVM-IgE/IgG4 ratios from baseline at 3, 6, and 12 months. These results suggest that ingestion of extensively heated egg by tolerant children might hasten the development of tolerance to unheated egg.

Egg Proteins in Medications and Vaccines

Medications and vaccines may have ingredients derived from egg. Patients should ensure that the clinicians and pharmacists caring for them are aware of their egg allergy, especially before receiving any new medication or vaccine. Influenza vaccines are derived from the extraembryonic fluid of chicken embryos inoculated with specific types of influenza virus. The vaccines typically contain measurable quantities of residual OVA. OVA levels in influenza vaccines vary between manufacturers and also between batches from the same manufacturer; from barely detectable to as high as 42 μg/mL.[80] There are few published data on the risk of allergic reaction to influenza vaccine in individuals with egg allergy.[81,82] Immediate allergic reactions, including anaphylaxis, have been reported in patients with egg allergy after influenza vaccination.[83–85] In a population survey of 48 million people undergoing influenza vaccination, there were only 11 reports of anaphylaxis, although none had a known prior history of egg allergy, suggesting an alternative allergen.[81] Several procedures have been proposed to safely vaccinate patients with a history of a severe hypersensitivity reaction to egg.[86–88]

The yellow fever vaccine is prepared in egg embryos, and allergic reactions to this vaccine have been reported.[89] This vaccination is required for travelers entering several countries in areas where yellow fever is endemic. In a small study, a reduced intradermal dose of the yellow fever vaccine induced protective antibody responses in individuals with egg allergy.[90]

In contrast, the measles, mumps, and rubella (MMR) vaccine is not contraindicated for children with egg allergy, although the measles vaccine is produced in a culture of chicken embryo fibroblasts. Three large trials have shown the safety of the MMR vaccine in children with egg allergy.[91–93] Allergic reactions to these vaccines have been primarily attributed to the gelatin component.[94]

Two other areas of concern are lipid emulsions that contain egg (eg, propofol and intralipid) and use of egg lysozyme, an enzyme found in egg white, in pharmaceutical products. There are case reports of anaphylaxis to these products.[95–97]

Provision of Emergency Treatment

Identification of individuals with IgE-mediated egg allergy is important, because these patients are at risk for severe reactions. As with other forms of food allergy, the severity of symptoms in a given individual with egg allergy may vary considerably between reactions. In addition, the severity of an initial reaction does not predict the severity of subsequent reactions. Children with egg allergy are more likely to develop asthma, and concomitant asthma places patients at higher risk for severe allergic reactions to foods.[9] In a small study investigating whether children with egg allergy of varying severity could tolerate extensively heated forms of egg, 18% of children who reacted to extensively heated egg and 23% who reacted to lightly cooked egg required treatment with epinephrine.[79] In another series of 167 children that examined dietary advice and adherence in patients with egg allergy, the initial episode was a local reaction in 29%, a mild to moderate systemic reaction in 31%, and a severe systemic reaction in 18%.[98] Twenty percent of the children in this study had a subsequent reaction to egg that was more severe than the initial event. Children whose only apparent clinical manifestation of food allergy is atopic dermatitis may be at risk of an acute systemic reaction on reintroduction of that food after a period of elimination because atopic dermatitis may have IgE-mediated triggers.[4,5,13]

Accordingly, we suggest that individuals diagnosed with IgE-mediated egg allergy have an epinephrine autoinjector(s) available at all times.[6] In addition, these patients should have written anaphylaxis emergency action plans.

NATURAL HISTORY

Earlier studies indicated that tolerance to egg is achieved by most children with egg allergy, with resolution in 50% by age 3 years and in 66% by age 5 years.[99] However, a more recent study suggested that egg allergy is more persistent, predicting resolution in 4% by age 4 years, 12% by age 6 years, 37% by age 10 years, and 68% by age 16 years.[100] Whether these differing results are caused by population differences or a change in the natural history of egg allergy is unclear. Because most children do outgrow their egg allergy, periodic reevaluation is recommended.

Several prognostic indicators for the development of tolerance to egg have been identified. These indicators include lower level of egg-specific IgE,[70] faster rate of decline of egg-specific IgE level with time,[70] earlier age at diagnosis,[70] milder symptoms,[79,101] and smaller skin test wheal sizes.[99] Moreover, people who are tolerant to extensively heated egg may be more likely to outgrow the egg allergy. However, those who are allergic to extensively heated egg are more likely to have severe, and maybe lifelong, egg allergy.

FUTURE TREATMENTS

Currently, there are no treatments that can cure or provide long-term remission from food allergy. However, several treatment strategies are being investigated. These approaches are either allergen-specific or aimed at modulating the overall allergic response. Oral tolerance induction studies to food allergens are still experimental[102,103] and a few studies show promising results.[103–106] However, adverse reactions are common.[102,103] There is still uncertainty about whether oral immunotherapy (OIT) achieves true tolerance or transient desensitization (with recurrence of symptoms after discontinuation of therapy). There is a high probability of spontaneous tolerance development to egg, so it is unclear whether OIT changes the time course to the development of tolerance.

With recent reports indicating that extensively heated egg is tolerated by most patients with egg allergy and that the associated immunologic changes with continued ingestion of extensively heated egg seem favorable, incorporation of extensively heated egg in the diet may present a more natural form of immunotherapy. At this point, OIT is still considered investigational, and therefore is not recommended in routine clinical practice.

SUMMARY

Egg allergy is one of the most common food allergies in childhood and can induce a range of IgE-mediated and non–IgE-mediated disorders. A recent study has suggested that egg allergy is more persistent than was previously believed. Avoidance and preparation in case of allergic reactions caused by accidental exposures remain the cornerstones of management. Although there are currently no cures for food allergy, ongoing studies of OIT are showing promise.

REFERENCES

1. Sicherer SH, Sampson HA. 9. Food allergy. J Allergy Clin Immunol 2006; 117(2 Suppl Mini-primer):S470–5.
2. Eggesbo M, Botten G, Halvorsen R, et al. The prevalence of allergy to egg: a population-based study in young children. Allergy 2001;56(5):403–11.
3. Sampson HA. Role of immediate food hypersensitivity in the pathogenesis of atopic dermatitis. J Allergy Clin Immunol 1983;71(5):473–80.
4. Sampson HA, McCaskill CC. Food hypersensitivity and atopic dermatitis: evaluation of 113 patients. J Pediatr 1985;107(5):669–75.
5. Sampson HA, Scanlon SM. Natural history of food hypersensitivity in children with atopic dermatitis. J Pediatr 1989;115(1):23–7.
6. Rona RJ, Keil T, Summers C, et al. The prevalence of food allergy: a meta-analysis. J Allergy Clin Immunol 2007;120(3):638–46.
7. Roehr CC, Edenharter G, Reimann S, et al. Food allergy and non-allergic food hypersensitivity in children and adolescents. Clin Exp Allergy 2004;34(10):1534–41.
8. Madrigal BI, Alfaro AN, Jimenez CC, et al. Adverse reactions to food in daycare children. Rev Alerg Mex 1996;43(2):41–4.
9. Osterballe M, Hansen TK, Mortz CG, et al. The prevalence of food hypersensitivity in an unselected population of children and adults. Pediatr Allergy Immunol 2005;16(7):567–73.
10. Niggemann B, Sielaff B, Beyer K, et al. Outcome of double-blind, placebo-controlled food challenge tests in 107 children with atopic dermatitis. Clin Exp Allergy 1999;29(1):91–6.
11. Nickel R, Kulig M, Forster J, et al. Sensitization to hen's egg at the age of twelve months is predictive for allergic sensitization to common indoor and outdoor allergens at the age of three years. J Allergy Clin Immunol 1997;99(5):613–7.
12. Ricci G, Patrizi A, Baldi E, et al. Long-term follow-up of atopic dermatitis: retrospective analysis of related risk factors and association with concomitant allergic diseases. J Am Acad Dermatol 2006;55(5):765–71.
13. Hill DJ, Hosking CS, de Benedictis FM, et al. Confirmation of the association between high levels of immunoglobulin E food sensitization and eczema in infancy: an international study. Clin Exp Allergy 2008;38(1):161–8.
14. Heine RG, Laske N, Hill DJ. The diagnosis and management of egg allergy. Curr Allergy Asthma Rep 2006;6(2):145–52.
15. Bernhisel-Broadbent J, Dintzis HM, Dintzis RZ, et al. Allergenicity and antigenicity of chicken egg ovomucoid (Gal d III) compared with ovalbumin (Gal d I) in children with egg allergy and in mice. J Allergy Clin Immunol 1994;93(6):1047–59.
16. Miller H, Campbell DH. Skin test reactions to various chemical fractions of egg white and their possible clinical significance. J Allergy 1950;21(6):522–4.
17. Bleumink E, Young E. Studies on the atopic allergen in hen's egg. II. Further characterization of the skin-reactive fraction in egg-white; immuno-electrophoretic studies. Int Arch Allergy Appl Immunol 1971;40(1):72–88.
18. Cooke SK, Sampson HA. Allergenic properties of ovomucoid in man. J Immunol 1997;159(4):2026–32.
19. Astwood JD, Leach JN, Fuchs RL. Stability of food allergens to digestion in vitro. Nat Biotechnol 1996;14(10):1269–73.

20. Jarvinen KM, Beyer K, Vila L, et al. Specificity of IgE antibodies to sequential epitopes of hen's egg ovomucoid as a marker for persistence of egg allergy. Allergy 2007;62(7):758–65.
21. Honma K, Aoyagi M, Saito K, et al. Antigenic determinants on ovalbumin and ovomucoid: comparison of the specificity of IgG and IgE antibodies. Arerugi 1991;40(9):1167–75.
22. Matsuda T, Watanabe K, Nakamura R. Immunochemical and physical properties of peptic-digested ovomucoid. J Agric Food Chem 1983;31(5):942–6.
23. Takagi K, Teshima R, Okunuki H, et al. Kinetic analysis of pepsin digestion of chicken egg white ovomucoid and allergenic potential of pepsin fragments. Int Arch Allergy Immunol 2005;136(1):23–32.
24. Yamada K, Urisu A, Haga Y, et al. A case retaining contact urticaria against egg white after gaining tolerance to ingestion. Acta Paediatr Jpn 1997;39(1): 69–73.
25. Joo K, Kato Y. Assessment of allergenic activity of a heat-coagulated ovalbumin after in vivo digestion. Biosci Biotechnol Biochem 2006;70(3):591–7.
26. Elsayed S, Hammer AS, Kalvenes MB, et al. Antigenic and allergenic determinants of ovalbumin. I. Peptide mapping, cleavage at the methionyl peptide bonds and enzymic hydrolysis of native and carboxymethyl OA. Int Arch Allergy Appl Immunol 1986;79(1):101–7.
27. Ilchmann A, Burgdorf S, Scheurer S, et al. Glycation of a food allergen by the Maillard reaction enhances its T-cell immunogenicity: role of macrophage scavenger receptor class A type I and II. J Allergy Clin Immunol 2010;125(1): 175.e1-11–83.e1-11.
28. Quirce S, Maranon F, Umpierrez A, et al. Chicken serum albumin (Gal d 5*) is a partially heat-labile inhalant and food allergen implicated in the bird-egg syndrome. Allergy 2001;56(8):754–62.
29. Szepfalusi Z, Ebner C, Pandjaitan R, et al. Egg yolk alpha-livetin (chicken serum albumin) is a cross-reactive allergen in the bird-egg syndrome. J Allergy Clin Immunol 1994;93(5):932–42.
30. Boyano-Martinez T, Garcia-Ara C, Diaz-Pena JM, et al. Validity of specific IgE antibodies in children with egg allergy. Clin Exp Allergy 2001;31(9):1464–9.
31. Monti G, Muratore MC, Peltran A, et al. High incidence of adverse reactions to egg challenge on first known exposure in young atopic dermatitis children: predictive value of skin prick test and radioallergosorbent test to egg proteins. Clin Exp Allergy 2002;32(10):1515–9.
32. Hill DJ, Heine RG, Hosking CS, et al. IgE food sensitization in infants with eczema attending a dermatology department. J Pediatr 2007;151(4):359–63.
33. Vance GH, Grimshaw KE, Briggs R, et al. Serum ovalbumin-specific immunoglobulin G responses during pregnancy reflect maternal intake of dietary egg and relate to the development of allergy in early infancy. Clin Exp Allergy 2004;34(12):1855–61.
34. Palmer DJ, Gold MS, Makrides M. Effect of maternal egg consumption on breast milk ovalbumin concentration. Clin Exp Allergy 2008;38(7):1186–91.
35. Palmer DJ, Gold MS, Makrides M. Effect of cooked and raw egg consumption on ovalbumin content of human milk: a randomized, double-blind, cross-over trial. Clin Exp Allergy 2005;35(2):173–8.
36. Spergel JM, Mizoguchi E, Brewer JP, et al. Epicutaneous sensitization with protein antigen induces localized allergic dermatitis and hyperresponsiveness to methacholine after single exposure to aerosolized antigen in mice. J Clin Invest 1998;101(8):1614–22.

37. Oyoshi MK, Murphy GF, Geha RS. Filaggrin-deficient mice exhibit TH17-dominated skin inflammation and permissiveness to epicutaneous sensitization with protein antigen. J Allergy Clin Immunol 2009;124(3):485–93, 493.e1.
38. Colver AF, Nevantaus H, Macdougall CF, et al. Severe food-allergic reactions in children across the UK and Ireland, 1998–2000. Acta Paediatr 2005;94(6): 689–95.
39. Ross MP, Ferguson M, Street D, et al. Analysis of food-allergic and anaphylactic events in the National Electronic Injury Surveillance System. J Allergy Clin Immunol 2008;121(1):166–71.
40. Sampson HA, Mendelson L, Rosen JP. Fatal and near-fatal anaphylactic reactions to food in children and adolescents. N Engl J Med 1992;327(6):380–4.
41. Mehl A, Wahn U, Niggemann B. Anaphylactic reactions in children–a questionnaire-based survey in Germany. Allergy 2005;60(11):1440–5.
42. Macdougall CF, Cant AJ, Colver AF. How dangerous is food allergy in childhood? The incidence of severe and fatal allergic reactions across the UK and Ireland. Arch Dis Child 2002;86(4):236–9.
43. Eigenmann PA. Anaphylactic reactions to raw eggs after negative challenges with cooked eggs. J Allergy Clin Immunol 2000;105(3):587–8.
44. Escudero C, Quirce S, Fernandez-Nieto M, et al. Egg white proteins as inhalant allergens associated with baker's asthma. Allergy 2003;58(7):616–20.
45. Mandallaz MM, de Weck AL, Dahinden CA. Bird-egg syndrome. Cross-reactivity between bird antigens and egg-yolk livetins in IgE-mediated hypersensitivity. Int Arch Allergy Appl Immunol 1988;87(2):143–50.
46. Tewari A, Du Toit G, Lack G. The difficulties of diagnosing food-dependent exercise-induced anaphylaxis in childhood – a case study and review. Pediatr Allergy Immunol 2006;17(2):157–60.
47. Lever R, MacDonald C, Waugh P, et al. Randomised controlled trial of advice on an egg exclusion diet in young children with atopic eczema and sensitivity to eggs. Pediatr Allergy Immunol 1998;9(1):13–9.
48. Werfel T, Ballmer-Weber B, Eigenmann PA, et al. Eczematous reactions to food in atopic eczema: position paper of the EAACI and GA2LEN. Allergy 2007;62(7): 723–8.
49. Breuer K, Heratizadeh A, Wulf A, et al. Late eczematous reactions to food in children with atopic dermatitis. Clin Exp Allergy 2004;34(5):817–24.
50. Tariq SM, Matthews SM, Hakim EA, et al. Egg allergy in infancy predicts respiratory allergic disease by 4 years of age. Pediatr Allergy Immunol 2000;11(3): 162–7.
51. Liacouras CA, Spergel JM, Ruchelli E, et al. Eosinophilic esophagitis: a 10-year experience in 381 children. Clin Gastroenterol Hepatol 2005;3(12):1198–206.
52. Spergel JM, Beausoleil JL, Mascarenhas M, et al. The use of skin prick tests and patch tests to identify causative foods in eosinophilic esophagitis. J Allergy Clin Immunol 2002;109(2):363–8.
53. Noel RJ, Putnam PE, Rothenberg ME. Eosinophilic esophagitis. N Engl J Med 2004;351(9):940–1.
54. Spergel JM, Brown-Whitehorn TF, Beausoleil JL, et al. 14 years of eosinophilic esophagitis: clinical features and prognosis. J Pediatr Gastroenterol Nutr 2009;48(1):30–6.
55. Kondo M, Fukao T, Omoya K, et al. Protein-losing enteropathy associated with egg allergy in a 5-month-old boy. J Investig Allergol Clin Immunol 2008;18(1):63–6.
56. Benhamou AH, Caubet JC, Eigenmann PA, et al. State of the art and new horizons in the diagnosis and management of egg allergy. Allergy 2010;65(3):283–9.

57. Verstege A, Mehl A, Rolinck-Werninghaus C, et al. The predictive value of the skin prick test weal size for the outcome of oral food challenges. Clin Exp Allergy 2005;35(9):1220–6.
58. Hill DJ, Heine RG, Hosking CS. The diagnostic value of skin prick testing in children with food allergy. Pediatr Allergy Immunol 2004;15(5):435–41.
59. Sporik R, Hill DJ, Hosking CS. Specificity of allergen skin testing in predicting positive open food challenges to milk, egg and peanut in children. Clin Exp Allergy 2000;30(11):1540–6.
60. Caffarelli C, Cavagni G, Giordano S, et al. Relationship between oral challenges with previously uningested egg and egg-specific IgE antibodies and skin prick tests in infants with food allergy. J Allergy Clin Immunol 1995;95(6):1215–20.
61. Sampson HA. Utility of food-specific IgE concentrations in predicting symptomatic food allergy. J Allergy Clin Immunol 2001;107(5):891–6.
62. Perry TT, Matsui EC, Kay Conover-Walker M, et al. The relationship of allergen-specific IgE levels and oral food challenge outcome. J Allergy Clin Immunol 2004;114(1):144–9.
63. Roehr CC, Reibel S, Ziegert M, et al. Atopy patch tests, together with determination of specific IgE levels, reduce the need for oral food challenges in children with atopic dermatitis. J Allergy Clin Immunol 2001;107(3):548–53.
64. Sampson HA, Ho DG. Relationship between food-specific IgE concentrations and the risk of positive food challenges in children and adolescents. J Allergy Clin Immunol 1997;100(4):444–51.
65. Celik-Bilgili S, Mehl A, Verstege A, et al. The predictive value of specific immunoglobulin E levels in serum for the outcome of oral food challenges. Clin Exp Allergy 2005;35(3):268–73.
66. Osterballe M, Bindslev-Jensen C. Threshold levels in food challenge and specific IgE in patients with egg allergy: is there a relationship? J Allergy Clin Immunol 2003;112(1):196–201.
67. Komata T, Soderstrom L, Borres MP, et al. The predictive relationship of food-specific serum IgE concentrations to challenge outcomes for egg and milk varies by patient age. J Allergy Clin Immunol 2007;119(5):1272–4.
68. Benhamou AH, Zamora SA, Eigenmann PA. Correlation between specific immunoglobulin E levels and the severity of reactions in egg allergic patients. Pediatr Allergy Immunol 2008;19(2):173–9.
69. Ando H, Moverare R, Kondo Y, et al. Utility of ovomucoid-specific IgE concentrations in predicting symptomatic egg allergy. J Allergy Clin Immunol 2008; 122(3):583–8.
70. Shek LP, Soderstrom L, Ahlstedt S, et al. Determination of food specific IgE levels over time can predict the development of tolerance in cow's milk and hen's egg allergy. J Allergy Clin Immunol 2004;114(2):387–91.
71. Langeland T. A clinical and immunological study of allergy to hen's egg white. VI. Occurrence of proteins cross-reacting with allergens in hen's egg white as studied in egg white from turkey, duck, goose, seagull, and in hen egg yolk, and hen and chicken sera and flesh. Allergy 1983;38(6):399–412.
72. Alessandri C, Calvani M Jr, Rosengart L, et al. Anaphylaxis to quail egg. Allergy 2005;60(1):128–9.
73. Mofidi S. Nutritional management of pediatric food hypersensitivity. Pediatrics 2003;111(6 Pt 3):1645–53.
74. United States Food Allergen Labeling and Consumer Protection Act of 2004.
75. Ford LS, Taylor SL, Pacenza R, et al. Food allergen advisory labeling and product contamination with egg, milk, and peanut. J Allergy Clin Immunol 2010;126(2):384–5.

76. Urisu A, Ando H, Morita Y, et al. Allergenic activity of heated and ovomucoid-depleted egg white. J Allergy Clin Immunol 1997;100(2):171–6.
77. Des Roches A, Nguyen M, Paradis L, et al. Tolerance to cooked egg in an egg allergic population. Allergy 2006;61(7):900–1.
78. Konstantinou GN, Giavi S, Kalobatsou A, et al. Consumption of heat-treated egg by children allergic or sensitized to egg can affect the natural course of egg allergy: hypothesis-generating observations. J Allergy Clin Immunol 2008; 122(2):414–5.
79. Lemon-Mule H, Sampson HA, Sicherer SH, et al. Immunologic changes in children with egg allergy ingesting extensively heated egg. J Allergy Clin Immunol 2008;122(5):977.e1–983.e1.
80. Chaloupka I, Schuler A, Marschall M, et al. Comparative analysis of six European influenza vaccines. Eur J Clin Microbiol Infect Dis 1996;15(2):121–7.
81. Retailliau HF, Curtis AC, Storr G, et al. Illness after influenza vaccination reported through a nationwide surveillance system, 1976–1977. Am J Epidemiol 1980; 111(3):270–8.
82. Bierman CW, Shapiro GG, Pierson WE, et al. Safety of influenza vaccination in allergic children. J Infect Dis 1977;136(Suppl):S652–5.
83. Ratner B, Untracht S. Egg allergy in children; incidence and evaluation in relation to chick-embryo-propagated vaccines. AMA Am J Dis Child 1952;83(3): 309–16.
84. Anolik R, Spiegel W, Posner M, et al. Influenza vaccine testing in egg sensitive patients. Ann Allergy 1992;68(1):69.
85. Miller JR, Orgel HA, Meltzer EO. The safety of egg-containing vaccines for egg-allergic patients. J Allergy Clin Immunol 1983;71(6):568–73.
86. James JM, Zeiger RS, Lester MR, et al. Safe administration of influenza vaccine to patients with egg allergy. J Pediatr 1998;133(5):624–8.
87. Chung EY, Huang L, Schneider L. Safety of influenza vaccine administration in egg-allergic patients. Pediatrics 2010;125(5):e1024–30.
88. Kelso JM. Administration of influenza vaccines to patients with egg allergy. J Allergy Clin Immunol 2010;125(4):800–2.
89. Kelso JM, Mootrey GT, Tsai TF. Anaphylaxis from yellow fever vaccine. J Allergy Clin Immunol 1999;103(4):698–701.
90. Roukens AH, Vossen AC, van Dissel JT, et al. Reduced intradermal test dose of yellow fever vaccine induces protective immunity in individuals with egg allergy. Vaccine 2009;27(18):2408–9.
91. Fasano MB, Wood RA, Cooke SK, et al. Egg hypersensitivity and adverse reactions to measles, mumps, and rubella vaccine. J Pediatr 1992;120(6): 878–81.
92. Freigang B, Jadavji TP, Freigang DW. Lack of adverse reactions to measles, mumps, and rubella vaccine in egg-allergic children. Ann Allergy 1994;73(6):486–8.
93. Aickin R, Hill D, Kemp A. Measles immunisation in children with allergy to egg. BMJ 1994;309(6949):223–5.
94. Pool V, Braun MM, Kelso JM, et al. Prevalence of anti-gelatin IgE antibodies in people with anaphylaxis after measles-mumps rubella vaccine in the United States. Pediatrics 2002;110(6):e71.
95. Hofer KN, McCarthy MW, Buck ML, et al. Possible anaphylaxis after propofol in a child with food allergy. Ann Pharmacother 2003;37(3):398–401.
96. Buchman AL, Ament ME. Comparative hypersensitivity in intravenous lipid emulsions. JPEN J Parenter Enteral Nutr 1991;15(3):345–6.

97. Artesani MC, Donnanno S, Cavagni G, et al. Egg sensitization caused by immediate hypersensitivity reaction to drug-containing lysozyme. Ann Allergy Asthma Immunol 2008;101(1):105.
98. Allen CW, Kemp AS, Campbell DE. Dietary advice, dietary adherence and the acquisition of tolerance in egg-allergic children: a 5-yr follow-up. Pediatr Allergy Immunol 2009;20(3):213–8.
99. Boyano-Martinez T, Garcia-Ara C, Diaz-Pena JM, et al. Prediction of tolerance on the basis of quantification of egg white-specific IgE antibodies in children with egg allergy. J Allergy Clin Immunol 2002;110(2):304–9.
100. Savage JH, Matsui EC, Skripak JM, et al. The natural history of egg allergy. J Allergy Clin Immunol 2007;120(6):1413–7.
101. Ford RP, Taylor B. Natural history of egg hypersensitivity. Arch Dis Child 1982; 57(9):649–52.
102. Beyer K, Wahn U. Oral immunotherapy for food allergy in children. Curr Opin Allergy Clin Immunol 2008;8(6):553–6.
103. Burks AW, Jones SM. Egg oral immunotherapy in non-anaphylactic children with egg allergy: follow-up. J Allergy Clin Immunol 2008;121(1):270–1.
104. Buchanan AD, Green TD, Jones SM, et al. Egg oral immunotherapy in nonanaphylactic children with egg allergy. J Allergy Clin Immunol 2007;119(1):199–205.
105. Patriarca G, Nucera E, Roncallo C, et al. Oral desensitizing treatment in food allergy: clinical and immunological results. Aliment Pharmacol Ther 2003; 17(3):459–65.
106. Staden U, Rolinck-Werninghaus C, Brewe F, et al. Specific oral tolerance induction in food allergy in children: efficacy and clinical patterns of reaction. Allergy 2007;62(11):1261–9.

Peanut Allergy

Jonathan O'B Hourihane, MB, DM, FRCPI

KEYWORDS

- *Arachis hypogea* • Atopic disorders
- Oral induction of tolerance • Peanut

HISTORY OF PEANUT CULTIVATION

Peanut (*Arachis hypogea*) is a native South American legume that has been valued for many centuries. Peanut kernels have been found in Peruvian archaeological sites demonstrating organized agriculture 10,000 years ago.[1,2] In contrast, the absence of peanuts from Greek and Roman remains and writings and pre-Columbian Old World records, strongly suggests that peanut was unknown to these early European civilizations. By the time the Conquistadores arrived in South America, the Incas felt that peanuts were "a luxury of the rich and curious (rather than) a food for the poor."[3] This high status of peanut in the South American diet contrasts with reports of customs on Hispaniola, Columbus's landfall in the New World. Fernandez (1535) noted "It [peanut] is a healthy food but it is not eaten by Christians unless they are unmarried males or children or slaves or common people. Its consumption among the Indians is very common."[4]

Peanut cultivation spread with the conquest of Central and North America and was introduced to Africa as a food for slaves. Today it is a significant cash crop particularly in West Africa. Up to the nineteenth century, peanut was used in North America as a food for slaves, poor whites, and increasingly as food for animals. In our time, the largest producers of peanuts (India and China) grow peanuts largely for animal rather than human consumption. The growth of peanut as a cash crop occurred in North America on the back of 2 developments: the American Civil War and mechanization of vegetable oil production. Peanuts were grown extensively in the southern United States before the Civil War. Its use as an easily transportable high-energy food increased during the Civil War and spread to northern cities. It is difficult to say when peanut and peanut butter appeared in significant amounts in Europe. However, by the 1970s, peanut had become a common food in the United Kingdom, in both its nut and butter forms. The United States produces 8 billion kg per annum.[5]

Conflict of interest: I have helped develop a patented desktop calculator for predicting the outcome of food challenge but I have no personal financial stake in its commercialization.

Department of Paediatrics and Child Health, Clinical Investigations Unit, Cork University Hospital, University College Cork, Wilton, Cork, Ireland
E-mail address: J.Hourihane@ucc.ie

Pediatr Clin N Am 58 (2011) 445–458
doi:10.1016/j.pcl.2011.02.004 **pediatric.theclinics.com**
0031-3955/11/$ – see front matter

BOTANY AND BIOLOGY OF PEANUT AND PEANUT PROTEINS

Peanut is the fruit of the legume *Arachis hypogea*. It is also know as the goober nut or earth nut, and more commonly as a groundnut. The German for peanut is erdnusse (groundnut). It is called a groundnut because the seed pod initially appears on the branches of the plant and as it increases in weight the branch bends and the dependent pods become buried in the soil where they mature before harvesting. Peanut is a high protein food, 24% by weight and is therefore comparable with cheese, fish, and beef. Most of peanut's 49% fat content is unsaturated making it an attractive and stable source of oil for human consumption. Fiber levels are comparable with wholemeal bread (1.5 g/100 g).

Peanuts contain ~25% protein. The major peanut proteins to which most North American and northern European individuals develop an allergic reaction are Ara h1, Ara h 2 and Ara h3, respectively[6,7] but in southern Europe Ara h 8 and Ara h 9 are more dominant (**Table 1** for summary).[8] The allergens in peanut have been studied intensively for more than 20 years, seeking to find a biochemical basis for the severity of peanut allergy and to explore whether protein modifications result in reduced allergenicity. Although neither aspiration has been fully satisfied much has been learned.

Efforts have been made to reduce the allergenicity of major peanut allergens, particularly Ara h 2, with in vitro studies showing significant reductions in IgE binding and in basophil histamine release.[9] However, modification of peanut proteins may alter its botanic function and it does not address the broad diversity of allergenic proteins that exist in peanut plants, where elimination of one will probably not eliminate the allergenic potential of other proteins.

EPIDEMIOLOGY

Peanut allergy seems to develop early in life with most affected children in the United States and the United Kingdom developing symptoms before the age of 2 years.[10,11]

Table 1
Botanic and immunologic profiles of major peanut allergens

Protein	Molecular Weight and Botanic Function	Clinical Relevance
Ara h1	63.5 kDa, vicillin storage protein	Heat stable
Ara h 2	17.5 kDa, vicillin storage protein, trypsin inhibitor	Heat stable, more commonly associated with severe clinical reactions than other peanut proteins
Ara h 3/4	60 kDa, 11S globulin, seed storage protein	—
Ara h5	15 kDa, profilin	Commonly associated with cross-sensitization with other plant allergens but probably of little relevance to clinical reactivity
Ara h6	15 kDa 2S albumin	Moderate homology with Ara h 2. IgE to Ara h6 persists with time
Ara h8	16.9 kDa, Bet v1 homolog	Probably most significant as being responsible for cross-reactivity with birch pollen analogs
Ara h 9	Lipid transfer protein	Low prevalence of recognition in American and northern European populations, more commonly recognized in southern Europe

Data from Refs.[6–8]

The age of exposure and age of first reaction to peanut have both decreased in recent years in the United States.[11]

Family studies have shown that peanut allergy is more common in first-degree relatives of children with peanut allergy than in the general population.[12–14] It remains uncertain if this can solely be explained by a shared genetic background[15,16] or also reflects environmental factors that are shared in families.

The known international variation in peanut allergen recognition probably reflects alternative cooking and intercultural feeding practices that may increase or decrease peanut's in vitro allergenicity (**Fig. 1**).[17–19] In addition, timing of its first introduction into the diet affects prevalence as clearly demonstrated when comparing peanut prevalence between genetically similar but geographically separate Jewish populations (Israel vs United Kingdom) with different feeding practices.[20]

Serologic studies have shown that the diversity of IgE recognition of peanut proteins is more associated with clinical outcome than recognition of individual proteins[21,22] although recognition of Ara h 2 is repeatedly shown to be associated with more severe (mostly respiratory) symptoms.[7] It has also been shown that Ara h 2 sensitivity is more likely to be associated with reactivity in formal challenge than recognition of Ara h 8, which probably reflects Bet v1-related cross-reactivity.[6] At the present time, the most useful predictors of persistence after the first 2 years of life are a maximum wheal size of >6 mm for the peanut skin prick test (SPT) or a peanut-specific IgE >3 kilounits of antibody (kUA)/L.[23]

Cellular-based assays of T-cell recognition of peanut peptides, and of IgE and IgG, G_1 and IgG_4 diversity, tend to show that there is a diverse spectrum of reactivity with no particular pattern of antibody production that could easily predict severity in a way that is clinical useful.[24–28] Combination scores that account for both dose and clinical reaction during food challenge have been associated with specific IgE levels[27,29] but there remains the problem that reactivity in a formal food challenge is not strongly linked with reported reaction severity in community reactions (reactions in the field).[29]

PEANUT ALLERGY IS A MARKER FOR OTHER ATOPIC DISORDERS

Individuals with peanut allergy are almost universally atopic in other ways, with rates of asthma, atopic dermatitis (AD), and rhinitis that are higher than the general population.

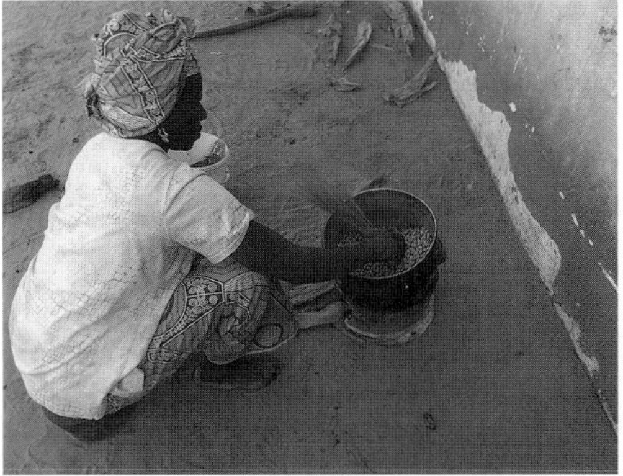

Fig. 1. Different cooking methods alter peanut's in vitro allergenicity in different ways. Boiling reduces IgE binding, roasting increases it. This woman in Keneba, Gambia, is dry roasting peanut kernels. (*Courtesy of* Dr Kerry Jones, Medical Research Council Laboratories, Keneba; with permission.)

In the United Kingdom, monoallergy to peanut is a rare finding, with less than 5% of cases showing no other sensitization.[10] This can be a good clue to the diagnosis when meeting a new referral for evaluation. In addition, it has been known for 2 decades that asthma, particularly poorly controlled asthma, is associated with fatal outcome in food allergy, particularly peanut allergy,[30] and conversely that an existing diagnosis of peanut allergy is associated with worse respiratory outcomes in asthmatic children.[31,32] Furthermore, children with peanut allergy who are clinically considered to have outgrown preexisting asthma continue to show increased levels of exhaled nitric oxide (eNO), implying persisting inflammation in the airway.[33] In view of these data, it is considered best practice to ensure optimal asthma control as a key part of managing peanut allergy (see later discussion). Similarly AD is a common clinical finding in children with peanut allergy. AD is considered the earliest marker of atopic predisposition.

Much higher odds of developing peanut allergy has been found if a mother (retrospectively recalled at 5–7 years) had applied skin creams containing peanut oil to infant skin.[34] Experimental work showed application of peanut to both intact and especially to abraded mouse skin caused migration of Langerhans cells out of the skin and to systemic sensitization, as measurable by increased serum peanut-specific IgE, and a T_h2 biased cytokine profile.[35]

An interesting observational study from the United Kingdom has suggested that compared with control families (no food allergy) and families with a child at high risk for but not actually demonstrating peanut allergy (the index child had egg allergy), families with a child with peanut allergy were more likely to consume peanut and especially peanut butter in the home, with a dose-response relationship evident between nonoral exposure to peanut and having peanut allergy.[36]

PREVALENCE OF PEANUT SENSITIZATION AND CONFIRMED ALLERGY

At present, there are estimates that up to 9% and 11% of North American and British children of 8 years or older[6,37] and 8.9% of Australian infants of 12 months of age (K. Allen, personal communication, 2010) are sensitized to peanut although less than half of these children can be proved to be allergic to peanut by food challenge (see later discussion). In contrast the Early Prevention of Asthma and Allergy in Childhood (EPAAC) study found that in infants aged 1 to 2 years with moderate AD, sensitization to peanut could be found in more than 20% of children.[38] It is unclear whether this is primary sensitization or cross-reactive sensitization with birch pollen and other plant allergens that may have been encountered by the inhaled route before oral exposure to peanut.

Several studies suggest a steady increase in the prevalence of peanut allergy from the mid-1990s. For example, at 3 to 4 years of age, the Isle of Wight cohort born in 1989 had a 1.3% peanut sensitization prevalence and a 0.6% prevalence of actual clinical peanut allergy. No formal diagnostic challenges were performed.[39] Subsequent birth cohort studies from the Isle of Wight[40] and a cross-sectional 2-center study from the UK mainland showed the rate of peanut allergy (proved by challenge) had increased to 1.8% by 2005.[41]

Population-based studies that result in a gold standard diagnostic double-blind, placebo-controlled, food challenge are less common in the United States but self-reported surveys conducted by telephone in the United States have shown similar figures and a similar increase from 0.4% in 1997 to 1.4% in 2008.[42] The 2005/2006 National Health and Nutrition Examination Survey study reported an estimate prevalence of peanut allergy of 1.3%.[43]

PATTERNS OF CLINICAL REACTIVITY

The diagnosis of peanut allergy is simple to make in the presence of known exposure to peanuts and a stereotypical reaction (**Table 2**). Reactions typically start soon after exposure and it is usually possible to identify peanut in the food eaten[10,11] Most reactions to peanut are benign and are survived. However, peanut is overwhelmingly and disproportionately represented in case series of severe and fatal outcomes, particularly in community-based retrospective surveys of deaths and severe allergic reactions.[30,44,45] Methodologically there may be biased reporting of reactions when peanut is implicated compared with more unusual foods that are not recognized by emergency staff as allergens or foods that are considered more mundane such as milk and egg.

DIAGNOSIS OF PEANUT ALLERGY

As shown in **Table 2** the features of a peanut allergic reaction are simple to distinguish as reactions are typical and are usually similar in individuals who have repeat reactions and in formal challenge settings. Observed variation in reactions with time[46] may be caused by the onset of asthma, dose variation, or extrinsic factors such as exercise, infection, and other cofactors.[47]

Although the double-blind, placebo-controlled food challenge is considered the gold standard for diagnosis, it is logistically demanding and time consuming. Therefore, an open food challenge is acceptable in most settings, especially for young children. Most peanut challenges are well tolerated; most children (>90%) who react to the challenge do not need epinephrine, even with conservative criteria for intervention.[48,49] Families respond favorably to food challenges, even when they result in a reaction.[50] Although a formal food challenge is not possible in all diagnostic settings, more than half of the individuals who undergo a food challenge do not react, even if their SPT or serum IgE level suggests the presence of a peanut allergy.[6,51]

Several investigators have developed specific values for SPT (>6–8 mm in most reports) or peanut-specific serum IgE levels (>14–15 kUA/L) that would indicate a likely

Table 2
Clinical reactivity to peanut is stereotyped

A Likely Case of Peanut Allergy	A Case Unlikely to be Caused by Peanut Allergy
First known exposure to peanut or previous known peanut allergy	Multiple previous episodes of safe consumption of peanut
Multiple allergic disorders Asthma AD Rhinitis Food allergies (especially egg allergy)	No other allergic disorders identified
Stereotyped reaction Rapid onset (minutes) Predominant cutaneous and respiratory symptoms Urticaria/angioedema Rhinoconjuctivitis Wheezing	Atypical reaction Slow onset (hours, even overnight) Headache/joint pains Nonurticarial skin rashes
Low (relative) dose of peanut consumed	High (relative) dose of peanut consumed
Peanut usually easily identifiable in implicated meal/snack	Peanut implicated in retrospect

positive reaction during an oral food challenge.[52] Although these may be useful in deciding if a diagnostic challenge is necessary or can be postponed, they do not add greatly to the scenario of a carefully taken history that characterizes a reaction as likely to have been caused by peanut, with a positive SPT or specific IgE level that might be less than the decision point. In clinical practice, a typical history (see **Table 2**) and supportive tests mean a true diagnosis of peanut allergy is likely to be present in 85% of cases.[10] Therefore it is not immediately and automatically necessary to challenge every child who presents with a history of reactivity to peanut. Research protocols may demand challenges but routine clinical practice is now more commonly using challenges to determine if peanut allergy has resolved. It is now possible to use more subtle assessments that combine the effects of known predictors of challenge outcome with others whose effect has been difficult to quantify, such as age and sex.[53]

RESOLUTION AND RECURRENCE OF PEANUT ALLERGY

Bock and Atkins'[54] famous paper in 1988 reported follow-up of 42 children with a positive double-blind, placebo-controlled food challenge. Four died and none of the survivors outgrew their sensitivity to peanut during follow-up. Our group's case-control study in the mid-1990s showed that peanut allergy could not be demonstrated in 20% of children with broadly similar reports of index reactions.[55] This group had not been established based on an initial double-blind, placebo-controlled food challenge but later studies, based on initial double-blind, placebo-controlled food challenge, found a near identical rate of resolution[56] and it is now well established that peanut allergy can resolve. Negative follow-up challenges are more likely in those with low SPT and specific IgE levels, so it is worth measuring these on an annual or biannual basis to assess the likelihood that the allergic reaction is subsiding.

Peanut allergy may recur. Eight percent of children who initially had a positive oral food challenge but with time became tolerant (as shown by negative challenge) could not tolerate peanut in their diet after discharge.[57] It is possible that a half-day or full-day challenge protocol may be too short for some individuals who might experience temporary hyposensitization and who then revert to a reactive state when reexposed to peanut at home. It is therefore recommended that after passing an oral food challenge, peanut should be eaten regularly (but how regularly is not known).[58] Children who cannot reintroduce peanuts after a challenge should be offered extended follow-up and reconsidered for further peanut challenge at a later date. Children who have passed a peanut challenge should remain under clinical review until peanut is back in the diet and family life no longer has to factor in the rigors of peanut avoidance. At this stage, epinephrine autoinjectors can be withdrawn if there is no other indication for their retention (usually other food allergies).

EFFORTS TO PREVENT PEANUT ALLERGY

When peanut allergy emerged as a significant health care condition in the early 1990s major research efforts were already underway to establish the efficacy of avoidance diets in preventing allergic disorders, mainly relating to the outcome of asthma. Regulatory and professional advice for pregnant and nursing mothers and their infants to avoid peanut was issued in the United Kingdom and the United States in the late 1990s.[59] Irrespective of the quality of the evidence base for this advice, it is clear the advice had no definite effect on sensitization or allergy rates. This might be because the advice was unclear or being ignored[41] or that the general population or even merely the atopic population were not the correct target populations. The

American Academy of Pediatrics and the UK's Committee on Toxicity of Food both rescinded this advice in 2008 (although they did not specify what advice should be given instead).[60,61] A recent report hints that the advice might have been correct if it had been more strictly limited to high-risk families. A prospective follow-up of young infants (mean age 9 months) with milk or egg allergy (therefore considered high risk for peanut allergy) has shown that more than a quarter of such infants have peanut-specific IgE levels higher than 5 kUA/L. These infants were 3 times more likely to have been born to mothers who had consumed peanut while pregnant or breastfeeding. The effect may have been stronger for consumption during pregnancy than during breastfeeding.[62] This finding merits prospective replication to elucidate some way to identify and counsel women at risk of such an outcome in their offspring.

An intensive trial of early introduction of peanut into the diet of peanut-sensitized children is underway,[63] aiming to prevent peanut allergy.

CONSERVATIVE MANAGEMENT OF PEANUT ALLERGY

Peanut allergy can be fatal so the anxiety that peanut allergy causes can be considered useful if it elicits appropriate levels of caution. However, it is also known that families can react in extreme ways because of their fears of such a fatal outcome.[64] Many children with food allergies are home schooled in the United States,[65] although this is unusual elsewhere. One of the most important tools to manage food allergies, including a peanut allergy, is the engagement of an expert allergist. Comprehensive allergy care significantly reduces the rate of accidental exposure as well as severity progression.[66,67]

Up to 50% of children with peanut allergy develop sensitization to tree nuts[10,68] and they are more likely to develop sensitization to sesame than children with other food allergies.[69] For these reasons, planned review of sensitization to these and occasionally other food groups is good practice in children with peanut allergy. However, if such foods are already safely consumed testing is not required.

In some countries most children with peanut allergy get an epinephrine pen prescription, but in other countries a more cautious approach is taken. The practice in the United States of providing most if not all individuals with peanut allergy with an epinephrine pen is easily understood from a medicolegal perspective but can be criticized for being paternalistic and too conservative, or conversely too aggressive (in that most children with peanut allergy will never need them and the requirement to decide when to use them is a burden on caregivers, especially those who are not members of the index family). It is definitely expensive. More importantly, their prescription without parental training and support may cause additional anxiety.[70] However, our local experience suggests that proper education on the use of epinephrine kits decreases parental anxiety (>95% of respondents, A Dunngalvin, J Hourihane, unpublished data, 2009). There is a strong case, accepted by affected families, for other modalities of availability of epinephrine to be explored,[71] analogous to the proliferation of automated external defibrillators in public facilities.

THERAPEUTIC OPTIONS FOR PEANUT ALLERGY

Conservative and supportive management remain the cornerstones of medical care for individuals with peanut allergy. Peanut allergy is now a well-characterized condition with some identifiable risk factors for persistence and resolution (SPT and peanut-specific IgE levels, allergen sensitization profile) and for severity (certainly asthma and possibly eNO status and Ara h 2 sensitization status). However, the medical goals of a cure or even an attenuation of severity of peanut allergy have been elusive.

Table 3
What are the unresolved issues regarding oral induction of tolerance to peanut?

Unknowns	Options	Reason	Comment
Who should be offered treatment?	Everyone	Progression of severity is uncertain	Not logistically feasible
	Benign reactors	To prevent progression	This group is most likely to remit spontaneously
	Severe reactors	To prevent fatality	Fatal reactions are rare but are feared by nearly all families
			Quality of life may improve significantly
How long to treat?	2–3 years	Early effects of peanut OIT reflect those of inhalant immunotherapy	No data yet for any duration of treatment
	5 years	Comparable with venom intolerance	—
	Indefinitely	—	Families may not want to stop
How can treatment success be measured?	SPT, peanut-specific IgE	Easily done in routine practice	May not change during treatment
	DBPCFC	Not easily done in routine practice	Reaction severity in DBPCFC not strongly associated with reaction severity in the field
	Quality of life	Easy to measure	Not yet studied systematically in OIT trials
Where to treat?	Research centers	Experience of peanut OIT	Not geographically accessible to most patients
	Allergy centers	Experience of immunotherapy	Resource issues, personnel, and financial
	Private practice	Patient access	Likely massive demand, but safety, governance and insurance/reimbursement issues
What peanut preparation to use?	Whole peanut	Widely available	—
	Defatted peanut	Easily available	Easy to vary dose, but may not be identical to whole peanut
	Modified dominant peanut allergens	Ara h2 modification attenuates reactivity in vitro and in animal studies	Other unmodified allergens may become more relevant in exposures after OIT
How to manage protocol violations	Missed doses	? drop a dose level	Early reports suggest not a major problem
	Double doses	? continue or skip a dose	No data yet
	Intercurrent life and health events	Asthma, pregnancy new medications, and so forth	Viral illness has elicited breakthrough reactions during OIT
			No pregnancy data yet

Abbreviation: DBPCFC, double-blind placebo-controlled food challenge.

Injection immunotherapy is not well tolerated[72] and anti-IgE therapy has not translated into routine clinical practice after the promising early studies.[73] Trials are underway after promising animal studies of Chinese herbal remedies and peanut-based immunotherapy with bacterial vectors.[74,75] The current cutting edge of peanut allergy research is oral induction of tolerance (OIT). Groups in the United States, the United Kingdom, Australia, and Germany are committed to large programs of research aiming to deliver what would be the most important development in this field to date.[76]

Protocols are broadly similar and have been shared between some groups, indicating viability outside the developing centers.[77–80] Entry criteria have not always been a formal double-blind, placebo-controlled food challenge and severe reactors were not always included in the first trials. Early data indicate that more than half of the subjects, but not all of them, complete induction and retain remission during the maintenance phase. Reactions to OIT, mostly minor upper airway symptoms, are more common during induction than during the maintenance. More severe symptoms, such as chest symptoms are only present in 1.7% of reactions during induction, and decrease to 0.2% during maintenance.[78,79]

The first report of successful treatment was from the United Kingdom,[80] using a protocol developed at Duke University. In this first report 4 subjects were reported, 2 with a history of previous reactions to peanut and 2 without such a history but with peanut-specific IgE levels that would predict reactivity. All 4 subjects increased their threshold dose of defatted peanut flour by factors of between 48 and 478 times their threshold dose at entry.

Duke data suggest that the immunologic changes witnessed in peanut OIT reflect those seen in inhalant allergen immunotherapy, which can be discontinued after 3 to 5 years with persisting clinical efficacy for several years thereafter, which might suggest that peanut OIT treatment could be limited to a 3-year or 5-year time frame rather than continued indefinitely.[78] This remains unproved to date. Furthermore, although early data suggest that peanut OIT may have a place in the management of patients with peanut allergy, substantial issues remain to be addressed, including the feasibility of providing peanut OIT outside heavily resourced academic centers (**Table 3**). Although in an attempt to gain access to such therapies, patients from some countries (eg, Ireland) travel to other countries (United Kingdom), authorities in the United States have on more than one occasion advised that peanut OIT is not yet ready for routine clinical practice.[81] It will take time for experience of peanut OIT to build up in centers outside the vanguard of this advance.

SUMMARY

Peanut allergy is now a well-characterized condition with high levels of medical, regulatory, and public awareness. Disease-modifying therapeutic options are emerging but the best approach has not yet been established. Families affected by peanut allergy are vulnerable to extreme anxiety around peanut allergy and physicians must recognize this undesirable consequence of the explosion of information about peanut allergy in the last 2 decades. Prudent and supportive medical advice, risk assessment, family education, and training in rescue medication use form the basis for the management of peanut allergy. The immunologic and biochemical information with which physicians can characterize patients with peanut allergy using routinely available in vivo and in vitro tests has improved and will continue to evolve. Meanwhile, sufficient data on the feasibility, effectiveness, and safety of peanut OIT are awaited. This therapy is not ready for prime time yet.

ACKNOWLEDGMENTS

Most of the historical details on peanut's adoption as a major crop are taken from an article by R. Hammon in a symposium report: "Early History and Origin of Peanut", *Peanut, Culture and Uses: A Symposium*. American Peanut Research and Education Foundation, Stillwater (OH), 1973.

REFERENCES

1. Waldron RA. The peanut (*Arachis hypogea*) - its history, histology, physiology and utility. Penn Univ Bot Lab Contrib 1919;4:301–38.
2. Dillehay TD, Rossen J, Andres TC, et al. Preceramic adoption of peanut, squash, and cotton in northern Peru. Science 2007;316(5833):1890–3.
3. Garsilaso de la Vega. Primeras parte de los Commentarios Reales 1609, translated CR Markham. London: Hakluyt Soc Works 1871;2:360.
4. De Oviedo y Valdes GF. La historia general de la Indias. Seville (Spain);1535.
5. American Peanut Board. Available at: www.peanutsusa.com. Accessed November 28, 2010.
6. Nicolaou N, Poorafshar M, Murray C, et al. Allergy or tolerance in children sensitized to peanut: prevalence and differentiation using component-resolved diagnostics. J Allergy Clin Immunol 2010;125:191–7.
7. Asarnoj A, Moverare R, Ostblom E, et al. IgE to peanut allergen components: relation to peanut symptoms and pollen sensitization in 8-year-olds. Allergy 2010;65:1189–95.
8. Krause S, Reese G, Randow S, et al. Lipid transfer protein (Arah9) as a new peanut allergen relevant for a Mediterranean allergic population. J Allergy Clin Immunol 2009;124:771–8.
9. King N, Helm R, Stanley JS, et al. Allergenic characteristics of a modified peanut allergen. Mol Nutr Food Res 2005;49:963–71.
10. Hourihane JO, Kilburn SA, Dean TP, et al. Clinical characteristics of peanut allergy. Clin Exp Allergy 1997;27:634–9.
11. Green TD, LaBelle VS, Steele PH, et al. Clinical characteristics of peanut-allergic children: recent changes. Pediatrics 2007;120:1304–10.
12. Hourihane JO, Dean TP, Warner JO. Peanut allergy in relation to heredity, maternal diet, and other atopic diseases: results of a questionnaire survey, skin prick testing, and food challenges. BMJ 1996;313(7056):518–21.
13. Sicherer SH, Furlong TJ, Maes HH, et al. Genetics of peanut allergy: a twin study. J Allergy Clin Immunol 2000;106(1 Pt 1):53–6.
14. Liem JJ, Huq S, Kozyrskyj AL, et al. Should younger siblings of peanut-allergic children be assessed by an allergist before being fed peanut? Allergy Asthma Clin Immunol 2008;4:144–9.
15. Howell WM, Turner SJ, Hourihane JO, et al. HLA class II DRB1, DQB1 and DPB1 genotypic associations with peanut allergy: evidence from a family-based and case-control study. Clin Exp Allergy 1998;28(2):156–62.
16. Shreffler WG, Charlop-Powers Z, Sicherer SH. Lack of association of HLA class II alleles with peanut allergy. Ann Allergy Asthma Immunol 2006;96(6):865–9.
17. Maleki SJ, Kopper RA, Shin DS, et al. Structure of the major peanut allergen Arah1 may protect IgE-binding epitopes from degradation. J Immunol 2000; 164:5844–9.
18. Mondoulet L, Paty E, Drumare MF, et al. Influence of thermal processing on the allergenicity of peanut proteins. J Agric Food Chem 2005;53(11):4547–53.

19. Kopper RA, Odum NJ, Sen M, et al. Peanut protein allergens: the effect of roasting on solubility and allergenicity. Int Arch Allergy Immunol 2005;136:16–22.
20. Du Toit G, Katz Y, Sasieni P, et al. Early consumption of peanuts in infancy is associated with a low prevalence of peanut allergy. J Allergy Clin Immunol 2008;122: 984–91.
21. Lewis SA, Grimshaw EC, Warner JO, et al. The promiscuity of immunoglobulin E binding to peanut allergens, as determined by Western blotting, correlates with the severity of clinical symptoms. Clin Exp Allergy 2005;35:767–73.
22. Astier C, Morisset M, Roitel O, et al. Predictive value of skin prick tests using recombinant allergens for diagnosis of peanut allergy. J Allergy Clin Immunol 2006; 118(1):250–6.
23. Ho MH, Wong WH, Heine RG, et al. Early clinical predictors of remission of peanut allergy in children. J Allergy Clin Immunol 2008;121:731–6.
24. Kolopp-Sarda MN, Moneret-Vautrin DA, Gobert B, et al. Polyisotypic antipeanut-specific humoral responses in peanut-allergic individuals. Clin Exp Allergy 2001; 31(1):47–53.
25. Shreffler WG, Beyer K, Chu TT, et al. Microarray immunoassay: association of clinical history, in vitro IgE function, and heterogeneity of allergenic peanut epitopes. J Allergy Clin Immunol 2004;113:776–82.
26. Tay SS, Clark AT, Deighton J, et al. Patterns of immunoglobulin G responses to egg and peanut allergens are distinct: ovalbumin-specific immunoglobulin responses are ubiquitous, but peanut-specific immunoglobulin responses are up-regulated in peanut allergy. Clin Exp Allergy 2007;37(10):1512–8.
27. Flinterman AE, Knol EF, Lencer DA, et al. Peanut epitopes for IgE and IgG4 in peanut-sensitized children in relation to severity of peanut allergy. J Allergy Clin Immunol 2008;121(3):737–43.e10.
28. Scott-Taylor TH, Hourihane JO'B, Strobel S. Correlation of allergen-specific IgG subclass antibodies and T lymphocyte cytokine responses in children with multiple food allergies. Pediatr Allergy Immunol 2010;21(6):935–44.
29. Hourihane JO, Grimshaw KE, Lewis SA, et al. Does severity of low-dose, double-blind, placebo-controlled food challenges reflect severity of allergic reactions to peanut in the community? Clin Exp Allergy 2005;35(9):1227–33.
30. Sampson HA, Mendelson L, Rosen JP. Fatal and near-fatal anaphylactic reactions to food in children and adolescents. N Engl J Med 1992;327(6):380–4.
31. Roberts G, Patel N, Levi-Schaffer F, et al. Food allergy as a risk factor for life-threatening asthma in childhood: a case-controlled study. J Allergy Clin Immunol 2003;112(1):168–74.
32. Simpson AB, Yousef E, Hossain J. Association between peanut allergy and asthma morbidity. J Pediatr 2010;156:777–81.
33. Hughes JL, Brown T, Edgar JD, et al. Peanut allergy and allergic airways inflammation. Pediatr Allergy Immunol 2010;21(8):1107–13.
34. Lack G, Fox D, Northstone K, et al; Avon Longitudinal Study of Parents and Children Study Team. Factors associated with the development of peanut allergy in childhood. N Engl J Med 2003;348(11):977–85.
35. Strid J, Hourihane J, Kimber I, et al. Disruption of the stratum corneum allows potent epicutaneous immunization with protein antigens resulting in a dominant systemic Th2 response. Eur J Immunol 2004;34(8):2100–9.
36. Fox AT, Sasieni P, DuToit G, et al. Household peanut consumption as a risk factor for the development of peanut allergy. J Allergy Clin Immunol 2009;123:417–23.
37. Branum AM, Lukacs SL. Food allergy among children in the United States. Pediatrics 2009;124(6):1549–55.

38. Hill DJ, Hosking C, de Benedictis FM, et al. Confirmation of the association between high levels of immunoglobulin E food sensitization and eczema in infancy: an international study. Clin Exp Allergy 2008;38(1):161–8.
39. Tariq SM, Stevens M, Matthews S, et al. Cohort study of peanut and tree nut sensitisation by age of 4 years. BMJ 1996;313(7056):514–7.
40. Venter C, Hasan Arshad S, Grundy J, et al. Time trends in the prevalence of peanut allergy: three cohorts of children from the same geographical location in the UK. Allergy 2010;65(1):103–8.
41. Hourihane JO, Aiken R, Briggs R, et al. The impact of government advice to pregnant mothers regarding peanut avoidance on the prevalence of peanut allergy in United Kingdom children at school entry. J Allergy Clin Immunol 2007;119: 1197–202.
42. Sicherer SH, Muñoz-Furlong A, Godbold JH, et al. US prevalence of self-reported peanut, tree nut, and sesame allergy: 11-year follow-up. J Allergy Clin Immunol 2010;125(6):1322–6.
43. Liu AH, Jaramillo R, Sicherer SH, et al. National prevalence and for food allergy and relationship to asthma: results from the National Health and Nutrition Examination Survey 2005–2006. J Allergy Clin Immunol 2010;126(4): 798–806.e13.
44. Bock SA, Muñoz-Furlong A, Sampson HA. Further fatalities caused by anaphylactic reactions to food, 2001–2006. J Allergy Clin Immunol 2007;119(4): 1016–8.
45. Pumphrey RS, Gowland MH. Further fatal allergic reactions to food in the United Kingdom, 1999–2006. J Allergy Clin Immunol 2007;119(4):1018–9.
46. Vander Leek TK, Liu AH, Stefanski K, et al. The natural history of peanut allergy in young children and its association with serum peanut-specific IgE. J Pediatr 2000;137:749–55.
47. Hourihane JO'B, Knulst AC. Thresholds of allergenic proteins in foods. Toxicol Appl Pharmacol 2005;207(Suppl 2):152–6.
48. Järvinen KM, Amalanayagam S, Shreffler WG, et al. Epinephrine treatment is infrequent and biphasic reactions are rare in food-induced reactions during oral food challenges in children. J Allergy Clin Immunol 2009;124(6):1267–72.
49. Yanishevsky Y, Daly D, Cullinane C, et al. Differences in treatment of food challenge-induced reactions reflect physicians' protocols more than reaction severity. J Allergy Clin Immunol 2010;126(1):182.
50. DunnGalvin A, Cullinane C, Daly DA, et al. Longitudinal validity and responsiveness of the food allergy quality of life questionnaire - parent form in children 0-12 years following positive and negative food challenges. Clin Exp Allergy 2010; 40(3):476–85.
51. Kagan RS, Joseph L, Dufresne C, et al. Prevalence of peanut allergy in primary-school children in Montreal, Canada. J Allergy Clin Immunol 2003;112(6):1223–8.
52. Burks AW. Peanut allergy. Lancet 2008;371(9623):1538–46.
53. DunnGalvin A, Daly D, Cullinane C, et al. Highly accurate prediction of food challenge outcome using routinely available clinical data. J Allergy Clin Immunol, in press.
54. Bock SA, Atkins FM. The natural history of peanut allergy. J Allergy Clin Immunol 1989;83:900–4.
55. Hourihane JO'B, Roberts SA, Warner JO. Resolution of peanut allergy: case-control study. BMJ 1998;316(7140):1271–5.
56. Skolnick HS, Conover-Walker MK, Koerner CB, et al. The natural history of peanut allergy. J Allergy Clin Immunol 2001;107(2):367–74.

57. Fleischer DM, Conover-Walker MK, Christie L, et al. The natural progression of peanut allergy: resolution and the possibility of recurrence. J Allergy Clin Immunol 2003;112:183–9.
58. Byrne AM, Malka-Rais J, Burks AW, et al. How do we know when peanut and tree nut allergy have resolved, and how do we keep it resolved? Clin Exp Allergy 2010;40:1303–11.
59. Committee on Toxicity of Chemicals in Food, Consumer Products and the Environment (COT). Adverse reactions to food and food ingredients. London: COT; 2000. p. 91–7.
60. UK Department of Health. Revised government advice on consumption of peanut during pregnancy, breastfeeding, and early life and development of peanut allergy. Available at: www.dh.gov.uk/en/Healthcare/Children/Maternity/Maternalandinfantnutrition/DH_104490. Accessed August 19, 2009.
61. Greer FR, Sicherer SH, Burks AW, American Academy of Pediatrics Committee on Nutrition, American Academy of Pediatrics Section on Allergy and Immunology. Effects of early nutritional interventions on the development of atopic disease in infants and children: the role of maternal dietary restriction, breastfeeding, timing of introduction of complementary foods, and hydrolyzed formulas. Pediatrics 2008;121(1):183–91.
62. Sicherer SH, Wood RA, Stablein D, et al. Maternal consumption of peanut during pregnancy is associated with peanut sensitization in atopic infants. J Allergy Clin Immunol 2010;126(6):1191–7.
63. Available at: www.leapstudy.co.uk. Accessed December 8, 2010.
64. King RM, Knibb RC, Hourihane JO'B. Impact of peanut allergy on quality of life, stress and anxiety in the family. Allergy 2009;64(3):461–8.
65. Bollinger ME, Dahlquist LM, Mudd K, et al. The impact of food allergy on the daily activities of children and their families. Ann Allergy Asthma Immunol 2006;96(3):415–21.
66. Ewan PW, Clark AT. Efficacy of a management plan based on severity assessment in longitudinal and case-controlled studies of 747 children with nut allergy: proposal for good practice. Clin Exp Allergy 2005;35:751–6.
67. Kapoor S, Roberts G, Bynoe Y, et al. Influence of a multidisciplinary paediatric allergy clinic on parental knowledge and rate of subsequent allergic reactions. Allergy 2004;59:185–91.
68. Clark AT, Ewan PW. The development and progression of allergy to multiple nuts at different ages. Pediatr Allergy Immunol 2005;16:507–11.
69. Stutius L, Sheehan WJ, Rangsithienchai P, et al. Characterizing the relationship between sesame, coconut, and nut allergy in children. Pediatr Allergy Immunol 2010;21(8):1114–8.
70. Vickers DW, Maynard L, Ewan PW. Management of children with potential anaphylactic reactions in the community: a training package and proposal for good practice. Clin Exp Allergy 1997;27:898–903.
71. Norton L, Dunn Galvin A, Hourihane JO. Allergy rescue medication in schools: modeling a new approach. J Allergy Clin Immunol 2008;122(1):209–10.
72. Oppenheimer JJ, Nelson HS, Bock SA, et al. Treatment of peanut allergy with rush immunotherapy. J Allergy Clin Immunol 1992;90(2):256–62.
73. Leung DY, Sampson HA, Yunginger JW, et al. Effect of anti-IgE therapy in patients with peanut allergy. N Engl J Med 2003;348:986–93.
74. Srivastava KD, Qu C, Zhang T, et al. Food allergy herbal formula-2 silences peanut-induced anaphylaxis for a prolonged post treatment period via IFN-g-producing CD8+ T cells. J Allergy Clin Immunol 2009;123:443–51.

75. Frick OL, Teuber SS, Buchanan BB, et al. Allergen immunotherapy with heat-killed *Listeria* monocytogenes alleviates peanut and food-induced anaphylaxis in dogs. Allergy 2005;60(2):243–50.
76. Beyer K, Wahn U. Oral immunotherapy for food allergy in children. Curr Opin Allergy Clin Immunol 2008;8(6):553–6.
77. Blumchen K, Ulbricht H, Staden U, et al. Oral peanut immunotherapy in children with peanut anaphylaxis. J Allergy Clin Immunol 2010;126(1):83–91.e1.
78. Jones SM, Pons L, Roberts JL, et al. Clinical efficacy and immune regulation with peanut oral immunotherapy. J Allergy Clin Immunol 2009;124:292–300.
79. Hofmann AM, Scurlock AM, Jones SM, et al. Safety of a peanut oral immunotherapy protocol in children with peanut allergy. J Allergy Clin Immunol 2009;124:286–91.
80. Clark AT, Islam S, King Y, et al. Successful oral tolerance induction in severe peanut allergy. Allergy 2009;64(8):1218–20.
81. Thyagarajan A, Varshney P, Jones SM, et al. Peanut oral immunotherapy is not ready for clinical use. J Allergy Clin Immunol 2010;126:31–2.

Living with Food Allergy: Allergen Avoidance

Jennifer S. Kim, MD*, Scott H. Sicherer, MD

KEYWORDS

• Food allergy • Avoidance • Management

The primary treatment of food allergy is to avoid the culprit foods. This is a complex undertaking that requires education about reading the labels of manufactured products, understanding how to avoid cross-contact with allergens during food preparation, and communicating effectively with persons who are providing allergen-safe meals including relatives and restaurant personnel. Successful avoidance also requires a knowledge of nuances such as appropriate cleaning practices, an understanding of the risks of ingestion compared to skin contact or inhalation, that exposure could occur through unanticipated means such as through sharing utensils or passionate kissing, and that food may be a component of substances that are not ingested such as cosmetics, bath products, vaccines and medications. Here we review the necessary tools of avoidance that physicians and medical practitioners can use to guide their patients through the complexities of food avoidance.

IDENTIFYING AND PREPARING SAFE FOODS

Patients and parents must become adept in label reading, meal preparation, and communicating their needs to other cooks and food preparers. Consultation with a registered dietitian may be helpful to ensure nutritional adequacies when multiple foods are excluded from the diet.[1,2]

Food Labeling

In the United States, the Food Allergen Labeling and Consumer Protection Act (FALCPA) of 2004 went into effect from January 1, 2006. This law requires that the 8 major allergens, including milk, egg, peanut, tree nuts, fish, crustacean shellfish, wheat, and soy, be declared on ingredient labels using plain English words. The common names used to identify the foods may be listed within the ingredient list or in a separate statement (eg, "Contains...") in a type size no smaller than that used

Division of Allergy & Immunology, Mount Sinai School of Medicine, One Gustave L. Levy Place, Box 1198, New York, NY 10029-6574, USA
* Corresponding author.
E-mail address: jennifer.kim@mssm.edu

Pediatr Clin N Am 58 (2011) 459–470
doi:10.1016/j.pcl.2011.02.007 **pediatric.theclinics.com**
0031-3955/11/$ – see front matter

in the list of ingredients. The law also requires that the specific type of allergen within a category be named, such as almond (tree nuts) or cod (fish). FALCPA applies to foods manufactured in the United States as well as to packaged foods that are imported for sale and subject to regulation by the US Food and Drug Administration (FDA). FALCPA does not apply to meat, poultry, certain egg products (eg, whole eggs), or raw agricultural foods, such as fruits and vegetables.

Product labeling laws in other countries, such as Canada, Europe, Australia, and New Zealand, vary by terms, definitions, and food allergens (http://www.foodallergens.info/Manufac/Guidelines.html). For example, the European Union defines 12 major allergens, including all gluten-containing products (wheat, rye, barley, oats, spelt, and their hybridized strains), celery, mustard, and sesame seeds, as well as sulfites. Canada, Australia, and New Zealand also identify sesame and sulfites as allergens.

The FALCPA applies only to 8 major allergens. Other foods, such as sesame, may still be listed using ambiguous terms, such as flavors or spices, and may not be included in the "Contains..." statement. In addition, noncrustacean shellfishes, such as clams and scallops, are not included in the act. The manufacturer may need to be contacted to specify ingredients in some cases when vague terms are used to describe ingredients categorically rather than individually.

Updates on FALCPA are available from the Center for Food Safety and Applied Nutrition, a branch of the FDA.[3] The legislation was designed to help reduce allergic reactions and simplify allergy management.[4] However, FALCPA does not require the FDA to establish a threshold level for any food allergen. Thus, an allergen must be declared even when trace amounts of protein that are unlikely to trigger an allergic reaction are included. Hence, soy lecithin, a fatty substance commonly used as an additive, must be disclosed as soy under the FALCPA, although lecithin is considered to have little allergenicity.[5] However, soy oil and other highly processed and refined vegetable oils are potentially exempt because protein is removed from while processing.

The FALCPA does not regulate the use of advisory labeling, including statements describing the potential presence of unintentional ingredients in food products resulting from the manufacturing of the ingredients or the preparation and packaging of the food. Phrases that are used to indicate possible cross-contact with allergens include "may contain," "processed in a facility with," and "manufactured on shared equipment with." Advisory labeling terms also vary by country; for example, the United Kingdom uses "not suitable for allergy sufferers." These terms are applied voluntarily at the manufacturers' discretion. Unfortunately, advisory labeling is widespread; one study found that 17% of 20,241 supermarket products had such labeling.[6] There are obvious benefits to advisory labeling, but its use may be too broad, limiting choices for some less sensitive food-allergic individuals. There are reports indicating that allergic individuals sometimes choose to ignore the advisory statements.[7,8] Presumably, consumers making such choices generally tolerate those foods; nevertheless, serious reactions from cross-contact have been reported.[9]

Risk of cross-contact seems to be calculated by the consumer based on label terminology.[7] A survey of more than 600 shoppers, primarily parents of children with food allergy and consumers with food allergy, revealed that products labeled "made in a facility that processes peanut" were more likely to be purchased over those labeled "may contain peanut." However, when samples of 179 products with advisory labeling for peanut were assayed, 7% of the products were found to have detectable peanut protein. Detection of peanut protein, however, did not correlate with how the warning was stated. Thus, consumers should be educated that risk level cannot be stratified according to wording (eg, "packaged in a facility" or "manufactured on shared equipment" does not indicate less risk of allergen exposure than "may contain traces of").

Products with milk advisory labeling have also been evaluated for contamination levels.[10] Detectable milk was found in 42% of 81 products, a much higher incidence than that mentioned earlier for peanut.[7] Dark chocolate products carried particularly high risk; among 18 dark chocolate items, 78% had detectable milk protein. The amount of milk in one serving of these products was estimated to range between 0.027 and 620 mg of milk. As a reference, 1 mL of cow's milk contains about 33 mg of milk protein.

Another recent study[11] examined products with advisory labeling for milk, egg, or peanut, as well as similar products without any advisory declaration, including products labeled as using "Good Manufacturing Practices." Allergenic residue was found in 5.3% of products with advisory labeling and 1.9% of products without advisory statements. A higher percentage of foods from small companies was contaminated when compared with that from large companies (5.1% vs 0.75%), although this percentage included products with allergen amounts that were arguably less than the threshold levels (which themselves have not been substantively defined). Notably, peanut was not detected in any of the 120 products tested without advisory labels.

Teenagers and young adults with food allergy are particularly less likely to heed advisory labeling. In one study, among 174 adolescents and young adults with food allergy, 42% were willing to eat foods labeled as "may contain."[12]

The question remains for many practitioners and patients alike: do these foods with advisory labeling need to be avoided? Patients should be educated that the wording does not correlate with the degree of risk. Based on the studies outlined, there is a small but definite risk of allergen exposure in a minority of products with advisory labeling, with the exception of dark chocolate products, which demonstrated higher risks for milk protein contamination. For practical purposes, however, complete avoidance is most prudent. An improved understanding of the minimal dose needed to provoke an allergic reaction among individuals and within the population would help guide the food industry to develop more precise labeling practices.[13]

Managing Meals—Both Within and Outside the Home

Many factors may play into the individual's and family's decision to keep the allergenic food in or to exclude it completely from the home. These factors may include the ease of removal of the allergen from the home, the effect of such removal on other members of the family, the sensitivity of the food-allergic individual, and personal preference of the family. Regardless of the choice, principles of avoidance of cross-contact must be reviewed carefully with patients and families, so that they are able to make informed decisions on how to manage their households (**Box 1**).

Being able to dine outside the home is an important element for socialization. Restaurants can present challenges for food-allergic individuals.[16] Preparation and clear communication are important aspects of the process when food preparation is under someone else's purview. In order to assess food allergy knowledge in the food service industry, a study used telephone questionnaires, which were administered to 100 employees (eg, managers, servers, chefs) of various restaurants and food establishments in the New York City area.[17] Only 22% provided correct responses to all 5 questions (true or false) about food allergy. Misconceptions included believing that fryer heat would destroy allergens, that it was safe to consume allergens in small amounts, and that removal of allergen from a finished dish (eg, picking off nuts) was safe. Most employees responded that they considered a buffet safe if kept clean. Despite this response, more than 90% rated themselves as being at least

Box 1
Tips for food allergen avoidance tips at home

Utensils, cookware, glassware, storage containers, and other food preparation equipment

- Thoroughly clean before preparing or serving safe meals
- Prepare safe meal first to avoid inadvertent cross-contact
- Be aware of the potential for cross-contact with utensils, for example, a knife used to prepare peanut butter and jelly by a nonallergic child could introduce peanut allergen into an otherwise safe jar of jelly and subsequently cause a reaction in a peanut-allergic sibling eating the jelly.[14] Similarly, the same knife with peanut butter (unclean) may be placed in the dishwasher, where a young child may later come upon it while the dishwasher is open
- Designate specific containers for use by the allergic person only. For example, avoid sippy cup mix-ups by using a specific cup for the allergic child or using an obvious label

Refrigerator/freezer and kitchen pantry

- Keep food containers covered/sealed to prevent spill contamination
- Assign a specific shelf or cabinet for safe foods. Consider using color codes or tags for easy identification

Behaviors of family members

- Wash hands before and after meals but particularly before serving allergen-free meals and after ingestion of allergen
- Confine food consumption to specified dining areas or create allergen-free zones within the home
- Wipe down surfaces after preparation and ingestion of meals[a]
- For young children, unsafe foods should be kept out of reach both at the dinner table and when storing foods

[a] Studies have investigated only peanut butter, but cleaning tabletops with several standard cleansers was sufficient for removal of the peanut allergen.[15] Household cleaners (except dishwashing liquid) and commercial wipes effectively removed peanut allergens from tabletops. Both liquid and bar soaps, but not alcohol-based antibacterial gels, removed peanut allergens from adults' hands.

"comfortable" in providing a safe meal to a food-allergic customer. Therefore, patients should not assume that restaurant personnel understand food allergy or know what steps must be taken to guarantee that a meal is safe. Instead, consumers should review issues of cross-contact, potential hidden ingredients, and the nature of allergy with the relevant personnel preparing and serving their food; all persons handling the food should be involved. This review could prevent errors, such as a preparation worker adding butter to a food that appears dry. See **Box 2** for additional strategies.

Special considerations for travel

Allergic reactions to peanut and tree nuts have been reported on commercial airliners.[18–20] Studies of these events have relied on self-reported reactions to ingestion, skin contact, and inhalation, which inherently have biases. The degree of risk is thus very difficult to ascertain, but travelers with food allergies should avoid eating potentially unsafe airline foods, as with any restaurant-prepared meal. Bringing along allergen-free foods would be a safer option. Those traveling with young children may wish to inspect crevices around their seats for residual foods that might be picked up and ingested by toddlers. Some airlines may provide additional accommodations when requested in advance (eg, a flight where peanuts are not served).

Box 2
Tips for eating out

Before (prepare)

- Check the menu online to determine if there are feasible meal options
- Call ahead to gauge the restaurant's ability and willingness to accommodate customer's needs
- Carry preprinted cards with information about allergens and warnings about cross-contact (http://www.faiusa.org/?page_ID=D52D2E0F-0925-3542-FBD667C23A000523)
- Carry emergency medications, especially epinephrine

During (communicate)

- Communicate clearly and directly about food allergy. At a restaurant, the communicating personnel includes the wait staff, chef, and/or manager
- Ask about ingredients and method of preparation. Do not trust ingredient lists on menus at face value
- It is best to speak directly to the person making the food

High-risk places for cross-contact (avoid)

- Buffets
- Ice cream parlors
- Bakeries
- Asian restaurants (for peanut and tree nut allergies[16])
- Seafood restaurants (for fish and shellfish allergies)
- Deep fryers, in which oil is reused for different foods and thus may be contaminated by previously cooked foods
- Potlucks and parties where homemade dishes come from a variety of sources/preparers

Patients may be directed to http://www.foodallergy.org/section/managing-food-allergies, http://www.faiusa.org/?page=living_with_food_allergies, and http://cofargroup.org as resources.

Vacation choices, including all-inclusive resorts, cruises, and international travel, are circumstances in which advance planning is highly advised because these are situations in which others prepare most of, if not all, the meals. Potentially less-risky alternatives include accommodations where self-cooking is possible, that is, choosing rooms with kitchenettes, or to ship safe foods ahead to the vacation destination, if economically feasible.

ALLERGEN AVOIDANCE

Nuances of Exposure Risks

The standard of care for the management of food allergy has been strict allergen avoidance. This advice is based on the possibility that exposure could result in allergic reactions.[21,22] However, thresholds of clinical reactivity can vary dramatically among allergic individuals, and even within the same individual.[23–26] In addition, there has been the notion that strict avoidance hastens allergy recovery, but there are limited supportive data on this hypothesis. Recent studies challenge the assumption that strict avoidance is required.[27]

Studies now demonstrate that most children (70%–75%) with egg and milk allergies[28,29] tolerate extensively heated forms of these foods when baked into foods (ie, muffins, waffles). The practitioner should be aware that these studies were performed using recipes outlining a defined amount of allergen cooked at a specific temperature for an exact duration. It is more difficult to know the amount of allergen in commercially prepared foods, which may also vary among batches.

But severe reactions were noted among those patients[28,29] who did not tolerate the extensively heated forms of those foods. In fact, 20% to 35% of those who reacted to extensively heated egg or milk received epinephrine during these physician-supervised food challenges. Exposure to extensively heated forms of milk and egg is not advisable outside a medically supervised setting because of these risks.

There are exceptions for which strict avoidance is not necessarily prescribed despite a diagnosis of food allergy. In pollen-food allergy syndrome (oral allergy syndrome), heat, acid, and proteases break down the unstable allergen, allowing the ingestion of cooked and processed forms without symptoms. Allergists often allow patients with this syndrome to ingest the food[30] if symptoms are mild and limited to the mouth and throat.

Accordingly, clinician experience and discretion is imperative in tailoring avoidance recommendations to the patient's specific situation and degree of sensitivity.

Route of allergen exposure

The route of exposure plays a key role in the risk and severity of the allergic response. Food-allergic reactions predominantly occur following ingestion. It is important to emphasize to patients that life-threatening reactions (involving respiratory or cardiovascular systems) overwhelmingly occur with ingestion when compared with skin or casual airborne exposures. Even in the most highly sensitive individuals, skin or inhalational exposures typically induce limited reactions.[31,32] Misunderstanding this concept is likely to arouse anxiety.

In one study, 1 g of peanut butter was applied for 15 minutes to the intact skin of 281 children who were skin prick test positive to peanut.[33] The allergen challenge was positive in 41% of children, meaning 1 or more hives were present at the site. None of the children experienced a systemic reaction. The study was then extended with blinded placebo-controlled oral challenges within a subset of children. In the contact-positive group, 82% of children reacted to ingesting peanut (including some with life-threatening anaphylaxis), whereas in the contact-negative group, 50% reacted. This result suggests that contact urticaria to peanut is not uncommon among peanut-allergic children. Its presence, in fact, may indicate a higher likelihood of symptoms with ingestion. However, skin contact alone did not induce any systemic reactions in this cohort. Conceivably, perceived systemic reactions to contact exposures (without obvious ingestion) may be explained by inadvertent contact with the food leading to subsequent transfer of allergen from the hands to the mouth or other mucosal surfaces. Alternatively, symptoms may occur from anxiety of exposure.

Inhalational exposures must be differentiated from smells or odors of food. In a double-blind placebo-controlled study, 30 children with clinical histories of severe peanut allergy were challenged by being near and smelling peanut butter.[31] A 6-sq in area of peanut butter was placed 12 in from the children's faces for 10 minutes. No symptoms developed with smelling peanut butter, although there was a respiratory reaction to the placebo inhalant attributed afterward to anxiety.

Box 3
Pearls for allergen avoidance: answers to common questions from patients

Milk

Cow's milk and goat's milk are more than 90% cross-reactive.

Sheep's milk is not a safe alternative.

Shellfish is occasionally dipped in milk to reduce odors.

Kosher pareve products may contain small amounts of milk protein.

Egg

Measles-mumps-rubella vaccines may be given safely to egg-allergic individuals (and is recommended by the American Academy of Pediatrics).

Influenza vaccines may contain a small amount of egg, but recent studies indicate that they may be safely administered in graded doses to most children with egg allergy.[46–48]

Varicella (chicken pox) vaccines do not contain egg.

Peanut

Peanut is a legume (in the same family as beans such as soy). More than 90% of peanut-allergic individuals tolerate soy[49] as well as other legumes. But an exception is that there is a risk of cross-reaction between peanuts and lupine.

Having peanut allergy is associated with developing a tree nut allergy.

Studies[50] show that most allergic individuals can safely eat peanut oil that has been highly refined (but not cold-pressed, expeller-pressed, or extruded peanut oil).

Tree nuts

Cashews and pistachios are highly cross-reactive.[51] Mortadella may contain pistachios.

Walnuts and pecans are highly cross-reactive.[51]

Almonds and hazelnuts are cross-reactive.[51]

Coconut is characterized by the FDA as a tree nut, but allergy is uncommon.

Nutmeg, water chestnuts, and butternut squash are not tree nuts.

Fish and shellfish

Fish and shellfish proteins can become airborne during cooking.

Having an allergy to fish or shellfish is not a contraindication to the use of radiocontrast material.

Noncrustacean shellfish (eg, clams, mussels, oysters, squid) do not have to be identified under FALCPA.

Soy

Soybean, soy, and soya are interchangeable.

Most individuals allergic to soy can safely eat soy lecithin, which contains a trace amount of detectable soy protein.[52,53]

Most allergic individuals can safely eat soybean oil that has been highly refined (not cold-pressed, expeller-pressed, or extruded soybean oil).

Wheat

Spelt is considered allergenically similar to wheat.

Sesame seed

Allergies to other seeds (eg, poppy, sunflower, pumpkin, rapeseed, and flaxseed/linseed) are much less common than sesame allergy.

People who are allergic to one type of seed do not necessarily need to avoid all others, but individuals should consult their physician.

In contrast to odors, aerosolization of food particles can occur with cooking (boiling, steaming, frying) or processing (grating, shredding, grinding), which in turn may trigger symptoms. Food allergens are proteins (as opposed to fats or carbohydrates); thus, airborne food proteins can induce allergic reactions. In contrast, smell from a noncooking food, such as peanut butter, results from airborne volatile organic compounds given off continuously by foods; these compounds are not allergenic. In highly sensitive individuals, inhalational contact with aerosolized food proteins can induce asthmatic or respiratory reactions[32,34] and sometimes skin symptoms. These individuals should avoid situations in which aerosolized food may be inhaled, for example, being near steam and vapors from cooking or being in close proximity to grinding or other handling of the allergenic food.

The clinician should reassure patients and their families that contact and inhalational exposures, compared with ingestion, carry very low risk for inducing life-threatening reactions. Moreover, inhalational exposures to aerosolized food proteins should be differentiated from smells or odors. It has already been well established that the quality of life of families and patients with food allergy is significantly affected,[35–39] and thus, the practitioner can play a key role in allaying disproportionate fears, hence reducing anxiety.

A type of casual exposure that could result in systemic symptoms is contact with saliva through shared utensils and straws or by kissing. Food-allergic individuals should be warned that exposure may occur through kissing, specifically passionate kissing. Studies indicate that 5% to 16% of patients report reactions from kissing.[40,41] In order to determine the time course of peanut protein in saliva after a meal of peanut butter, one study used Ara h 1 as a marker protein.[42] Of 36 individuals, 30 had detectable levels of Ara h 1 at 5 minutes after ingesting 2 tablespoons of peanut butter. Of these 30 subjects, 26 (87%) had undetectable levels of the protein after 1 hour without any interventions (detection limit, 15–20 ng/mL). None had detectable levels several hours later following a subsequent peanut-free meal.

Interventions after a peanut butter meal were assessed in the same study, including brushing teeth, brushing and rinsing, rinsing, waiting then brushing, and waiting then

Table 1
Nonfood items in which food ingredients may be found

Nonfood Items	Potential Allergens
Vaccines	Milk, chicken, and gelatin proteins Egg (see **Box 3**)
Medications	Lactose: Some dry powder inhalers are prescribed for asthma,[54] although the level of milk protein contamination, if any, is unknown Oral medications (check labels, specifically inactive ingredients) Egg lecithin: propofol (general anesthetic) Risk of a reaction is presumed to be low Soy lecithin: certain inhalers Risk of a reaction seems very low[4,5] Egg lysozyme (enzyme found in egg white): nasal decongestants[55]
Cosmetics	Milk, tree nut oils, wheat, and soy[56,57]
Modeling Dough	Wheat
Finger Paints	Egg white
Latex Gloves	Casein (used as antistick agent)[58]
Alcoholic Beverages	Egg, cow's milk, and seafood (used as clarifying agents) Tree nut flavoring

chewing gum.[42] None of these interventions consistently resulted in undetectable levels, although detected levels were lower than the threshold levels reported to trigger reactions (<17 μg of peanut protein per 5 mL of saliva). The immediate interventions were less effective than those involving a waiting period. Results may also vary with other allergens or forms of peanut. There is one case report of a mild reaction to peanut (lip swelling and perioral pruritus) despite a 2-hour wait, brushing teeth, rinsing, and chewing gum.[43]

Food-allergic reactions from blood transfusions or semen are theoretically possible. Individual case reports can be found in the literature.[44,45] Possible explanations for allergic reactions include the reduction of plasma fractions in blood prepared for transfusion and recent ingestion by partners of large amounts of the allergen before intimate contact.

Additional pearls regarding allergen avoidance are provided in **Box 3**.

FOOD ALLERGENS IN NONFOOD ITEMS

Nonfood items may contain food ingredients, such as medications, vaccines, cosmetics, and craft supplies. See **Table 1** for specific examples.

SUMMARY

The everyday task of food avoidance presents challenges and uncertainties. Those affected by food allergy are constantly gauging risks associated with buying prepackaged foods, eating at restaurants, attending social functions, traveling, and other activities of daily life. US labeling laws have, for the most part, facilitated the ability to avoid allergens in packaged foods under FDA regulation, although interpretation of advisory labeling is more complex. Eating outside, at restaurants in particular, requires direct communication between the consumer and the food preparer. Care must be taken to avoid cross-contact. Patients must be aware of food allergens in unanticipated sources, such as vaccines and medications. Patients should be reminded that salivary transfer, which can occur through shared utensils and straws or passionate kissing, is also a concern. Implementing these tools of avoidance is essential to avoid serious allergic reactions, which can be life threatening. Medical practitioners play a key role in guiding patients through the difficulties of food avoidance.

REFERENCES

1. Lack G. Clinical practice. Food allergy. N Engl J Med 2008;359:1252–60.
2. Aldamiz-Echevarria L, Bilbao A, Andrade F, et al. Fatty acid deficiency profile in children with food allergy managed with elimination diets. Acta Paediatr 2008;97:1572–6.
3. Center for Food Safety and Applied Nutrition. Available at: www.cfsan.fda.gov. Accessed September 21, 2010.
4. Simons E, Weiss CC, Furlong TJ, et al. Impact of ingredient labeling practices on food allergic consumers. Ann Allergy Asthma Immunol 2005;95:426–8.
5. Awazuhara H, Kawai H, Baba M, et al. Antigenicity of the proteins in soy lecithin and soy oil in soybean allergy. Clin Exp Allergy 1998;28:1559–64.
6. Pieretti MM, Chung D, Pacenza R, et al. Audit of manufactured products: use of allergen advisory labels and identification of labeling ambiguities. J Allergy Clin Immunol 2009;124:337–41.

7. Hefle SL, Furlong TJ, Niemann L, et al. Consumer attitudes and risks associated with packaged foods having advisory labeling regarding the presence of peanuts. J Allergy Clin Immunol 2007;120:171–6.
8. Noimark L, Gardner J, Warner JO. Parents' attitudes when purchasing products for children with nut allergy: a UK perspective. Pediatr Allergy Immunol 2009;20: 500–4.
9. Jones RT, Squillace DL, Yunginger JW. Anaphylaxis in a milk-allergic child after ingestion of milk-contaminated kosher-pareve-labeled "dairy-free" dessert. Ann Allergy 1992;68:223–7.
10. Crotty MP, Taylor SL. Risks associated with foods having advisory milk labeling. J Allergy Clin Immunol 2010;125:935–7.
11. Ford LS, Taylor SL, Pacenza R, et al. Food allergen advisory labeling and product contamination with egg, milk, and peanut. J Allergy Clin Immunol 2010;126: 384–5.
12. Sampson MA, Munoz-Furlong A, Sicherer SH. Risk-taking and coping strategies of adolescents and young adults with food allergy. J Allergy Clin Immunol 2006; 117:1440.
13. Taylor SL, Baumert JL. Cross-contamination of foods and implications for food allergic patients. Curr Allergy Asthma Rep 2010;10:265–70.
14. Sicherer SH, Furlong TJ, Munoz-Furlong A, et al. A voluntary registry for peanut and tree nut allergy: characteristics of the first 5149 registrants. J Allergy Clin Immunol 2001;108:128–32.
15. Perry TT, Conover-Walker MK, Pome A, et al. Distribution of peanut allergen in the environment. J Allergy Clin Immunol 2004;113:973–6.
16. Furlong TJ, DeSimone J, Sicherer SH. Peanut and tree nut allergic reactions in restaurants and other food establishments. J Allergy Clin Immunol 2001;108: 867–70.
17. Ahuja R, Sicherer SH. Food-allergy management from the perspective of restaurant and food establishment personnel. Ann Allergy Asthma Immunol 2007;98: 344–8.
18. Sicherer SH, Furlong TJ, DeSimone J, et al. Self-reported allergic reactions to peanut on commercial airliners. J Allergy Clin Immunol 1999;104:186–9.
19. Comstock SS, DeMera R, Vega LC, et al. Allergic reactions to peanuts, tree nuts, and seeds aboard commercial airliners. Ann Allergy Asthma Immunol 2008;101:51–6.
20. Greenhawt MJ, McMorris MS, Furlong TJ. Self-reported allergic reactions to peanut and tree nuts occurring on commercial airlines. J Allergy Clin Immunol 2009;124:598–9.
21. Yu JW, Kagan R, Verreault N, et al. Accidental ingestions in children with peanut allergy. J Allergy Clin Immunol 2006;118:466–72.
22. Boyano-Martinez T, Garcia-Ara C, Pedrosa M, et al. Accidental allergic reactions in children allergic to cow's milk proteins. J Allergy Clin Immunol 2009;123:883–8.
23. Taylor SL, Hefle SL, Bindslev-Jensen C, et al. Factors affecting the determination of threshold doses for allergenic foods: how much is too much? J Allergy Clin Immunol 2002;109:24–30.
24. Taylor SL, Hefle SL, Bindslev-Jensen C, et al. A consensus protocol for the determination of the threshold doses for allergenic foods: how much is too much? Clin Exp Allergy 2004;34:689–95.
25. Sicherer SH, Morrow EH, Sampson HA. Dose-response in double-blind, placebo-controlled oral food challenges in children with atopic dermatitis. J Allergy Clin Immunol 2000;105:582–6.

26. Flinterman AE, Pasmans SG, Hoekstra MO, et al. Determination of no-observed-adverse-effect levels and eliciting doses in a representative group of peanut-sensitized children. J Allergy Clin Immunol 2006;117:448–54.
27. Kim JS, Sicherer S. Should food avoidance be strict in prevention and treatment of food allergy? Curr Opin Allergy Clin Immunol 2010;10:252–7.
28. Nowak-Wegrzyn A, Bloom KA, Sicherer SH, et al. Tolerance to extensively heated milk in children with cow's milk allergy. J Allergy Clin Immunol 2008; 122:342–7.
29. Lemon-Mule H, Sampson HA, Sicherer SH, et al. Immunologic changes in children with egg allergy ingesting extensively heated egg. J Allergy Clin Immunol 2008;122:977–83.
30. Ma S, Sicherer SH, Nowak-Wegrzyn A. A survey on the management of pollen-food allergy syndrome in allergy practices. J Allergy Clin Immunol 2003;112: 784–8.
31. Simonte SJ, Ma S, Mofidi S, et al. Relevance of casual contact with peanut butter in children with peanut allergy. J Allergy Clin Immunol 2003;112:180–2.
32. Roberts G, Golder N, Lack G. Bronchial challenges with aerosolized food in asthmatic, food-allergic children. Allergy 2002;57:713–7.
33. Wainstein BK, Kashef S, Ziegler M, et al. Frequency and significance of immediate contact reactions to peanut in peanut-sensitive children. Clin Exp Allergy 2007;37:839–45.
34. Tonnel AB, Tillie-Leblond I, Botelho AD, et al. Severe acute asthma associated with raw meat cutting. Ann Allergy Asthma Immunol 2009;102:348.
35. Sicherer SH, Noone SA, Munoz-Furlong A. The impact of childhood food allergy on quality of life. Ann Allergy Asthma Immunol 2001;87:461–4.
36. Marklund B, Ahlstedt S, Nordstrom G. Food hypersensitivity and quality of life. Curr Opin Allergy Clin Immunol 2007;7:279–87.
37. Avery NJ, King RM, Knight S, et al. Assessment of quality of life in children with peanut allergy. Pediatr Allergy Immunol 2003;14:378–82.
38. Bollinger ME, Dahlquist LM, Mudd K, et al. The impact of food allergy on the daily activities of children and their families. Ann Allergy Asthma Immunol 2006;96: 415–21.
39. Primeau MN, Kagan R, Joseph L, et al. The psychological burden of peanut allergy as perceived by adults with peanut allergy and the parents of peanut-allergic children. Clin Exp Allergy 2000;30:1135–43.
40. Hallett R, Haapanen LA, Teuber SS. Food allergies and kissing. N Engl J Med 2002;346:1833–4.
41. Eriksson NE, Moller C, Werner S, et al. The hazards of kissing when you are food allergic. A survey on the occurrence of kiss-induced allergic reactions among 1139 patients with self-reported food hypersensitivity. J Investig Allergol Clin Immunol 2003;13:149–54.
42. Maloney JM, Chapman MD, Sicherer SH. Peanut allergen exposure through saliva: assessment and interventions to reduce exposure. J Allergy Clin Immunol 2006;118:719–24.
43. Wuthrich B, Dascher M, Borelli S. Kiss-induced allergy to peanut. Allergy 2001; 56:913.
44. Bansal AS, Chee R, Nagendran V, et al. Dangerous liaison: sexually transmitted allergic reaction to Brazil nuts. J Investig Allergol Clin Immunol 2007; 17:189–91.
45. Arnold DM, Blajchman MA, Ditomasso J, et al. Passive transfer of peanut hypersensitivity by fresh frozen plasma. Arch Intern Med 2007;167:853–4.

46. Clark AT, Skypala I, Leech SC, et al. British Society for Allergy and Clinical Immunology guidelines for the management of egg allergy. Clin Exp Allergy 2010;40:1116–29.
47. Gagnon R, Primeau MN, Des Roches A, et al. Safe vaccination of patients with egg allergy with an adjuvanted pandemic H1N1 vaccine. J Allergy Clin Immunol 2010;126:317–23.
48. Chung EY, Huang L, Schneider L. Safety of influenza vaccine administration in egg-allergic patients. Pediatrics 2010;125:e1024–30.
49. Bernhisel-Broadbent J, Taylor S, Sampson HA. Cross-allergenicity in the legume botanical family in children with food hypersensitivity. II. Laboratory correlates. J Allergy Clin Immunol 1989;84:701–9.
50. Moneret-Vautrin DA, Kanny G. Update on threshold doses of food allergens: implications for patients and the food industry. Curr Opin Allergy Clin Immunol 2004;4:215–9.
51. Maloney JM, Rudengren M, Ahlstedt S, et al. The use of serum-specific IgE measurements for the diagnosis of peanut, tree nut, and seed allergy. J Allergy Clin Immunol 2008;122:145–51.
52. Gu X, Beardslee T, Zeece M, et al. Identification of IgE-binding proteins in soy lecithin. Int Arch Allergy Immunol 2001;126:218–25.
53. Palm M, Moneret-Vautrin DA, Kanny G, et al. Food allergy to egg and soy lecithins. Allergy 1999;54:1116–7.
54. Nowak-Wegrzyn A, Shapiro GG, Beyer K, et al. Contamination of dry powder inhalers for asthma with milk proteins containing lactose. J Allergy Clin Immunol 2004;113:558–60.
55. Artesani MC, Donnanno S, Cavagni G, et al. Egg sensitization caused by immediate hypersensitivity reaction to drug-containing lysozyme. Ann Allergy Asthma Immunol 2008;101:105.
56. Codreanu F, Morisset M, Cordebar V, et al. Risk of allergy to food proteins in topical medicinal agents and cosmetics. Eur Ann Allergy Clin Immunol 2006;38:126–30.
57. Wang J, Nowak-Wegrzyn A. Reactions of 2 young children with milk allergy after cutaneous exposure to milk-containing cosmetic products. Arch Pediatr Adolesc Med 2004;158:1089–90.
58. Ylitalo L, Makinen-Kiljunen S, Turjanmaa K, et al. Cow's milk casein, a hidden allergen in natural rubber latex gloves. J Allergy Clin Immunol 1999;104:177–80.

Managing Food Allergies in Schools and Camps

Kim Mudd, RN, MSN*, Robert A. Wood, MD

KEYWORDS

• Food allergies • School • Camp • Food allergy action plan

Managing food allergies in schools and camps involves a community approach. The goal is to create a safe environment that still allows for maximal growth and development of the food-allergic child. The process involves building a supportive structure based on education and planning and then dismantling the more restrictive components through constant revision. The product is an individualized strategy that not only meets the needs of a food-allergic child but also supports the development of a food-allergic adolescent.

THE PRESCHOOL-AGED FOOD-ALLERGIC CHILD

By the time the child reaches preschool age, most families and caregivers have a constructed a significant protective structure around their food-allergic child to prevent food exposures at home, and to a lesser extent at the homes of family and friends. The thought of sending a food-allergic child to preschool or day camp without their carefully orchestrated plans is daunting to most parents. Families are very anxious about the child's safety[1] although the level of anxiety is not necessarily related to the severity of previous reactions, the need to treat with epinephrine, or a food allergy–related hospital admission.[2] Despite the fact that many families of food-allergic children would prefer a food-free (or at least, allergen-free) preschool situation, a realistic goal is to create a safe environment. The key is to implement the necessary structure and restrictions to balance safety with a situation that allows for growth and development. The structure should include both preventive strategies and food allergy emergency treatment plans. The preventive plans may include more restrictive techniques such as peanut-free policies and/or allergen-free tables. The level of restriction should reflect the personality and the developmental stage of the food-allergic child.

Preschool-aged children are prone developmentally to food sharing and messy eating behaviors. Many exhibit hand-to-mouth activities, all of which put them at

Johns Hopkins Division of Pediatric Allergy and Immunology, Johns Hopkins Hospital, 600 North Wolfe Street, CMSC 1105, Baltimore, MD 21287, USA
* Corresponding author.
E-mail address: kmudd2@jhmi.edu

Pediatr Clin N Am 58 (2011) 471–480
doi:10.1016/j.pcl.2011.02.009 **pediatric.theclinics.com**
0031-3955/11/$ – see front matter

risk for inadvertent ingestion exposures. Creating a safe environment for preschool-aged food-allergic children starts with prevention techniques, such as appropriate avoidance measures, proper cleaning techniques, and a "No Food Sharing" policy. Most of the avoidance effort should focus on preventing allergen ingestion because the largest "risk" to any food-allergic individual is actually consuming an allergenic food. Details of avoidance measures including label reading and prevention of cross-contamination are discussed in detail elsewhere in this issue in the article by Kim and Sicherer. In general, any food consumed by a food-allergic child needs to be pre-approved or provided by the family of the food-allergic child, or checked by a caregiver well versed in food label reading and preparation. A shared cookie can circumvent all of the layers of pre-approval and planning, necessitating a "No Food Sharing" policy. This policy ideally should include all children, not only the food-allergic child. Planning also should include a contingency plan for impromptu "special treats" that may appear in a classroom at birthdays as well as the potential consumption of "nonfood items." For example, there is wheat in molding clay and egg in certain finger paints, and preschool-aged children may ingest these "nonfood items" during an art project.

Proper cleaning is another important part of the prevention strategy. Cleaning policies should reflect the evidence-based research on allergen removal. Food allergens can be effectively removed from eating surfaces with household cleaners such as soap and water, sanitizing wipes, and spray cleaners, using usual cleaning techniques. Allergens can also be removed from hands using soap and water or wipes.[3] Therefore, foods can be prepared and served in a safe manner using proper cleaning and hand-washing procedures. It is noteworthy that hand sanitizers such as antibacterial gels are not effective at removing allergens,[3] which means that for the purpose of "allergy cleaning," use of hand sanitizer is not an acceptable alternative to hand washing. Areas where children eat or play with must be properly cleaned before and after eating, and proper hand washing needs to be enforced.

Creating a safe environment also includes having people and plans to recognize a food-allergic reaction and initiate a treatment plan. In the event of a food allergy reaction, everyone responsible for the food-allergic child needs to be able to respond appropriately. Written food allergy emergency treatment plans include specific instructions on symptom recognition and treatment. Because it is not possible to predict the severity of a reaction based on a previous reaction,[4] it is prudent to prepare for a severe event. As shown in **Fig. 1**, a Food Allergy Action Plan lists potential symptoms matched with appropriate treatment including medications, doses, and monitoring plans.

Many preschool programs choose to implement "Peanut-Free" or "Peanut/Tree Nut-Free" policies. These food bans take several different forms, from allergen-safe tables in the cafeteria to school-wide, food-specific bans. There is evidence that school-wide "peanut-free guidelines" are successful in decreasing the amount of peanut present in lunches brought from home,[5] but it is not clear that the allergen-free guidelines actually result in fewer allergen exposures.[6] There is no agreement on the effectiveness or need for food bans (**Table 1**). In general, food bans and allergen-free seating may be helpful in preschool and early elementary school children, but are generally not necessary in upper elementary school-aged children.[6]

It is clear that it is not feasible to eliminate all allergenic foods from public venues including preschools, schools, and camps. The most commonsense approach to allergen avoidance is to tailor the allergen avoidance plan to the developmental age of the child. Most of the responsibility for establishing and maintaining a safe environment for the preschool-aged child obviously lies with the adults, but preschool-aged children can actively participate in managing their food allergy. These children can learn not to accept food from peers, and can be taught that not all foods are "safe." Although it is impossible to attain an allergen-free environment, a written food allergy emergency treatment plan, an increase in allergen awareness combined with hand washing, cleaning of eating surfaces, and high levels of supervision to prevent food sharing all work together to create a safe environment. Most of these measures also have a high level of "buy-in" from both allergic and nonallergic families. After all, everyone wants their children to have adequate supervision, clean hands, and a clean table when they eat.

SCHOOL-AGED CHILDREN

During the late preschool and early school years, children are more verbal and can follow rules such as "no sharing of food." As children and their peers develop an understanding of the potential implications of a food allergy diagnosis, a safe environment no longer requires the highly restrictive controls that were appropriate at the preschool level. Camp and school environments offer food-allergic children an opportunity to practice food allergy management skills. Involving children in the process of developing a plan for lunch, for a school field trip, or including them in the discussions about choosing a camp promotes shared responsibility. Children who observe this type of adaptive behavior are more likely to be ready to assume self-management.[1] Children who adopt a negative attitude that focuses on limitations imposed by their food allergy are more likely to be distressed by their food allergy as compared with children who adopt a positive perspective that focuses on strengths and coping strategies.[7] Children can become overwhelmed by the process or the lack of coping demonstrated by the adults in their life. Negative parental attitudes toward food allergy and maternal anxiety are related to greater child anxiety.[7] Children who have been "programmed to be anxious" by the adults in their lives have a level of anxiety surrounding their food allergy that is not concordant with the severity of their food allergy or frequency of reactions.[2] Some amount of caution is of course necessary to maintain vigilance. However, maladaptive behavior such as overresponding to perceived risk or anxiety that interferes with activity should be addressed with a health care professional.[7]

As with preschool-aged children, growth and development issues have to be balanced with safety. School-aged children do not need the same level of supervision and restriction as preschool-aged children, but they are not ready to manage their food allergies on their own. Most school-aged kids know and can follow the rules to avoid most food allergen exposures, but they still need support and supervision. Some parents are apprehensive about moving their food-allergic child from the relatively contained environment of preschool to the larger, more chaotic, less controlled environment of school. Everyone realizes that the plan that worked for the 2-hours-a-day, 3-days-a-week, preschool program is completely inadequate for the 5-days-a-week, day-long demands of kindergarten.

One of the revisions to the safety structure as children transition from preschool to school is the relaxing of food bans, allergen-free tables, and hand washing. At some point, having the entire student population wash up after lunch or snacks becomes an unrealistic expectation and having a food-allergic child sit at the "allergy table" becomes onerous. As children and their peers develop impulse control and understand the rationale for allergen avoidance, allowing food-allergic children to sit with their friends and supportive peers is much less socially isolating. One of the obvious concerns is that the lack of hand washing and sharing of table space will result in

Food Allergy Action Plan

Name: ______________________ **D.O.B.:** __/__/__

Allergy to: ______________________

Weight: ______ lbs. **Asthma:** ☐ Yes (higher risk for a severe reaction) ☐ No

Place Student's Picture Here

Extremely reactive to the following foods: ______________________
THEREFORE:
☐ If checked, give epinephrine immediately for ANY symptoms if the allergen was *likely* eaten.
☐ If checked, give epinephrine immediately if the allergen was *definitely* eaten, even if no symptoms are noted.

Any SEVERE SYMPTOMS after suspected or known ingestion:

One or more of the following:
LUNG: Short of breath, wheeze, repetitive cough
HEART: Pale, blue, faint, weak pulse, dizzy, confused
THROAT: Tight, hoarse, trouble breathing/swallowing
MOUTH: Obstructive swelling (tongue and/or lips)
SKIN: Many hives over body

Or **combination** of symptoms from different body areas:
SKIN: Hives, itchy rashes, swelling (e.g., eyes, lips)
GUT: Vomiting, crampy pain

→

1. **INJECT EPINEPHRINE IMMEDIATELY**
2. Call 911
3. Begin monitoring (see box below)
4. Give additional medications:*
   -Antihistamine
   -Inhaler (bronchodilator) if asthma

*Antihistamines & inhalers/bronchodilators are not to be depended upon to treat a severe reaction (anaphylaxis). USE EPINEPHRINE.

MILD SYMPTOMS ONLY:

MOUTH: Itchy mouth
SKIN: A few hives around mouth/face, mild itch
GUT: Mild nausea/discomfort

→

1. **GIVE ANTIHISTAMINE**
2. Stay with student; alert healthcare professionals and parent
3. If symptoms progress (see above), USE EPINEPHRINE
4. Begin monitoring (see box below)

Medications/Doses

Epinephrine (brand and dose): ______________________
Antihistamine (brand and dose): ______________________
Other (e.g., inhaler-bronchodilator if asthmatic): ______________________

Monitoring

Stay with student; alert healthcare professionals and parent. Tell rescue squad epinephrine was given; request an ambulance with epinephrine. Note time when epinephrine was administered. A second dose of epinephrine can be given 5 minutes or more after the first if symptoms persist or recur. For a severe reaction, consider keeping student lying on back with legs raised. Treat student even if parents cannot be reached. See back/attached for auto-injection technique.

Parent/Guardian Signature **Date** **Physician/Healthcare Provider Signature** **Date**

TURN FORM OVER **Form provided courtesy of FAAN (www.foodallergy.org) 7/2010**

Fig. 1. Food Allergy and Anaphylaxis Network food allergy action plan. Copyright © The Food Allergy and Anaphylaxis Network. Reprinted with permission. Available at: http://www.foodallergy.org/files/FAAP.pdf.

a "casual exposure" significant enough to cause a systemic reaction. The current research of casual types of exposures have focused on people with peanut allergy because peanut is a food staple in many nonallergic diets, peanut allergy is one of the most prevalent food allergies, and this allergy is responsible for more severe reactions than any other food.[4,8] One study looked at the amount of peanut protein present in samples collected from lunch tables, water fountains, desks, and food preparation areas in 6 different schools. None of the eating areas, food preparation areas, or desks had detectable peanut protein. In that same study, researchers tried to detect peanut protein in the air under several different conditions, including by an open peanut butter

EPIPEN Auto-Injector and EPIPEN Jr Auto-Injector Directions

- First, remove the EPIPEN Auto-Injector from the plastic carrying case
- Pull off the blue safety release cap
- Hold orange tip near outer thigh (always apply to thigh)
- Swing and firmly push orange tip against outer thigh. Hold on thigh for approximately 10 seconds. Remove the EPIPEN Auto-Injector and massage the area for 10 more seconds

EPIPEN 2-PAK® | EPIPEN Jr 2-PAK®
(Epinephrine) Auto-Injectors 0.3/0.15mg

DEY® and the Dey logo, EpiPen®, EpiPen 2-Pak®, and EpiPen Jr 2-Pak® are registered trademarks of Dey Pharma, L.P.

Twinject® 0.3 mg and Twinject® 0.15 mg Directions

Remove caps labeled "1" and "2."

Place rounded tip against outer thigh, press down hard until needle penetrates. Hold for 10 seconds, then remove.

SECOND DOSE ADMINISTRATION: If symptoms don't improve after 10 minutes, administer second dose:

Unscrew rounded tip. Pull syringe from barrel by holding blue collar at needle base.

Slide yellow collar off plunger.

Put needle into thigh through skin, push plunger down all the way, and remove.

Adrenaclick™ 0.3 mg and Adrenaclick™ 0.15 mg Directions

Remove GREY caps labeled "1" and "2."

Place RED rounded tip against outer thigh, press down hard until needle penetrates. Hold for 10 seconds, then remove.

A food allergy response kit should contain at least two doses of epinephrine, other medications as noted by the student's physician, and a copy of this Food Allergy Action Plan.

A kit must accompany the student if he/she is off school grounds (i.e., field trip).

Contacts

Call 911 (Rescue squad: (__)____-______) Doctor:__________ Phone: (__)____-______

Parent/Guardian:________________ Phone: (__)____-______

Other Emergency Contacts

Name/Relationship: ________________ Phone: (__)____-______

Name/Relationship: ________________ Phone: (__)____-______

Form provided courtesy of FAAN (www.foodallergy.org) 7/2010

Fig. 1. (*continued*)

jar and while nonallergic subjects ate peanut butter and jelly sandwiches. Airborne peanut protein was not detectable.[3] When peanut-allergic children, many of whom had reported reactions to inhaled peanut, were purposely exposed to inhaled peanut fumes, none of the children experienced a respiratory or systemic reaction.[9] Other studies have looked at reactions in children with known peanut sensitivity who had peanut butter applied directly to their skin. It turns out that the skin is a fairly effective barrier. None of the children experienced a systemic reaction, even those who developed a rash at the site where the peanut protein was applied.[9,10] The consensus is that

Table 1
Pro/con food bans

PRO	CON
"Loaded Gun" argument: reduce the chance of exposure	"No peanut detectors" to enforce food bans
Young children cannot bear responsibility of avoiding allergens	Causes an undue burden on children without a peanut allergy
Food contamination of shared equipment resulting in contact exposures	"Slippery Slope" argument: if you ban peanuts, why not ban other allergy foods
Food sharing is a common behavior in children	"False Sense of Security" argument
School bullying difficult to control	Schools should prepare students for the "real world"
"Community responsibility" approach to safety	Feelings of divisiveness

Adapted from Young MC, Munoz-Furlong A, Sicherer SH. Management of food allergies in school: a perspective for allergists. J Allergy Clin Immunol 2009;124(2):178; with permission.

90% of highly peanut-allergic children would not experience a systemic or respiratory reaction with "casual contact" to peanut.[9] The lack of evidence to support measurable amounts of allergens from casual exposures does not negate a common sense approach to allergen avoidance. Activities that involve allergenic foods (eg, peanut butter bird feeders, wheat-containing modeling clay, using pudding as finger paint, churning butter, using peanuts in the classroom as a counting aid) should not technically involve food ingestion, but putting food-allergic children in such a situation lacks common sense.

Another repercussion of the transition from preschool to school is the issue of bullying. Bullying behavior has become a major concern in school-aged children. Bullying behaviors include "direct bullying" such as verbal abuse or physical aggression, and "relational victimization" such as intentionally excluding someone or targeting someone as a scapegoat.[11] "Cyber bullying" is a relatively new phenomenon that includes threatening behaviors and behaviors that are meant to embarrass or socially exclude someone through e-mail, cell phone or text messages, Twitter, Facebook, and Internet sites.[12] The actual number of kids who are bullied is uncertain, but it is clear that children with food allergies are not immune to bullying behavior.[13] Bullying behaviors in the school setting should be addressed directly with school officials, as many schools have antibullying policies. In addition, parents need to be aware of the role of electronic technology in cyber bullying.[12]

It is clear that camp facilities and schools need comprehensive plans for managing food allergies in community settings. The Food Allergy and Anaphylaxis Network developed a set of guidelines useful in creating plans (Available at http://www.foodallergy.org/page/school-guidelines-for-managing-students-with-food-allergies). To date, 12 US states have adopted statewide guidelines to establish standards of care and current best practices. These guidelines are to meant assist local school systems in developing policies and procedures to provide consistent and safe care to food-allergic students. A current listing on the State guidelines is available at http://www.foodallergy.org/page/statewideguidelines-for-schools. The existing guidelines and policies are used as a framework to create an Individualized Health Care Plan (IHCP). According to the US National Association of School Nurses Position Statement, the IHCP is to specify the health care services required for students who have health care needs that "affect or have the potential to affect safe and optimal school attendance and academic performance." These written plans are developed collaboratively by the school nurse with input from the student, family, health care providers, and school staff. IHCPs are used to manage the potential risks associated with food allergy, to facilitate communication, and to coordinate and evaluate the care specified. The plans are dynamic documents that are meant to be evaluated and revised (as appropriate) on a yearly basis. The IHCP should include plans for allergen avoidance measures that focus on ingestion prevention and noningestion-type exposures that have the potential to expose food-allergic individuals to significant amounts of allergens. Because it is impossible to eliminate the potential risk of an allergen exposure, IHCPs need to specify food allergy emergency actions in the classroom, cafeteria, gymnasium, and playground, on field trips, and for extracurricular events; epinephrine administration and storage; student self-carrying of medications; emergency medical system activation; and transportation issues.

Some situations require more than an IHCP. Section 504 of the US Rehabilitation Act of 1973 is a piece of civil rights law that prohibits discrimination against individuals with disabilities in public and private programs and activities that receive financial assistance from the federal government. The Americans with Disabilities Act (ADA) prohibits discrimination against individuals with disabilities (including food allergy) and extends this protection to the full range of state and local government services, programs, or activities regardless of whether they receive federal assistance. In general, 504 Plans are used when food allergy discrimination has the potential to affect a food-allergic student's education. 504 Plans are legal documents with the backing of the US Department of Education, Office of Civil Rights.

Several other countries support the goals of The Food Allergy and Anaphylaxis Alliance to promote country-specific guidelines and policies to manage students with food allergy in schools and other child care settings. Countries including Sweden, China, Italy, Germany, Israel, New Zealand, The Netherlands, and Japan have food allergy management, education, and anaphylaxis forms available in many different languages (available at http://www.FoodAllergyAlliance.org). Anaphylaxis Canada (available at http://www.anaphylaxis.ca) has a resource section for schools that details a "Safe4kids" program, which includes sample policies, a Handbook for School Boards, and Anaphylaxis Alert Forms. The Quebec Food Allergy Association (available at http://www.aqaa.qc.ca/accueil.asp) provides similar information, guidance, and forms in French. The Department of Education and Skills in the United Kingdom has published a document *Managing Medicines an Schools and Early Years Settings* (available at http://www.anaphylaxis.org.uk/information/Schools/information-for-schools.aspx), which delineates the roles of local authorities, health trusts, and schools to create policies that support children with medical needs.

Even with the best avoidance plan in place, food-allergic reactions inevitably happen. In one study of food-allergic reactions in schools and preschools, close to 20% of the children experienced a food-allergic reaction in the school setting.[14] Plans are only as good as their implementation, and there are multiple cases of deficient plans or plans written and not followed in food-allergic emergencies.[6,15] The school needs time to write, revise, and initiate the plan. Frequently some amount of training is necessary. School nurses and teachers are not usually available in the summer, and trying to initiate a meeting and write a plan in the weeks before the school year can be challenging. The conversation about a written food allergy plan needs to be initiated well in advance of the school year. Therefore, it is suggested that food-allergic families need to plan to meet with the school nurse and school administration before everyone leaves for the summer holiday. A second meeting before the school year begins is helpful to ensure that training is completed, medications are in place, and the plan is clear before the food-allergic child walks through the door. It is important that plans are in place before the school year starts. Imagine the potential disaster if an uninformed teacher promises the class a sundae bar or pizza day as a reward for project completion and then has to pull the plug because of a student's food allergy.

Camps and their staff need access to the same type of information that goes into preparing an IHCP. According to the Food Allergy and Anaphylaxis Network's Guidelines for Managing Food Allergies at Camp (available at http://www.foodallergy.org/section/guidelines), families should inform the camp director of the food allergies early in the process in order to give the camp time to hire and/or train appropriate personnel. As with schools, all of the people who will be responsible for the food-allergic child need to be aware of the food allergy and the proper steps to avoid food allergy reactions, as well as how to respond in the event of a food-related reaction.

As children enter late elementary and middle school years, they need to build on their management skills with the goal of progressing toward independence. At this age, children should be responsible enough to self-carry auto-injectors and make appropriate food choices outside the home setting. Many food-allergic children are ready to self-administer epinephrine by age 8 or 10 years. By age 12 or 13, children need to be well on their way to recognizing symptoms and initiating a food allergy emergency treatment plan, including self-administration of epinephrine. These skills need to be in place before food-allergic children can attain the independence they desire in the teenage years.

TEENAGED FOOD-ALLERGIC INDIVIDUALS

The teenage years can be challenging. After all, being a teen or young adult is one of the risk factors of death from food-induced anaphylaxis (**Box 1**).[16] During this time of transition adolescents spend more of their time with friends, exploring their independence, and taking risk. The development of this peer network is an important goal of adolescence. The support from friends is important in protecting adolescents from bullying. High levels of support from friends seem to have a protective effect from the negative impact of bullying behaviors.[11] However, the very same peer group can put negative pressure on adolescent behavior. Adolescents and young adults are more concerned about fitting in with their peer group than with having a food-

Box 1
Risk factors for fatal anaphylaxis

- Teen or young adult
- Asthma
- Peanut, tree nut, or seafood allergy
- Delay in administration of epinephrine
- Eating restaurant food
- Reactions that do not involve skin symptoms
- Denying symptoms
- Concurrent intake of alcohol
- Reliance on oral antihistamines to treat symptoms of anaphylaxis
- Lack of reaction management education from health care providers

allergic reaction, and they balance safety with quality of life issues.[17] Because teens have a poor perception of their health needs and a sense of invulnerability,[18] they can make bad decisions. In one study of food-allergic adolescents and young adults, more than half of the adolescents reported trying a food that they knew contained a known allergen.[19] In another study, a majority of teens reported checking food labels only on "new" foods and routinely trying foods that likely contain food allergens.[13] Teens and college-aged students report trying food allergens despite a history of anaphylaxis.[18]

Even when they know what the "right" or expected behavior should be, teens will still balance safety with convenience. When asked about carrying self-injectable epinephrine, two-thirds reported carrying epinephrine "at all times." This same group actually had epinephrine available mainly during times of travel or eating out and not during social events like parties and dances or sport events, or when carrying the epinephrine was inconvenient because of tight clothing.[19] A study of food-allergic college-age individuals showed an alarmingly low number of young adults who had self-injectable epinephrine available on campus.[18]

By the time food-allergic children reach high school, the structure of the food allergy management plan has been condensed to a few vital parts consisting of education and support. Teens need appropriate knowledge about their food allergy and potential implications, because they will use the available information to assess the risk and make informed decisions.[17] In addition, teens want their peers to know about food allergy and they identify classmates, friends, and teachers as the "most needy group" for education.[19] It is obvious that sharing specific information on a teen's food allergy with the entire school or camp would likely be viewed as an invasion of privacy by the teen. However, teens want their peers to know about the potential seriousness of food-allergic reactions,[13] and sharing general information about food allergen avoidance, symptom recognition, and emergency plans helps establish a social safety net at school, at camp, and in other social situations. There are Web sites maintained by groups such as the Food Allergy and Anaphylaxis Network that are specifically designed for food-allergic teens (http://www.fanteen.org). These social networking sites give teens an opportunity to share their experiences and learn about food allergies from their peers.

Teens also need healthy, adaptive coping, planning, and food allergy management skills that they can take into adulthood.[17] These skills are developed over time, with support and practice in an environment where the teens feel as though they can succeed. The school environment and camp experience lend themselves to practicing skills that teens need. By the time teens reach high school, they should be mastering the ability to make safe food selections in a variety of settings. These teens should be active participants in the conversation with the school cafeteria or the camp kitchen staff, and should also begin practicing the "art of compromise." For example, if a teen wants to attend a school-related social event, is the parent going to contact the organizers to check for safe foods, or is the teen? If the teen chooses not to check the venue for safe foods, then is the teen going to bring his or her own safe foods? If bringing food is not an acceptable option and eating out of a common bowl is unacceptable, then the teen could agree to attend the event but not eat. Encouraging active participation allows the teen to practice planning and adaptive behaviors, fosters independence, and addresses the dreaded awkward social situation that a food reaction can cause.

Managing food allergy in any setting involves education and a team to establish and maintain a safe environment with food-allergic individuals. The process should create a dynamic structure that evolves as food-allergic individuals acquire confidence in their knowledge, and an ability to manage their food allergy and become self-sufficient. The ultimate goal is a support system that transitions the very young food-allergic child through age-appropriate developmental stages and culminates in an empowered food-allergic individual.

REFERENCES

1. Williams NA, Parra GR, Elkin TD. Parenting children with food allergies; preliminary development of a measure assessing child-rearing behaviors in the context of pediatric food allergy. Ann Allergy Asthma Immunol 2009;103:140–5.
2. Cummings AJ, Knibb RC, Erlewyn-Lajeunesse M, et al. Management of nut allergy influences quality of life and anxiety in children and their mothers. Pediatr Allergy Immunol 2010;21:586–94.
3. Perry TT, Conover-Walker MK, Pomes A, et al. Distribution of peanut allergen in the environment. J Allergy Clin Immunol 2004;113(5):973–6.
4. Wang J, Sampson HA. Food anaphylaxis. Clin Exp Allergy 2007;37:651–60.
5. Banerjee DK, Kagan RS, Turnbull E, et al. Peanut-free guidelines reduce school lunch peanut contents. Arch Dis Child 2007;92:980–2.
6. Young MC, Munoz-Furlong A, Sicherer SH. Management of food allergies in school: a perspective for allergists. J Allergy Clin Immunol 2009;124(2):175–82.
7. LeBovidge JS, Strauch H, Kalish LA, et al. Assessment of psychological distress among children and adolescents with food allergy. J Allergy Clin Immunol 2009; 124(6):1282–8.
8. Yu JW, Kagan R, Verreault N, et al. Accidental ingestions in children with peanut allergy. J Allergy Clin Immunol 2006;118(2):466–72.
9. Simonte SJ, Ma S, Mofidi S, et al. Relevance of casual contact with peanut butter in children with peanut allergy. J Allergy Clin Immunol 2003;112(1):180–2.
10. Wainstein BK, Kashef S, Ziegler M, et al. Frequency and significance of immediate contact reactions to peanut in peanut-sensitive children. Clin Exp Allergy 2007;37(6):839–45.
11. Rothon C, Head J, Klineberg E, et al. Can social support protect bullied adolescents from adverse outcomes? A prospective study on the effects of bullying on the educational achievement and mental health of adolescents at secondary schools in East London. J Adolesc 2010. [Epub ahead of print]. DOI: 10.1016/j.adolescence.2010.02.007.
12. Mishna F, Cook C, Gadalla T, et al. Cyber bullying behaviors among middle school and high school student. Am J Orthopsychiatry 2010;80(3):362–74.
13. Monks H, Gowland MH, MacKenzie H, et al. How do teenagers manage their food allergies? Clin Exp Allergy 2010;40:1533–40.
14. Nowak-Wegrzyn A, Conover-Walker M, Wood R. Food-allergic reactions in schools and preschools. Arch Pediatr Adolesc Med 2001;155:790–5.
15. Pulcini JM, Sease KK, Marshall GD. Disparity between the presence and the absence of food allergy action plans in one school district. Allergy Asthma Proc 2010;31(2):141–6.
16. Munoz-Furlong A, Weiss CC. Characteristics of food-allergic patients placing them at risk for a fatal anaphylactic episode. Curr Allergy Asthma Rep 2009;9(1):57–63.
17. MacKenzie H, Roberts G, Van Laar D, et al. Teenagers' experience of living with food hypersensitivity: a qualitative study. Pediatr Allergy Immunol 2009;21:595–602.
18. Greenhawt MJ, Singer AM, Baptist AP. Food allergy and food allergy attitudes among college students. J Allergy Clin Immunol 2009;124(2):323–7.
19. Sampson M, Munoz-Furlong A, Sicherer SH. Risk-taking and coping strategies of adolescents and young adults with food allergy. J Allergy Clin Immunol 2006; 117(6):1440–5.

Can Food Allergy Be Prevented? The Current Evidence

George Du Toit, FRCPCH (UK)*, Gideon Lack, FRCPCH (UK)

KEYWORDS

• Food allergy • Prevention • IgE • At-risk populations

The prevalence of IgE-mediated food allergy has increased in the last 2 decades, with approximately 3–6% of children in the developed world being affected[1–6]; however, the increase in food allergy is best described for peanut allergy (PA).[2,7,8] Although genetic factors are important in the development of food allergy,[9] the increase in food allergy has occurred in a short period and is therefore unlikely to be the result of germline genetic changes alone. It seems plausible that 1 or more environmental exposure(s), or lack of exposure(s), may through epigenetic changes result in the interruption of the default immunologic state of tolerance to food. Strategies aimed at the prevention of food allergy are therefore required: primary prevention strategies seek to prevent the onset of IgE sensitization; secondary prevention seeks to interrupt the development of food allergy in IgE-sensitized children; and tertiary prevention seeks to reduce the expression of end-organ allergic disease in children with established food allergy.

This article highlights important conclusions of the many reviews in this field and adds to current evidence.

METHODOLOGICAL CHALLENGES

The fact that no single intervention, or combination of interventions, is able to repeatedly show a strong protective effect against food allergy reflects either on the interventions themselves or the study methods used to measure them. This section examines the methodological concerns that complicate the interpretation of these studies (summarized in **Table 1**).

A major limitation of many food allergy prevention studies lies in the study design; linked to this are the necessary ethical limitations that apply to allergy prevention, particularly when applied to the in-utero environment and in early childhood. For

Division of Asthma, Allergy and Lung Biology, Guy's and St Thomas' National Health Service Foundation Trust, the Medical Research Council and Asthma UK Centre in Allergic Mechanisms of Asthma, King's College London, London, UK
* Corresponding author.
E-mail address: george.dutoit@kcl.ac.uk

Pediatr Clin N Am 58 (2011) 481–509
doi:10.1016/j.pcl.2011.02.002 **pediatric.theclinics.com**
0031-3955/11/$ – see front matter

Table 1
Methodological issues known to complicate the interpretation of studies aimed at the prevention of food allergy

Issue	Problem	Recommended Approach
Study design	Most studies in this field are observational studies	Randomized double-blind, placebo-controlled (RDBPC) trials reduce unmeasured and unknown sources of bias
Reverse causality	Early signs of suspected allergic disease (eg, eczema) may influence feeding patterns	Although challenging (and not always possible), trials should adopt RDBPC methodologies
Randomization	There are necessary ethical restraints that surround nutritional intervention studies in infancy	Breastfeeding should always be encouraged. Studies that wish to assess the effect of complementary feeding can then randomize breastfed children, from 4 months onwards and when exclusive breastfeeding no longer satisfies the infant
Blinding of dietary interventions	It may prove difficult to blind the dietary intervention/s	Some dietary interventions cannot be blinded
Determination of food allergy	Few studies make use of oral food challenges (OFCs) for the diagnosis of food allergy. The diagnosis of food allergy may therefore be inadequate both at study entry and exit. Too many studies rely on allergy testing (SPT and/or Sp-IgE) for the determination of food allergy	Aim to perform OFCs in all participants. For children who do not undergo OFCs, a priori diagnostic algorithms (which make use of the combination of history, examination, skin prick testing, and Sp-IgE) are required to reach a best possible diagnosis
Surrogate markers	IgE sensitization, eczema, asthma and rhinitis are often used as surrogate markers for food allergy	As above
Natural history of food allergy	Tolerance is anticipated for many, but not all, childhood food allergies	Account for natural remission rate of food allergy before assessing for a study effect
Nomenclature	There is insufficient consensus with respect to the terminology used for common allergic conditions, particularly in early childhood. Definitions of generic terms such as allergy or atopy are open to variability	Consensus with respect to the allergy nomenclature will facilitate research in this field
Determination of diet	The determination of food consumptions is usually by retrospective food frequency questionnaires (FFQs), which are prone to many forms of bias	Use should be made of prospective food diaries, which have been validated for context, language, and consistency

Dietary variables and measurement thereof	Few dietary analyses consider all variables; these include age of introduction, quantity ingested (individual and cumulative quantity), frequency of exposure, variability of allergens, and allergen processing and concomitant breastfeeding at time of commencing complementary feeds	Well-designed validated tools are required to accurately record all dietary variables
Definitions: weaning	Use of the term weaning is not consistent and indicates the introduction of solid foods only	WHO recommends that the term weaning should be replaced by the term complementary feeding. which incorporates any nutrient-containing food or liquid (other than breast milk) given to young children
Differing patterns of complementary feeding	Endless permutations make study effects difficult to compare (eg, many exclusively breastfed infants receive early top-up infant feeds with cow's milk formula)	Studies need to try to capture the following dietary variables: dose, timing, recurrence of exposure, variability of allergens, and allergen quality such as degree of processing
Outcome classifications	Many studies refer generically to allergy: allergic disease may encompass 1 or more of asthma, eczema, and hay fever. Definitions for each of these conditions are also open to great variability	A priori clinically validated definitions required
High-risk markers	Many studies are aimed at high-risk atopic populations; such populations are difficult to define	Studies should include entire study populations (ie, both low and high risk). At-risk populations should be defined a priori. Better at-risk markers are required
Separation of specific effects when interventions are combined	Multiple interventions are often studied at different time points. For example, probiotic administration may be administered to mother (during pregnancy and/or breastfeeding) and/or newborn infant. This strategy makes it difficult to determine the specific effect of each intervention at each time point	Preliminary proof-of-concept studies need to separate the effects of each intervention
Introduction of complementary feeds is associated with multiple variables	The early introduction of solid foods has been associated with cultural and socioeconomic factors as well as specific factors such as maternal age, formula feeding, and maternal smoking	Regression analysis should control for as many relevant confounders as possible, especially in observational studies. This strategy highlights the need for randomized controlled studies
Monitoring adherence	Monitoring of adherence to dietary interventions is difficult	Better tools for monitoring dietary adherence are required

example, strict ethical restrictions surround randomization of infants to anything but breast milk.

A second major limitation of studies in this field is the phenotypic description of food allergy. Few studies make use of food challenge diagnostic procedures; although tolerance is adequately determined by open food challenge, the gold standard for the determination of food allergy is the double-blind, placebo-controlled food challenge; these challenges are laborious and sometimes difficult to perform, particularly in young children. In addition, entry-level oral challenges cannot be performed in those children assigned to the avoidance arm of intervention studies, with the consequence that the true allergic phenotype of such infants at time of enrolment or exit from studies remains uncertain. This limitation is particularly problematic for the diagnosis of cow's milk allergy, which is a common, and frequently studied, childhood allergy.

The most frequently used surrogate marker for the determination of food allergy is the determination of IgE sensitization by skin prick test (SPT) results and/or serum specific IgE (sp-IgE) measurement. Although IgE-mediated food allergy requires a state of sensitization, most sensitized children are not food allergic. Many variables are also associated with the determination of sp-IgE and SPT, which further limit the use of this surrogate marker.

Eczema is also a commonly used surrogate, which itself has many limitations. Although eczema is strongly associated with food allergy, the 2 are not synonymous, as evidenced by studies that show an improvement in eczema but not in food allergy. Without proper study randomization it is often difficult to establish if studies that show protection against the development of eczema are showing the treatment thereof (ie, tertiary prevention, as opposed to primary prevention). Many studies do not adequately assess eczema severity; there is therefore a risk that beneficial effects are restricted to mild eczema, which runs a transient course, when compared with moderate to severe eczema. Similar limitations hold true for the use of asthma and rhinoconjunctivitis as food allergy surrogates.

Additional limitations of the surrogate markers used arise because of the inconsistencies in nomenclature used and difficulties in accurately diagnosing these conditions. For example, wheezing in infancy does not always mean that the child has asthma. Moreover, lung function is difficult to measure in infants.

There are many other limitations to studies in this field. For example, nutritional interventions are prone to both selection bias and reverse causality. Such bias may arise when atopic families (if aware of public health recommendations) are motivated to alter maternal and/or infant dietary practices. The effects of reverse causality are highlighted in various studies and for different allergic outcomes. For example, in the Avon Longitudinal Study of Parents and Children (ALSPAC) study,[10] a history of an allergic reaction to peanut is associated with prolonged breastfeeding. However, when adjusted for infantile eczema by regression analysis, there was no effect of breastfeeding on the development of PA. This phenomenon is also true for asthma; Fussman and colleagues,[11] in a large (n = 696) international study, reported that reverse causation negates the finding that the consumption of cow's milk is associated with asthma, as shown by the finding that the presence of asthma in the months before assessment led to a reduction in further exposure to cow's milk. Likewise, Lowe and colleagues,[12] in a prospective birth cohort of 620 infants, reported that early symptoms of eczema prolong the duration of exclusive breastfeeding.

Childhood food allergies are dynamic, with the general trend being for resolution of many, but not all, food allergies during the first decade of life (a time course sometimes referred to as the food allergic march). Other atopic conditions such as childhood eczema and asthma also share unique natural histories. Study planning should therefore take these natural histories into account when planning the introduction of interventions as well as when measuring potential outcomes.

The inclusion of a placebo in nutritional studies is not always practical, or safe. For example, in the LEAP (Learning Early about Allergy to Peanut) peanut intervention study[13] a placebo snack is not used for safety reasons. If it were possible to create an equivalent peanut placebo, children consuming the placebo snack might be at risk of consuming peanut-containing foods (to which they might unknowingly be allergic). In addition to representing a major safety concern this action would nullify any immunologic consequence that may have resulted from the avoidance of peanut.

Study interventions should be safe for both mother and child. Safety concerns have nonetheless arisen in select studies. For example, dietary interventions have been noted to compromise fetal and maternal well-being,[14] and probiotics have been shown to increase rates of sensitization and allergic outcomes in separate studies.[15]

Many interventions are introduced to both mother and child. This strategy complicates the understanding of specific study effects because it is unclear whether the immunologic effects were achieved prenatally or postnatally or whether effects should be attributed to a single or multiple factors.

The determination of dietary intake is usually performed by food frequency questionnaires (FFQs); FFQs are known to be subject to substantial forms of bias. Studies do not always make use of validated FFQs, a complex but important undertaking. FFQs do not always assess all relevant dietary variables, such as age of introduction, recurrence of exposure, quantity (single and cumulative) of exposure, variability of allergens eaten, and allergen processing. In addition, it is often difficult to disguise those questions that relate to the specific food/s of interest. Prospective food diaries are cumbersome because they demand detailed information and effort on the part of parents. It is particularly difficult to measure food allergen exposure that occurs via routes other than the oral route (eg, through an abraded skin barrier). For example, the nursing mother who ingests peanut butter is also likely to transfer this allergen to the infant through kiss and touch contact.[16–19] In addition, it is often the nursing mother who determines consumption patterns within the household, which further increases (or decreases) the opportunity for environmental food allergen exposure to foods that the mother likes (or dislikes). A different problem arises if the intervention is one of avoidance, because the elimination of 1 or more foods from the diet is likely to affect the diet. Such changes may be anticipated and therefore measured, or unknown and missed.

Many studies in this field are aimed at at-risk children; however, at-risk populations are difficult to define. For example, approximately 10% of children without an allergic first-degree relative develop allergic disease, compared with 20% to 30% with single allergic heredity (parent or sibling) and 40% to 50% with double allergic heredity.[20–22] In addition, the definition of the term atopy is inconsistent.

Observational study designs (ie, most studies in this field) are particularly vulnerable to bias from both unmeasured, and unknown, sources; study hypotheses would ideally be assessed using only randomized placebo-controlled, double-blind studies.

ONSET OF SENSITIZATION AND FOOD ALLERGY

It remains unclear when prevention strategies should be implemented. Prerequisites for the development of food allergy (particularly in genetically susceptible individuals) are believed to include allergen exposure, uptake, recognition, and processing. It is therefore important to determine whether sensitization occurs in-utero or afterwards. That in-utero sensitization to foods is possible is suggested by the early detection of sp-IgE[23] and clinical presentation of IgE-mediated food allergies within the first few days of life[24] (but usually within the first years of life). This finding is also true for non–IgE-mediated food-induced immunologic reactions such as colitis induced by cow's milk protein,[25] eosinophilic esophogitis,[26] and colitis induced by food protein.[27]

The fetal immune system is sufficiently mature and able to respond to both food allergens and aeroallergens. It has also been shown that food allergens and aeroallergens can pass transplacentally. The analysis of sp-IgE to foods in cord blood has been restricted to occasional studies. Two large birth cohort studies were unable to show measurable food sp-IgE in cord blood, even in those children who subsequently developed clinical or immunologic food sensitization.[10,28]

Summary

There is no firm evidence to support the hypothesis that sensitization and allergy to foods commences in-utero.

MATERNAL DIET (DURING PREGNANCY AND/OR BREASTFEEDING) AND THE PREVENTION OF FOOD ALLERGY

This section examines the effect of maternal diet during pregnancy and/or lactation on the development of food allergy.

There are studies that assess the effects with respect to allergy prevention through maternal dietary avoidance of 1 or more common food allergens during pregnancy and/or lactation.[29–31] Kramer and Kakuma[32] in a Cochrane review assessed the evidence for allergy prevention through prescribing an antigen avoidance diet during lactation. Three trials were included involving 209 women; findings suggest a strong protective effect of maternal antigen avoidance on the incidence of atopic eczema during the child's first 12 to 18 months of life. The investigators note the methodological shortcomings in all 3 trials and argue for caution in applying these results; in particular, the high incidence of atopic eczema in the control groups is of concern and may be explained by non-blinding or de-blinding of the examining physicians. One trial reported that a restricted diet (egg and cow's milk) during pregnancy was associated with a small but statistically significant lower mean gestational weight gain and there were trends toward increased preterm delivery and lower birth weight. Given the uncertainty of these findings, and potential safety concerns, no allergy organizations recommend the avoidance of either egg or milk during pregnancy. The American Academy of Pediatrics[33] and the UK Government Department of Health[34] had previously suggested that at-risk families may wish to avoid peanut; these recommendations have been withdrawn, like in many organizations that offer similar, nonrestrictive, dietary recommendations for the prevention of allergy.[23,35–37] Two large prospective birth cohort studies, one based on the Isle of Wight, UK[38] and the ALSPAC[10] study, showed no effect of maternal peanut consumption in pregnancy or lactation on the development of immunologic or clinical reaction to peanuts on follow-up at 4 to 6 years of age. Likewise Fox and colleagues,[19] in a questionnaire-based study, found no effect of maternal peanut consumption during pregnancy or lactation. More recently, 2 studies have suggested that peanut exposure during pregnancy and lactation may be associated with higher rates of PA; however, these studies made use of less rigorous methodologies.[39,40]

There are studies that examine the role of dietary patterns on other allergic disease outcome. For example, the protective effects against childhood wheezing associated with a Mediterranean diet[41] are largely a result of dietary effects in pregnancy.[42] In the ALSPAC UK birth cohort,[43] health-conscious dietary patterns were positively associated with eczema, total IgE, forced expiratory volume after 1 second, and forced expiratory flow, and negatively associated with early wheezing and asthma. The processed dietary pattern was positively associated with early wheezing and negatively associated with atopy and forced vital capacity; however, when controlling for confounders, these effects were substantially attenuated and became nonsignificant, suggesting that in this cohort dietary patterns in pregnancy did not predict asthma and related outcomes in the offspring.[43]

Breast milk contains low concentrations of dietary proteins, which are present in maternal serum such as gliadin,[44] peanut, β-lactoglobulin, and ovalbumin.[45,46] β-Lactoglobulin is found in the breast milk of as many as 95% of mothers consuming cow's milk during lactation.[47] Whether at-risk infants are protected by the many beneficial immunologic properties of breast milk or put at risk by this low-dose allergen exposure is an ongoing debate. No studies have modified maternal diet during lactation only. There are studies that modify the maternal diet during both pregnancy and lactation. Neither the study by Hattevig and colleagues[48] nor the study by Herrmann and colleagues[49] reported a protective role against infant food allergy through maternal dietary avoidance of cow's milk, egg, and fish during either pregnancy or both pregnancy and lactation. However, the study by Herrmann and colleagues[49] did note effects for eczema.

Summary

There is little evidence to suggest that manipulation of the maternal diet during pregnancy and/or breastfeeding has any protective effect on the development of food allergy; preventative effects are noted for eczema. Such strategies have been shown to potentially compromise the nutritional well-being of both mother and child.

COMPLEMENTARY INFANT FEEDING AND THE PREVENTION OF FOOD ALLERGY

This section examines the effect of complementary feeding on the development of food allergy. The World Health Organization (WHO) now recommends that the term weaning be replaced by the term complementary feeding, which incorporates any nutrient-containing food or liquid other than breast milk.

Exclusive Breastfeeding Versus Mixed Feeding/Complementary Feeding

Although there is universal consensus that breast milk remains unchallenged as the milk of choice for all infants, there is conflicting advice with respect to the age at which complementary feeding should occur. Whereas most allergy/gastrointestinal opinion leaders suggest that complementary feeding may occur (if the infant is ready) from 4 months of age onwards[23,35–37] WHO recommends that complementary feeding should occur only after 6 months of age.[50]

Breast milk provides a rich and favorable source of important immune-regulating substances such as immunoglobulins, lactoferrin, lysozymes, oligosaccharides, long-chain fatty acids, cytokines, nucleotides, hormones, antioxidants, and maternal immune cells. The importance of these factors was shown by Verhasselt and colleagues,[51] who investigated whether the exposure of lactating mice to an airborne allergen affects asthma development in progeny; they found that airborne antigens were efficiently transferred from the mother to the neonate through milk and that tolerance induction did not require the transfer of immunoglobulins. Breastfeeding-induced tolerance relied on the presence of transforming growth factor β (TGF-β) during lactation, was mediated by regulatory CD4+ T lymphocytes, and depended on TGF-β signaling in T cells.[51] Breast milk may affect other processes capable of directly influencing allergic disease expression such as food antigen absorption and processing. It is frustrating therefore that breastfeeding rates remain below WHO targets.

Studies that support a protective effect of breastfeeding over cow's milk formulae date back to the 1930s, when Grulee and Sanford,[52] in a large (n ≈ 20,000) observational study, reported a protective effect with respect to the development of eczema in the first 12 to 48 months of life. A systematic review of 12 prospective studies (8183 infants) found that exclusive breastfeeding in the first months of life is associated with reduced rates of subsequent asthma (odds ratio [OR] 0.70; 95% confidence interval [CI] 0.60–0.81).[53] Many, but not all, of the observational studies that followed supported these early findings. Nonetheless, there is a consensus among reviews in the field that breastfeeding offers at least some protection against the development of allergy.[53–55] For example, Muraro and colleagues[54] suggest an overall protective effect (for at-risk children) of exclusive breastfeeding during the first 3 months of life on atopic eczema, asthma, but not childhood allergic rhinitis. Although the protective effects are most consistent for eczema, the underlying immunologic mechanisms to explain this phenomenon remain unclear. In support of those previous studies that report a protective effect of breastfeeding over asthma is the observational study from Australia by Oddy and colleagues.[56] These investigators followed a large cohort (n = 2602) of children (enrolled before birth) and reported a protective effect for asthma (strict diagnostic criteria used) and atopy (positive reaction to common aeroallergens) at 6 years of age. After adjustment for sex, prematurity, and maternal smoking during pregnancy, they found that exclusive breastfeeding for less than 4 months was associated with an increased risk for current asthma (ie, there is a substantial reduction in risk of childhood allergy [asthma and atopy] at 6 years of age if infants are exclusively breastfed for at least the first 4 months of life); it may also be that the benefits of breastfeeding persist into the teenage years. Saarinen and Kajosaari,[57] in an observational community-based study, reported early (less eczema and food allergy at 1–3 years of age) and late (respiratory allergy at 17 years of age) effects in infants who were exclusively breastfed for 6 months compared with those who were breastfed for 3 months or less.

No studies report a clear benefit of breastfeeding over cow's milk formula on the development of food allergy; this is true even for premature infants (with an increased gut permeability and an immature gut immune system). Lucas and colleagues,[58] in a large (n = 777) randomized interventional study of premature infants, compared the effect of human milk, standard preterm formula, and nutrient-enriched preterm formula. At 18 months after term there was no difference in the incidence of allergic reactions between dietary groups. However, in the subgroup of infants with a family history of atopy, those infants who received preterm formula rather than human milk had a significantly greater risk of developing 1 or more atopic conditions (notably eczema) by 18 months. Furthermore, De Jong and colleagues[59] in a large (n = 1693) randomized intervention study (the BOKAAL study) found that early (first 3 days of life) high-dose exposure to cow's milk (as frequently occurs in nurseries) was not associated with an increase in allergic disease or symptoms. In addition, no increase between the groups was found in sensitization or allergy to cow's milk (up to 5 years of age).

There are observational studies that controversially report an increased risk for the development of allergic disorders in breastfed infants. Sears and colleagues[60] in a large (n = 1037 children) observational study followed children until 21 years of age. These investigators found that breastfeeding (for at least 4 weeks) does not protect against childhood atopy and asthma. Significantly more breastfed children were atopic to common aeroallergens at age 13 years than non-breastfed children. Breastfeeding also increased the likelihood of current asthma at age 9 years and at age 21 years. Findings were similar when breastfeeding was considered over longer periods (8–12 weeks). However, there are many criticisms of this study; these include that data for breastfeeding were retrospectively gathered when infants were age 3 years; definitions for atopic heredity included parental atopy only, hence adjustments were not made for eczema or sibling atopy. The number of exclusively breastfed children in this study was low, with nonsignificant findings when considering the effects of exclusive breastfeeding only. Likewise, Bergmann and colleagues,[61] in the large Multicentre Allergy Study observational birth cohort (n = 1314 infants born in 1990), found that each month of breastfeeding increased the risk of developing atopic eczema in the first 7 years by approximately 3%. It was noted that breastfeeding persisted for longer if at least 1 parent had eczema, the mother was older, did not smoke in pregnancy, and the family had a high social status. Whereas many studies report the greatest benefit for the prevention of allergies lies with at-risk groups, this study suggests that breastfeeding does not prevent eczema in children with a genetic risk. However, multiple regression analysis cannot exclude reverse causation (ie, mothers may extend exclusive breastfeeding and duration of breastfeeding once infants develop eczema). Isolauri and colleagues[62] observed that atopic eczema in exclusively breastfed infants improved when breastfeeding was stopped, which suggests that the protective effect may be caused by the reduction in allergic disease expression (tertiary prevention) rather than primary prevention. However, this finding cannot easily be assessed because this study did not include controls to confirm that this effect was caused by the cessation of breastfeeding Hence, these studies suggest that prolonged breastfeeding could maintain eczema, at least in some infants, and that cessation of breastfeeding acts to treat the eczema as opposed to prevent it.

As detailed earlier, there are many potential mechanisms by which breastfeeding may reduce allergic outcomes. Alternatively, breastfeeding may serve as a surrogate for other important factors, the most obvious of which is the absence of complementary feeding (see definition in earlier discussion). Prospective birth cohorts that show a preventive effect of breastfeeding on allergy report prolonged breastfeeding (>4–6 months) and late introduction of solids (>4–6 months).[54] Most studies in this field consider weaning to be the introduction of solid foods only. However, the biophysical properties of allergens are complex and there is no reason to believe that the allergenic potential of liquid feeds is different from that of solid or semisolid feeds. For example, both cow's milk and hen's egg allergy (EA) are common childhood allergies despite being ingested as liquid and solid, respectively. It is therefore arbitrary to restrict the usage of the term weaning to solids. An infant who is breastfed while receiving cow's milk formula supplementation is no more or less weaned than a breastfed infant who is fed rice cereal mixed with expressed breast milk.

Kramer and Kakuma[63] performed a systematic review of the available evidence concerning the effects of exclusive breastfeeding for 6 months versus exclusive breastfeeding for 3 to 4 months followed by mixed breastfeeding (complementary liquid or solid foods with continued breastfeeding) to 6 months, on eczema, asthma, and other atopic outcomes. This extensive review covers 20 independent, observational studies. These investigators were unable to establish evidence for a significant reduction in the risk of atopic eczema, asthma, or other atopic outcomes amongst those infants who were exclusively breastfed for 6 months compared with those exclusively breastfed for only 3 to 4 months followed by mixed feeding.

Summary

Evidence suggests that exclusive breastfeeding offers some protection against eczema and asthma, but not food allergy, when compared with cow's milk protein formulas. Observational studies that report an increase in allergic disease because of breastfeeding are prone to reverse causality. Studies in this area suffer from true randomization because of necessary ethical limitations.

Cow's Milk Hydrolysates and Other Milk Formulas

The Cochrane review by Osborn and Sinn[64] found no evidence to support feeding with a hydrolyzed formula for the prevention of allergy compared with exclusive breast-feeding. For high-risk infants who are unable to breastfeed there seems to be a consensus among reviews that the use of hydrolyzed milk formula offers at least some protection against allergic disease, and in particular eczema.[54] Although these findings are reflected in recent summary papers,[65–67] in view of methodological concerns and inconsistency of findings, Osborn and Sinn[64] recommend for future research in this field that large, well-designed trials should be used, comparing formulas containing partially hydrolyzed whey or extensively hydrolyzed casein with cow's milk formulas. One such study is the German Infant Nutritional Interventional (GINI) Study.[68] This is a large (n = 2252) randomized multicenter study in which Von Berg and colleagues allocated at-risk infants to 1 of 4 milks (cow's milk formula, partially or extensively hydrolyzed whey formula, or extensively hydrolyzed casein formula). Overall, a significant reduction in the incidence of atopic dermatitis was achieved in this study using the hydrolyzed formula; the preventive effect of partially hydrolyzed whey formula and extensively hydrolyzed casein formula on allergic manifestations (defined as physician's diagnosis of atopic dermatitis, food allergy/intolerance, and allergic urticaria; asthma and rhinitis were added at the later time points) and atopic dermatitis found in the 2 previous analyses at age 1 year and until 3 years have been confirmed at age 6 years in both the intention-to-treat and the per-protocol analyses.[69] The results found with extensively hydrolyzed whey formula in this 6-year analysis are interesting; until 3 years, this formula showed only a small preventive effect that never reached significance, whereas at age 6 years it showed a preventive late-onset effect on atopic dermatitis and allergic anifestations in the per protocol population similar to that of the other 2 hydrolysates and a considerable, although not significant, effect on rhinitis. The GINI study is ongoing.

Although the clinical benefits reported by the GINI study[69] are convincing, it remains unclear whether dietary modification has prevented allergic disease. The challenge in interpreting these findings lies in the relationship between eczema and cow's milk allergy, because the preventative effect of select formula may simply show tertiary prevention (ie, eczema treatment, as opposed to the prevention of eczema). The GINI study was not able to clearly define the end point of food allergy by double-blind, placebo-controlled food challenge (because many parents declined). Thus, the reduction in eczema could be caused by a true preventative effect of infant dietary modification or alternatively it could reflect the beneficial effect of removing cow's milk protein from the diet of infants with eczema and milk allergy. It is difficult to separate these effects when the study intervention (modified formula) is introduced at, or before, the expected age of onset of eczema. In addition, the GINI study does not include the findings of the breastfed infants (n = 945) in the analysis (because this group differed significantly from the formula-fed group).

Soy Formula and Other Mammalian Milks and the Prevention of Allergy

Soy formulas have long been used as cow's milk formula alternatives. Osborn and Sinn,[70] in a recent Cochrane review, concluded that, on current evidence, the use of soy formulae could not be recommended for the prevention of allergy or food intolerance in infants at high risk. No study reported an increase in soy allergy. There is also no evidence to support the use of other mammalian milks for the prevention of food allergy.

Summary

There is evidence that for high-risk infants who are unable to exclusively breastfeed the use of hydrolyzed infant formula may protect against the development of allergic disease, particularly eczema. It may be that protective effects better reflect tertiary prevention (ie, reduction of disease expression in infants with preexisting milk allergy) rather than true primary prevention. Overall, with 1 notable exception, the studies suggest a priority of an extensively hydrolyzed formula over a partially hydrolyzed formula.

Complementary Feeding (with Solid Foods)

Before 2001, WHO recommended that infants be exclusively breastfed for between 4 and 6 months, with the introduction of complementary foods thereafter. In 2001, after expert consultation and the systematic review by Kramer and Kakuma,[63] the recommended period of exclusive breastfeeding was extended to the first 6 months of life. Advice in this regard is conflicting, with other allergy organizations recommending exclusive breastfeeding for between 4 and 6 months. Since 1975, there has been a significant trend in developed countries for the later introduction of solid foods. For example, in the United Kingdom, the proportion of infants given solids by 8 weeks of age decreased from 49% in 1975 to 24% in 1980 and 1985 and 19% in 1990.[34] This decrease has coincided with a 3-fold increase in allergy in children. Reasons for differences in complementary feeding are complex and early weaning has been associated with cultural and socioeconomic factors, as well as specific factors such as maternal age, formula feeding, and maternal smoking. All of these factors need to be controlled for in study analyses.

A review of the evidence of the relationship between the early (defined as <4 months of age) introduction of solid foods to infants and the development of allergic disease was recently performed by Tarini and colleagues.[71] Thirteen studies met their criteria for review, of which only one was controlled. Studies were not limited to at-risk study populations. These investigators conclude that there is insufficient evidence to suggest that, on its own, the early introduction of solids to infants is associated with an increased risk of asthma, food allergy, allergic rhinitis, or animal allergies. Tarini and colleagues note the consistent association between the persistence of eczema and the introduction of solid foods before age 4 months that is supported by long-term follow-up studies and the dose-dependent nature of the association.

Reverse causality has been proposed as an explanation for many of the study findings in this field. There are 2 studies that may be less severely affected by the effects of reverse causality. The first study by Fergusson and colleagues[72] was performed in New Zealand in 1977 (ie, before the publication of WHO weaning recommendations); feeding practices would not therefore have been influenced by these recommendations. These investigators report a 2.9-times greater risk of chronic or recurrent eczema amongst children fed 4 or more solids before 4 months of age compared with those not fed solids before 4 months of age. This difference was still apparent at 10 years of age. However, individually, exposure to cow's milk, egg, cereals, vegetables, meat products, or fruit did not increase the risk for the development of atopic dermatitis.[72] Zutavern and colleagues[73] studied a large population-based, multicenter cohort; they controlled for the effects of reverse causality and assessed the effect of early life diet on allergy outcomes. No measurements were made for sensitization to foods or food allergy. There was no evidence for a protective effect of late introduction of solids on the development of preschool wheezing, transient wheezing, atopy, or eczema. On the contrary, there was a statistically significant increased risk of eczema in relation to late introduction of egg and milk. The late introduction of egg was also associated with a nonsignificant increased risk of preschool wheezing.

A common finding in these studies is that the introduction of 4 or more foods during the first 4 months of life may increase allergic outcomes but not increase risk for the development of food allergy. Whereas the influence of complementary feeding with solid foods during the fifth or sixth month of life is less clear, complementary feeding after the age of 6 months seems not to influence allergic outcomes. Why 4 or more, as opposed to 1, 2, or 3 foods, would confer an increased risk is unclear, but may simply reflect a greater opportunity for the food-allergic infant to encounter an allergen to which they are allergic. A later section covers in greater detail studies that relate to the early introduction of single common food allergens such as egg[74] and peanut.[5,13]

Summary

Observational studies suggest that complementary feeding with 4 or more solid foods in the first 4 months of life may increase the risk of developing allergic disease (but not food allergy). There is no evidence that delaying the introduction of solid foods beyond 4 months of age is protective, and some evidence suggests that the delayed introduction of solids may promote allergies.

COMBINED MATERNAL AND INFANT DIETARY MEASURES AND THE PREVENTION OF FOOD ALLERGY

It seems intuitive that of all interventions aimed at the prevention of food allergy the combined approach should offer the greatest hope because it covers the many routes of allergen exposure at times of immune vulnerability and pliability. The past 2 decades have witnessed a trend to allergen avoidance, with early calls to support this[75]; however, more recently many have questioned the wisdom of strict allergen modification in the diet of pregnant and breastfeeding women and the newborn diet.[36,76–79]

Kramer and Kakuma,[32] in a Cochrane review, assess the evidence for the prevention of allergic disease through maternal dietary antigen avoidance during pregnancy or lactation, or both. Their analysis finds that the prescription of an antigen avoidance diet to a high-risk woman during pregnancy is unlikely to substantially reduce her child's risk of atopic disease. These investigators warn against the potential dangerous nutritional consequences of overzealous and unsupervised dietary restrictions. However, they do acknowledge that the prescription of an antigen avoidance diet (to high-risk women) during lactation may reduce the child's risk of developing atopic eczema, but better trials are needed.

Of the existing studies in this field, 2 pioneering randomized studies adopt a multi-intervention approach (in both mother and child) with subsequent long-term blinded follow-up. Clinical assessments were robust in both these studies. Zeiger and Heller[80] report a significant reduction in milk sensitization and eczema before age 2 years but no differences for food allergy, atopic dermatitis, allergic rhinitis, asthma, any atopic disease, lung function, food or aeroallergen sensitization, or serum IgE level, at 7 years of age. The early dietary differences were almost entirely caused by cow's milk allergy, so it is not surprising that the early differences between the 2 groups were not sustained, and disappeared by 2 years of age. No difference in skin prick testing or sp-IgE was shown for the other food allergens tested, including peanut, which was the most common skin- test–positive food allergen at 7 years of age, indicating that the beneficial effect of the dietary interventions was mainly in reducing allergy to cow's milk.

Arshad and colleagues[38] also reported that allergic disease (asthma, atopy, rhinitis, eczema) could be reduced, at least for the first 8 years of life, by combined food and house dust mite allergen avoidance in infancy. These investigators recruited infants at high risk of atopy and randomized them to either a prophylactic (n = 58) or control (n = 62) group. Infants in the prophylactic group were either breastfed (with the mother on a low-allergen diet) or given an extensively hydrolyzed formula. The control group followed standard UK Department of Health advice. Repeated measurement analysis, adjusted for all relevant confounding variables, confirmed a preventive effect on asthma, atopic dermatitis, rhinitis, and atopy. The protective effects were primarily observed in the subgroup of children with persistent disease (symptoms at all visits) and in those with evidence of allergic sensitization. Study powering did not allow for the assessment of food allergy at 8 years of age, but earlier transient effects show some protection, at least for cow's milk allergy. The specific preventative contribution of the dietary and aeroallergen interventions is unclear.

Summary

There are randomized trials that adopt a multi-intervention approach (ie, dietary modification of both maternal diet during pregnancy and lactation and infant diet) that report a reduction in allergic disease. Although findings in 1 study were transient and no longer observed at 7 years of age, in a second study the effects in allergy reduction were still observed at 8 years of age. The effects with respect to a reduction in food allergy seem to predominantly apply to cow's milk allergy. Caution is required before the recommendation of such interventions because of the potential for nutritional compromise in both mother and child.

ROUTES OF SENSITIZATION, CROSS-SENSITIZATION, ORAL TOLERANCE INDUCTION, AND INTERVENTIONAL STUDIES IN THIS FIELD

Sensitization Through the Skin

Until recently, preventive strategies focused on oral exposure to foods. However, the oral route of exposure is not the only route because exposure to food allergens may occur through aerosolized allergen exposure (eg, fish and milk cooking vapors) or via the skin.[16–18]

In animal models, the application of egg white[81,82] and peanut[83] onto abraded skin has led to IgE sensitization. These observations support the occupational health findings in humans that sensitization may occur through contact with the skin, particularly through abraded skin.

The ALSPAC study[10] followed a large cohort of children (n = 13,971) from birth. The results of this study show a positive association between PA and eczema, and an even greater association with an oozing or crusting skin rash. There was an increased use of preparations using peanut oil in children with PA; almost 91% of the children with PA had been exposed topically to creams containing *Arachis* oil in the first 6 months of life and more children with PA were exposed to significantly more preparations containing *Arachis* oil than were controls.

Although the ALSPAC study raised the possibility that exposure to low doses of peanut antigen through inflamed skin causes allergic sensitization, exposure to topical preparations may represent only 1 component of environmental exposure. For example, cutaneous contact may occur when a tolerant household member eats allergen-containing food and then touches or kisses someone naive to that allergen or when the infant touches a surface contaminated with peanut.[16–18] After peanut butter has been consumed, there is residual detectable Ara h 1 on the hands or in saliva, despite washing the hands or cleaning the teeth; there are thus many opportunities for an infant to experience cutaneous allergen exposure in households in which peanut-containing foods are consumed. That peanut is bioavailable after only skin contact is clear from studies showing that cutaneous exposure to peanut causes contact reactions in 33% of patients.[84] Fox and colleagues[19] found that total weekly household peanut consumption during the first year of life is significantly higher for infants who developed PA than for those who did not. The median household peanut consumption is more than 10 times greater in these cases than in high-risk controls. These investigators reported a dose-response relationship between household peanut consumption and the risk of later PA that is unaffected by maternal peanut consumption during pregnancy and lactation. Furthermore, the household peanut consumption in the controls with EA is significantly lower than that of the low-risk controls. Children with EA are at high risk of developing PA, so these data suggest that reduced or absent levels of household peanut consumption may exert a protective effect.[19,85]

Oral Tolerance Induction

There is a significant body of evidence with respect to oral tolerance induction in animal models in which a single oral dose of antigen was sufficient to induce tolerance, a phenomenon that has been reported for different antigens and in different experimental models.[86–88] The data are consistent, uniformly showing that a single dose of oral protein administration effectively causes immunologic tolerance and prevents the expression of related clinical disease. Furthermore, oral tolerance to peanut in mice has been shown to be antigen-specific (ie, tolerizing doses of peanut did not promote tolerance to ovalbumin and vice versa).[86]

In humans, 1 previous study showed a nonsignificant trend toward increased peanut consumption during pregnancy in mothers of children who developed PA.[85] Fox and colleagues[19] showed a significant increase in maternal consumption of peanuts during pregnancy and lactation in mothers of children who develop PA; however, after adjusting for household peanut consumption, maternal consumption becomes insignificant. It seems the increased maternal consumption during pregnancy and lactation is merely a marker of high household peanut consumption: mothers in households with high peanut consumption are more likely to eat peanut because of its availability. However, this maternal consumption seems to be irrelevant.

Ecological data suggest that African, Asian, and Middle Eastern countries where peanuts are consumed throughout pregnancy and early childhood have low rates of PA compared with Western, industrialized societies such as the United Kingdom and United States, where PA is high despite peanut avoidance during pregnancy and infancy.[1,5,89,90] Our cross-sectional data[5] on the prevalence of PA and peanut consumption in the United Kingdom and Israel lends weight to the hypothesis that early and frequent oral exposure to peanut may facilitate the tolerance to peanut. Using a questionnaire-based study of 8600 schoolchildren, we found that the prevalence of PA is 10-fold higher in Jewish children in the United Kingdom compared with that seen in Jewish children in Israel (1.85% and 0.17%, respectively). These differences cannot be explained by differences in age, sex, ancestry, atopy, or socioeconomic class. After adjustment for atopy, other food allergies, age, and sex, the relative risk (RR) for PA in the United Kingdom remained high at 5.8 (95% CI 2.8–11.8), whereas the RRs for egg and milk allergy were low, at 1.3 (95% CI 0.9–1.9) and 1.8 (95% CI 1–3.1), respectively, suggesting an allergen-specific effect. The biggest difference in PA was observed in primary schools (in children aged 4–12 years), where the prevalence was 2.05% in the United Kingdom and 0.12% in Israel (P<.001). Even after adjustment, the RR for PA among UK primary schoolchildren was 9.8 (95% CI 3.1–30.5). Even confining the analysis to the high-risk subgroup of children with a stringent diagnosis of eczema, the difference in PA between countries remained high (6.5% in the United Kingdom and 0.8% in Israel, P = .024). The most obvious difference in the diet of infants in both populations occurs in the introduction of peanut; Israeli infants are introduced to peanut during early weaning and continue to eat peanut more frequently and in higher amounts than UK infants, who avoid peanut, as per Department of Health recommendations. The difference between PA in United Kingdom and Israeli infants cannot be accounted for by differences in atopy, social class, ancestry, weaning, or methods of peanut processing in the 2 countries. These findings raise the question of whether early and frequent ingestion of high-dose peanut protein during infancy might prevent the development of PA through tolerance induction.

This study[5] also found a greater prevalence of sesame allergy (SA) in the United Kingdom (0.79% vs 0.13% in Israel), with the latter being similar to that reported in Israel in 2002.[91] The lower levels of SA in Israel could also be explained by higher consumption of sesame observed in Israeli infants. The differences in tree nut allergy between the 2 populations cannot be accounted for by differences in consumption of tree nut.

There are no interventional studies that examine the potential role of oral tolerance induction to foods in childhood. There is 1 adult human study showing that feeding keyhole limpet hemocyanin (KLH) results in immunologic tolerance to KLH antigen.[92] Interventional studies under way that aim to further examine these associations using rigorous study designs. Examples include the National Institutes of Health/Immune Tolerance Network-sponsored interventional study (LEAP study)[13] and the Enquiring About Tolerance (EAT) study.[93] The LEAP study seeks to compare 2 strategies for the prevention of PA in high-risk infants: participants were stratified into 2 groups based on SPT results for peanut:, a first group with a wheal diameter of 0 mm (SPT-negative stratum, n = 542) and a second group with a wheal diameter of 1, 2, 3, or 4 mm (SPT-positive stratum, n = 98). Participants in each stratum were randomly assigned to receive a peanut-containing snack or to avoid peanut. Whereas half the infants carefully avoid peanut, the other half regularly eat peanut (6 g of peanut protein/wk). The prevalence of PA is compared at age 5 years (visit 60 months = V60) by oral challenge to peanut and is powered at 89% to detect the difference between a 9.04% rate in the avoidance group and a 2% rate in the consumption group within the negative stratum. Immunologic assays are performed to identify the mechanisms that underpin antigen-specific oral tolerance induction. Study findings are due in 2014.

The EAT study[93] is a randomized controlled trial testing the hypothesis that the introduction of 6 allergenic foods (cow's milk, egg, fish, wheat, sesame, and peanut) into the diet of infants from 3 months of age, alongside continued breastfeeding, results in a reduced prevalence of food allergies by 3 years of age. The study is recruiting from an unselected UK population over 2 years, with study results due in 2015.

There are observational studies to other foods that lend weight to the hypothesis of tolerance induction through early oral exposure. More than 20 years ago, Saarinen and Kajosaari[57] in a population-based observational study assessed the effect of fish and citrus consumption during the first year of life. These investigators found no difference in the cumulative incidence of fish and citrus allergy at 3 years of age between children with fish introduced early or late (after age 1 year). The reaction earlier in life of the children introduced to fish earlier suggests a delay in allergy presentation rather than protection from allergy. However, fish is not only a common food allergen but also a rich source of antiinflammatory omega-3 polyunsaturated fatty acids (PUFAs).

More recently, studies have assessed the influence between early introduction of, and allergy to, wheat and egg. Poole and colleagues[94] reported that delaying the initial exposure to cereal grains until after 6 months of age may increase the risk of developing IgE-mediated wheat allergy. Using a more stringent methodology, Koplin and colleagues recorded parental responses on infant feeding (73% response rate), and potential confounding factors, before SPT for egg white had been performed (to minimize bias in parental responses). Egg-sensitized infants were then offered an egg oral food challenge to definitively diagnose EA. Multiple logistic regression was used to investigate associations between diet and EA adjusted for possible confounding factors. Compared with the introduction at 4 to 6 months of age, introducing egg into the diet later was associated with higher risks of EA. At age 4 to 6 months, first exposure as cooked egg reduced the risk of EA compared with first exposure as egg in baked goods. Duration of breastfeeding and age at introduction of solids were not associated with EA.

There may be lessons to be learnt for the prevention of food allergy when assessing studies concerning celiac disease; although celiac disease is not an IgE-mediated allergy the disease processes are analogous in the sense that it is a gut disorder in genetically predisposed people in whom an immunologic response is raised to a commonly consumed food protein. In the last few years, epidemiologic studies have strongly suggested that the timing of the introduction of gluten, as well as the pattern of breastfeeding (ie, reduced prevalence if cereal grains introduced while still breastfed), may play an important role in the subsequent development of celiac disease.[95] An ongoing interventional study is examining this question further.[96]

Summary

Recent observational and animal studies have raised the question whether sensitization to food antigens may occur via the cutaneous route. There is a body of literature (in animal models) that reports the effect of tolerance induction after early high-dose food allergen consumption. There are also observational data in humans to suggest that the early introduction of peanut, cereal grains, and egg is not associated with an increased prevalence of allergy to these foods and may possibly serve as a means of inducing oral tolerance to that protein; however, randomized interventional trials are needed to definitively answer these questions and to guide public health strategies. In the interim, international consensus does not support allergen avoidance as a strategy for the primary prevention of food allergy.

UNPASTEURIZED MILK AND THE USE OF PROBIOTICS AND PREBIOTICS

It is hypothesized that the increase in allergic disease may be caused by a relative lack of microbial stimulation of the infant gut immune system, often referred to as the hygiene hypothesis. Limited evidence for the hygiene hypothesis exists with respect to food allergy. A Norwegian birth cohort study showed that birth through a cesarean section was associated with a 7-fold increased risk of parental perceived reactions to eggs, fish, or nuts.[97] For infants whose mothers were allergic, there was also a 4-fold increased risk of confirmed EA in this study. A recent meta-analysis on the relationship between cesarean delivery and atopic outcome[98] found 6 studies that confirmed a mild effect of cesarean delivery increasing the risk of food allergy or food atopy (OR 1.32; 95% CI 1.12–0.55). One explanation is that early colonization of the infant by colonic microflora protects against the development of allergic disease. However, other explanations are possible: cesarean sections are more common in firstborns (therefore there may be a sibling effect); alternatively, the primary effect might be on reducing eczema rather than food allergy. Another possible explanation for the effect of cesarean sections is that they are associated with high maternal age, which has been shown to be a possible risk factor for food allergy in a case-control study.[99]

There are studies that investigate the role of other dietary or related immune-modulating factors associated with the anthropophosphic lifestyle and their effect on rates of allergic disease. For example, observations from rural environments suggest an inverse association between consumption of farm-produced dairy products and the prevalence of allergic disease. More specifically, Waser and colleagues[100] reported that the consumption of farm milk may offer protection against asthma and allergy. These associations are independent of farm-related coexposures, and other farm-produced products were not independently related to any allergy-related health outcome. Similarly, Perkin and Strachan[101] reported that unpasteurized milk may be a modifiable influence on allergic sensitization in children. The effect was seen in all children, independent of farming status.

Other strategies have sought to alter the commensal gut flora either directly through the administration of living microorganisms (probiotics), or indirectly through the provision of nondigestible growth-enhancing substrates (prebiotics). One study assessed the effects of prebiotics on allergy prevention,[102] in which 134 of 152 infants (68 in placebo, 66 in intervention group) completed the follow-up period; significant lower cumulative incidences for possible allergic outcomes such as atopic dermatitis, recurrent wheezing, and allergic urticaria in the intervention group compared with the placebo group were noted.[102]

There are many studies that investigate the role of probiotics on the prevention and treatment of allergies; however, many variables are associated with such studies. For example, different probiotic strains have been studied, at different doses, and with different treatment regimens. Not all studies treat both mother (during pregnancy and/or breastfeeding) and child, and the viability of probiotic organisms is not always detailed. Hence, clinical trial results from 1 probiotic strain in 1 population cannot be automatically generalized to other strains or to different populations. There is also great variability with respect to patient groups recruited. A recent meta-analysis found evidence for the use of probiotics for the treatment of eczema, but the evidence regarding the role of probiotics for the prevention of eczema is described as weak.[103]

Whether probiotic-induced microbiota changes (and associated clinical effects) persist after administration ceases remains unclear.

It has been shown that infant formulae that are fortified with prebiotics can bias the microbiota to more closely resemble that of breast milk (the so-called bifidogenic effect). The clinical correlates of these changes, at least with respect to allergy, remain unclear. Whether the many reviews in this field will yield different findings when more recent studies are included in the analyses of pooled data remains to be seen.

Summary

Observational studies suggest that the consumption of unpasteurized milk may reduce the prevalence of allergic sensitization and disease; however, there are safety concerns regarding consumption of unpasteurized milk and this cannot therefore be recommended for the prevention of food allergy. Study findings are inconsistent with respect to the use of prebiotics and probiotics for the prevention of allergy.

NUTRITIONAL SUPPLEMENTS

There are ecological observations that note geographic differences in allergy prevalence; such changes have been linked with regional dietary practices and/or environmental factors (eg, sunlight and its subsequent influence on metabolic factors). In recent years, there has been a focus on the role of vitamins, antioxidants, and vegetables, as well as fatty acid intake, on the prevention or treatment of allergies.[104,105]

Fatty Acids

Dietary lipids, especially n-3 and n-6 long-chain PUFAs (LCPUFA), regulate immune function, and may modify the adherence of microbes in the mucosal, thereby contributing to host-microbe interactions. Studies in this field report a positive effect with respect to the prevention of allergic outcomes (sensitization,[106] eczema,[107] and asthma[108]). However, the outcomes are inconsistent.[109] For example. Dunstan and colleagues,[110] in a small randomized controlled trial of omega-3 fatty acids administered prenatally in high dose to atopic women, reported a reduction in both hen's egg sensitization and severe eczema (at 1 year of age).[111] However, Peat and colleagues,[112] in a large randomized controlled trial (n = 616 children), reported only a positive allergy-preventive effect through fatty acid supplementation for the outcomes for dust mite sensitization and the atopic cough. However, the study intervention was of low dose and was introduced at only 36 weeks' gestation. In addition, many of the infants did not have direct dietary supplementation until 6 months postnatal age (ie, there was only limited perinatal intervention in this study). Oral food challenges were not performed. Kull and colleagues[113] showed, after controlling for confounding factors (parental allergy and early onset eczema or wheeze), that regular fish (a rich source of omega-3 fatty acids) consumption during the first year of life was associated with a reduced risk for allergic sensitization to foods (by age 4 years). Oral food challenges were not performed. It is unclear whether such an effect could be explained by oral tolerance induction (as discussed earlier) to food proteins or whether omega-3 fatty acids could have a generic antiallergy effect. Negative study findings include those by Marks,[114] who in a randomized, placebo-controlled trial found that a reduction in exposure to house dust mite allergens and modification of dietary fatty acids (in the first 5 years of life) did not reduce the risk of asthma or allergic disease at 5 years of age in at-risk children. These negative findings corroborate the negative results of previous studies trialing environmental modifications to reduce asthma in children.[115] Despite these conflicting findings, many infant formulas are supplemented with LCPUFAs (such as arachidonic acid and docosahexaenoic acid). The ability of these fatty acids to exert immunologic effects has been shown[116]; however, the clinical benefits with respect to allergy outcomes require further investigation.

Vitamins

Dietary vitamins have potent immune-modulating effects.[117,118] The most notable example of a clear epigenetic effect of a vitamin at risk of subsequent allergic disease is evident in a mouse model in which Hollingsworth and colleagues[119] reported that folate (a dietary methyl donor) supplementation in pregnancy induces hypermethylation (silencing) of regulatory genes in lung tissue, leading to the development of allergic airway disease and associated allergic responses: this effect was also transmitted to subsequent generations. In humans, 1 study reported that folate supplements in pregnancy are associated with increased childhood wheezing[120]; another found the opposite relationship.[121] It has been possible to study the effect of vitamin supplementation in young children with respect to allergy outcomes, because many countries advocate routine vitamin supplementation during early childhood. Separate studies in Finland[118] and the United States[122] have observed an increased association between vitamin D supplementation in infancy and atopic disease. However, study outcomes were restricted to rhinitis in adulthood in the first study, and select subgroups in the second study: asthma (in black children) and food allergies (as defined by a medical professional) in the exclusively formula-fed population. Kull and colleagues[123] in a large (n = 4089) prospective birth cohort investigated the association between the supplementation of vitamins A and D (administered in either a water-based or peanut-oil–based vehicle) during the first year of life, and the outcome of allergic disease up to 4 years of age. Children supplemented with vitamins A and D in the water-soluble vehicle during the first year of life had an almost 2-fold increased risk of asthma, food hypersensitivity (determined by parental questionnaire), and sensitization (to common food and airborne allergens) at age 4 years, when compared with those receiving vitamins in peanut oil. There are various possible explanations for these findings. Vitamin A and/or D may protect against the risk of developing allergy. The study findings then hinge on better absorption of vitamin A and D from the oil-based vehicle than from a water-based vehicle. Alternatively, vitamin A and/or D increase the risk for the development of allergy. The absorption of vitamin A and/or D then needs to be superior when the vitamins are administered in the water-based vehicle. Systemic uptake was not measured. The rates of allergy in the 2 study groups were not compared with children who had not received vitamin supplementation at all as only 2% of children in this cohort did not receive vitamin supplementation at all. It may also be that vitamin A and/or D has no effect on allergy outcomes and the effects observed are caused by the use of peanut oil. However, the fatty acids in peanut oil are strongly biased toward the proinflammatory omega-6 fatty acids in a ratio of omega-6/omega-3 fatty acids of 34:1. Were this effect to be significant, a higher rate of allergy would be expected in the group of children who received the oil-based supplement.

Vitamin D deficiency (VDD) has previously been linked with allergic disease; more specifically atopic dermatitis[124] and recurrent wheeze,[124,125] In 2007, Camargo and colleagues[126] first implicated this deficiency as a potential risk factor for food allergy because of similar epidemiologic trends for UV-B exposure and VDD, and evidence of a striking north-south gradient in the prescription of epinephrine autoinjectors (used as a proxy for food allergy and/or anaphylaxis) in the United States. There are significant differences in UV-B exposure; levels of 25-hydroxyvitamin D (25 [OH]D) fluctuate with season (lowest in winter and highest in summer) and latitude (inversely with distance from the equator). The epinephrine autoinjector finding was recently replicated by Mullins and colleagues[127] and extended to hospitalizations for anaphylaxis in Australia; these investigators also reported similar findings using a different surrogate for food allergy, namely the use of hypoallergenic infant formulae.[128] Moreover, north-south differences in the United States have been reported for both emergency department visits and hospitalizations for food allergy.[129,130] Several studies have described that food allergy is more commonly reported in children born in seasons of low UV-B intensity.[131–133] Risk factors for VDD, such as obesity and race, have been associated with food allergen sensitization. For example, the prevalence of obesity (a risk factor for VDD[134] and associated with decreased bioavailability of vitamin D metabolites[135]) has increased in children and adults in the past 20 years. Potentially further implicating VDD in the development of food allergy is the observation that obesity/overweight status in children between 2 and 5 years of age is a risk factor for food allergen sensitization relative to normal-weight peers.[136] In addition, characteristic racial variations in VDD (attributed to the effect of skin pigment on UV-B penetration essential for 25[OH]D synthesis) parallel food allergy and sensitization[137] because the prevalence of both conditions are highest among African Americans, followed by Hispanics and then non-Hispanic whites. The potential mechanisms for the hypothesized link between sunshine, vitamin D, and food allergy in children have been further analyzed in a review by Vassallo and Camargo.[138]

More direct studies in this field need to proceed with caution, particularly during pregnancy, when fat-soluble vitamins A, D, and E have the potential to either increase or disease or have other adverse effects.

Summary

Randomized controlled studies provide conflicting results with respect to LCPUFA supplementation for the prevention of allergy. Studies that show a positive effect do so for different allergic disease outcomes. Observational studies that examine the effect of vitamin A and D supplementation during the first year of life suggest an increased rate of sensitization and allergy at 4 years of age, but only when administered in water-soluble vehicles; it remains unclear why vitamin A and D supplementation in different vehicles exerts such different clinical effects. It may be that VDD, induced through decreased UV-B exposure, obesity, or factors related to ethnicity, is associated with increased food allergy or surrogates thereof; whether early life supplementation with vitamin D acts to prevent the development of allergy needs to be trialed in safe randomized studies.

Antioxidants

Antioxidants such as vitamins C and E, β-carotene, zinc, and selenium are free-radical scavengers shown to decrease inflammatory processes. Recent dietary changes include decreasing intake of foods containing these compounds (eg, fresh fruit and vegetables). There are no interventional studies that assess the effect of antioxidant supplementation on the prevention of food allergy; however, ecological observations, suggest that the higher intake of fresh fruit and vegetables in certain European countries is associated with a decreased prevalence of food allergy.[139] In addition, there is preliminary evidence in children[140,141] and adults[142,143] to suggest that high antioxidant intake (in select subgroups) may influence respiratory diseases such as wheeze or hay fever.

Trace Elements

Low cord blood selenium and iron have been associated with a higher subsequent risk of persistent wheeze for the former and both wheeze and eczema for the latter.[144]

Summary

Ecological observations, and preliminary studies, suggest that a higher intake of foods rich in antioxidants may confer protection against allergy outcomes. However, further randomized interventional studies are required.

NEW POTENTIAL STRATEGIES FOR THE PREVENTION OF FOOD ALLERGY

In addition to the studies detailed earlier, other approaches are being investigated to prevent the onset or progression of food allergy. Given that an abraded skin barrier such as that found in eczema may be an important route of food allergen sensitization, trials that adopt a rigorous approach to the treatment of infantile eczema are needed; Fukuie and colleagues,[145] using a retrospective methodology, recently explored the relationship between serum IgE levels and proactive treatment with corticosteroid creams in 45 patients with moderate to severe atopic dermatitis. In a 2-year period, 25 proactive and 20 reactive patients were followed; at baseline, their SCORAD (Scoring Atopic Dermatitis) scores were similar at 82.2 and 79.5 for proactive and reactive patients, respectively. Their serum IgE levels were 2442 and 2081 IU/mL, respectively. Serum IgE was significantly decreased in the proactive group at 24 months ($P<.01$). Moreover, the food-specific IgE levels for egg white and cow's milk were significantly decreased in the proactive group ($P = .004$ and $P = .016$, respectively). Saprophytic mycobacteria such as *Mycobacterium vaccae* are potent type 1 immunostimulants and have also been trialed as candidates for the modulation of allergic disease. Studies into the alleviation of childhood eczema symptoms have proved disappointing.[146] A similar approach has also been trialed using intestinal helminthic infections. There is ongoing research into the use of novel immune-modifying agents such as vaccines and/or vaccine adjuvants. With respect to the use of adjuvants, CpG oligonucleotides might offer an alternative to conventional immunotherapy in preventing, and potentially reversing, Th2-biased immune deregulation (which leads to allergy).

SUMMARY

The natural history of food allergy suggests plasticity within the developing immune system as many common food allergies (such as egg and milk allergy) are outgrown. The switch from a state of allergy to tolerance may even occur during the first few years of life. Turcanu and colleagues[147] reported that the resolution of PA is accompanied by a reversal of the Th2-skewed to Th1-skewed, allergen-specific, immune response. These findings are encouraging because they raise the possibility that immune responses are susceptible to prevention strategies.

The conventional wisdom is that early exposure to allergenic food proteins during pregnancy, lactation, or infancy leads to food allergies, and that prevention strategies should aim to eliminate allergenic food proteins during these periods of immunologic vulnerability, especially in at-risk subgroups. There is some evidence to support the use of dietary interventions in at-risk pregnant and/or lactating women, but benefits are largely restricted to the outcome of mild atopic eczema and are not uniformly achieved. There is also a risk that these interventions may compromise maternal and fetal nutrition. Breastfeeding for at least the first 4 months of life offers some protection against allergic disease (eczema and asthma) but the protective effect of exclusive breastfeeding beyond 4 months of age is uncertain. For at-risk infants who are not exclusively breastfed, or who require supplementation of breastfeeding, the use of extensively hydrolyzed formula offers some protection against the development of allergy (eczema and possibly asthma). The findings of dietary interventions with products such as s LCPUFAs, antioxidants, prebiotics and probiotics, and vitamin supplementation, are unclear or inconsistent, with some having potential safety issues, and can therefore not be broadly recommended.

Future studies need to overcome the many methodological challenges detailed in this article. Better markers are required to identify at-risk populations, because not all children who develop food allergies are born to atopic families. With current advances in gene-environment interactions, future studies may be aimed at interventions of specifically defined groups of children, whose genotyping identifies them as being at risk.

REFERENCES

1. Shek LP, Cabrera-Morales EA, Soh SE, et al. A population-based questionnaire survey on the prevalence of peanut, tree nut, and shellfish allergy in 2 Asian populations. J Allergy Clin Immunol 2010;126:324–31, 331.e1–7.
2. Sicherer SH, Munoz-Furlong A, Godbold JH, et al. US prevalence of self-reported peanut, tree nut, and sesame allergy: 11-year follow-up. J Allergy Clin Immunol 2010;125:1322–6.

3. Venter C, Pereira B, Grundy J, et al. Prevalence of sensitization reported and objectively assessed food hypersensitivity amongst six-year-old children: a population-based study. Pediatr Allergy Immunol 2006;17:356–63.
4. Venter C, Pereira B, Grundy J, et al. Incidence of parentally reported and clinically diagnosed food hypersensitivity in the first year of life. J Allergy Clin Immunol 2006;117:1118–24.
5. Du Toit G, Katz Y, Sasieni P, et al. Early consumption of peanuts in infancy is associated with a low prevalence of peanut allergy. J Allergy Clin Immunol 2008;122:984–91.
6. Liu AH, Jaramillo R, Sicherer SH, et al. National prevalence and risk factors for food allergy and relationship to asthma: results from the National Health and Nutrition Examination Survey 2005–2006. J Allergy Clin Immunol 2010;126:798–806.
7. Ben-Shoshan M, Harrington DW, Soller L, et al. A population-based study on peanut, tree nut, fish, shellfish, and sesame allergy prevalence in Canada. J Allergy Clin Immunol 2010;125:1327–35.
8. Ben-Shoshan M, Harrington DW, Soller L, et al. Rising prevalence of allergy to peanut in children: data from 2 sequential cohorts. J Allergy Clin Immunol 2002;110:784–9.
9. Sicherer SH, Furlong TJ, Maes HH, et al. Genetics of peanut allergy: a twin study. J Allergy Clin Immunol 2000;106:53–6.
10. Lack G, Fox D, Northstone K, et al. Factors associated with the development of peanut allergy in childhood. N Engl J Med 2003;348:977–85.
11. Fussman C, Todem D, Forster J, et al. Cow's milk exposure and asthma in a newborn cohort: repeated ascertainment indicates reverse causation. J Asthma 2007;44:99–105.
12. Lowe AJ, Carlin JB, Bennett CM, et al. Atopic disease and breast-feeding–cause or consequence? J Allergy Clin Immunol 2006;117:682–7.
13. Learning early about allergy to peanut (LEAP study) 2007. Available at: http://www.clinicaltrials.gov/ct2/show/NCT00329784. Accessed February 24, 2011. [Internet Communication].
14. Zeiger RS. Food allergen avoidance in the prevention of food allergy in infants and children. Pediatrics 2003;111:1662–71.
15. Boyle RJ, Robins-Browne RM, Tang ML. Probiotic use in clinical practice: what are the risks? Am J Clin Nutr 2006;83:1256–64.
16. Nolan RC, de Leon MP, Rolland JM, et al. What's in a kiss: peanut allergen transmission as a sensitizer? J Allergy Clin Immunol 2007;119:755.
17. Maloney JM, Chapman MD, Sicherer SH. Peanut allergen exposure through saliva: assessment and interventions to reduce exposure. J Allergy Clin Immunol 2006;118:719–24.
18. Perry TT, Conover-Walker MK, Pomes A, et al. Distribution of peanut allergen in the environment. J Allergy Clin Immunol 2004;113:973–6.
19. Fox AT, Sasieni P, Du TG, et al. Household peanut consumption as a risk factor for the development of peanut allergy. J Allergy Clin Immunol 2009;123:417–23.
20. Arshad SH, Kurukulaaratchy RJ, Fenn M, et al. Early life risk factors for current wheeze, asthma, and bronchial hyperresponsiveness at 10 years of age. Chest 2005;127:502–8.
21. Bergmann RL, Edenharter G, Bergmann KE, et al. Predictability of early atopy by cord blood-IgE and parental history. Clin Exp Allergy 1997;27:752–60.
22. Hansen LG, Halken S, Host A, et al. Prediction of allergy from family history and cord blood IgE levels. A follow-up at the age of 5 years. Cord blood IgE. IV. Pediatr Allergy Immunol 1993;4:34–40.

23. Greer FR, Sicherer SH, Burks AW. Effects of early nutritional interventions on the development of atopic disease in infants and children: the role of maternal dietary restriction, breastfeeding, timing of introduction of complementary foods, and hydrolyzed formulas. Pediatrics 2008;121:183–91.
24. Swart JF, Ultee K. Rectal bleeding in a preterm infant as a symptom of allergic colitis. Eur J Pediatr 2003;162:55–6.
25. Machida HM, Catto Cith AG, Gall DG, et al. Allergic colitis in infancy: clinical and pathologic aspects. J Pediatr Gastroenterol Nutr 1994;19:22–6.
26. Pentiuk SP, Miller CK, Kaul A. Eosinophilic esophagitis in infants and toddlers. Dysphagia 2007;22:44–8.
27. Sicherer SH, Eigenmann PA, Sampson HA. Clinical features of food protein-induced enterocolitis syndrome. J Pediatr 1998;133:214–9.
28. Hide DW, Matthews S, Tariq S, et al. Allergen avoidance in infancy and allergy at 4 years of age. Allergy 1996;51:89–93.
29. Falth-Magnusson K, Kjellman NI. Development of atopic disease in babies whose mothers were receiving exclusion diet during pregnancy–a randomized study. J Allergy Clin Immunol 1987;80:868–75.
30. Falth-Magnusson K, Kjellman NI. Allergy prevention by maternal elimination diet during late pregnancy–a 5-year follow-up of a randomized study. J Allergy Clin Immunol 1992;89:709–13.
31. Lilja G, Dannaeus A, Foucard T, et al. Effects of maternal diet during late pregnancy and lactation on the development of atopic diseases in infants up to 18 months of age–in-vivo results. Clin Exp Allergy 1989;19:473–9.
32. Kramer MS, Kakuma R. Maternal dietary antigen avoidance during pregnancy or lactation, or both, for preventing or treating atopic disease in the child. Cochrane Database Syst Rev 2006;3:CD000133.
33. American Academy of Pediatrics Committee on Nutrition. Pediatric nutrition handbook. Elk Grove (CA); 2004.
34. COMA Working Group on the Weaning Diet. Weaning and the weaning diet [report]; 2007. London. 1-1-1994.
35. Infant Feeding Advice: Australasian Society of Allergy and Immunology. Available at: http://www.allergy.org.au/content/view/350/287/. Accessed May 28, 2009. [Internet Communication].
36. Agostoni C, et al. Complementary feeding: a commentary by the ESPGHAN Committee on Nutrition. J Pediatr Gastroenterol Nutr 2008;46:99–110.
37. Boyce JA, Assa'ad A, Burks AW, et al; NIAID-Sponsored Expert Panel. Guidelines for the diagnosis and management of food allergy in the United States: report of the NIAID-sponsored expert panel. J Allergy Clin Immunol 2010;126: S1–58.
38. Arshad SH, Bateman B, Sadeghnejad A, et al. Prevention of allergic disease during childhood by allergen avoidance: the Isle of Wight prevention study. J Allergy Clin Immunol 2007;119:307–13.
39. Sicherer SH, Wood RA, Stablein D, et al. Maternal consumption of peanut during pregnancy is associated with peanut sensitization in atopic infants. J Allergy Clin Immunol 2010;126(6):1191–7.
40. DesRoches A, Infante-Rivard C, Paradis L, et al. Peanut allergy: is maternal transmission of antigens during pregnancy and breastfeeding a risk factor? J Investig Allergol Clin Immunol 2010;20:289–94.
41. Castro-Rodriguez JA, Garcia-Marcos L, Alfonseda Rojas JD, et al. Mediterranean diet as a protective factor for wheezing in preschool children. J Pediatr 2008;152:823–8, 828.e1–2.

42. Chatzi L, Torrent M, Romieu I, et al. Mediterranean diet in pregnancy is protective for wheeze and atopy in childhood. Thorax 2008;63:507–13.
43. Shaheen SO, Northstone K, Newson RB, et al. Dietary patterns in pregnancy and respiratory and atopic outcomes in childhood. Thorax 2009;64:411–7.
44. Chirdo FG, Rumbo M, Anon MC, et al. Presence of high levels of non-degraded gliadin in breast milk from healthy mothers. Scand J Gastroenterol 1998;33: 1186–92.
45. Palmer DJ, Makrides M. Diet of lactating women and allergic reactions in their infants. Curr Opin Clin Nutr Metab Care 2006;9:284–8.
46. Vadas P, Wai Y, Burks W, et al. Detection of peanut allergens in breast milk of lactating women. JAMA 2001;285:1746–8.
47. Host A, Halken S. A prospective study of cow milk allergy in Danish infants during the first 3 years of life. Clinical course in relation to clinical and immunological type of hypersensitivity reaction. Allergy 1990;45:587–96.
48. Hattevig G, Kjellman B, Sigurs N, et al. The effect of maternal avoidance of eggs, cow's milk, and fish during lactation on the development of IgE, IgG, and IgA antibodies in infants. J Allergy Clin Immunol 1990;85:108–15.
49. Herrmann ME, Dannemann A, Grüters A, et al. Prospective study of the atopy preventive effect of maternal avoidance of milk and eggs during pregnancy and lactation. Eur J Pediatr 1996;155:770–4.
50. World Health Organization, Breastfeeding Recommendations. 2010. Available at: http://www.who.int/topics/breastfeeding/en/. Accessed December 1, 2010. [Internet Communication].
51. Verhasselt V, Milcent V, Cazareth J, et al. Breast milk-mediated transfer of an antigen induces tolerance and protection from allergic asthma. Nat Med 2008; 14:170–5.
52. Grulee CG, Sanford HN. The influence of breast and artificial feeding on infantile eczema. J Pediatr 1930;9:223–5.
53. Gdalevich M, Mimouni D, David M, et al. Breast-feeding and the onset of atopic dermatitis in childhood: a systematic review and meta-analysis of prospective studies. J Am Acad Dermatol 2001;45:520–7.
54. Muraro A, Dreborg S, Halken S, et al. Dietary prevention of allergic diseases in infants and small children. Part III: Critical review of published peer-reviewed observational and interventional studies and final recommendations. Pediatr Allergy Immunol 2004;15:291–307.
55. Khakoo A, Lack G. Preventing food allergy. Curr Allergy Asthma Rep 2004;4: 36–42.
56. Oddy WH, de Klerk NH, Sly PD, et al. The effects of respiratory infections, atopy, and breastfeeding on childhood asthma. Eur Respir J 2002;19:899–905.
57. Saarinen UM, Kajosaari M. Does dietary elimination in infancy prevent or only postpone a food allergy? A study of fish and citrus allergy in 375 children. Lancet 1980;1:166–7.
58. Lucas A, Brooke OG, Morley R, et al. Early diet of preterm infants and development of allergic or atopic disease: randomised prospective study. BMJ 1990; 300:837–40.
59. de Jong MH, Scharp-Van Der Linden VT, Aalberse R, et al. The effect of brief neonatal exposure to cows' milk on atopic symptoms up to age 5. Arch Dis Child 2002;86:365–9.
60. Sears MR, Greene JM, Willan AR, et al. Long-term relation between breastfeeding and development of atopy and asthma in children and young adults: a longitudinal study. Lancet 2002;360:901–7.

61. Bergmann RL, Diepgen TL, Kuss O, et al. Breastfeeding duration is a risk factor for atopic eczema. Clin Exp Allergy 2002;32:205–9.
62. Isolauri E, Tahvanainen A, Peltola T, et al. Breast-feeding of allergic infants. J Pediatr 1999;134:27–32.
63. Kramer MS, Kakuma R. The optimal duration of exclusive breastfeeding: a systematic review. Adv Exp Med Biol 2004;554:63–77.
64. Osborn DA, Sinn J. Formulas containing hydrolysed protein for prevention of allergy and food intolerance in infants. Cochrane Database Syst Rev 2003;4: CD003664.
65. Fiocchi A, Brozek J, Schünemann H, et al. World Allergy Organization (WAO) Diagnosis and Rationale for Action against Cow's Milk Allergy (DRACMA) Guidelines. Pediatr Allergy Immunol 2010;21(Suppl 21):1–125.
66. Høst A, Halken S, Muraro A, et al. Dietary prevention of allergic diseases in infants and small children. Pediatr Allergy Immunol 2008;19:1–4.
67. du Toit G, Meyer R, Shah N, et al. Identifying and managing cow's milk protein allergy. Arch Dis Child Educ Pract Ed 2010;95:134–44.
68. von Berg A, Filipiak-Pittroff B, Krämer U, et al. Preventive effect of hydrolyzed infant formulas persists until age 6 years: long-term results from the German Infant Nutritional Intervention Study (GINI). J Allergy Clin Immunol 2008;121: 1442–7.
69. von Berg A, Koletzko S, Filipiak-Pittroff B, et al. Certain hydrolyzed formulas reduce the incidence of atopic dermatitis but not that of asthma: three-year results of the German Infant Nutritional Intervention Study. J Allergy Clin Immunol 2007;119:718–25.
70. Osborn DA, Sinn J. Soy formula for prevention of allergy and food intolerance in infants. Cochrane Database Syst Rev 2006;4:CD003741.
71. Tarini BA, Carroll AE, Sox CM, et al. Systematic review of the relationship between early introduction of solid foods to infants and the development of allergic disease. Arch Pediatr Adolesc Med 2006;160:502–7.
72. Fergusson DM, Horwood LJ, Shannon FT. Early solid feeding and recurrent childhood eczema: a 10-year longitudinal study. Pediatrics 1990;86:541–6.
73. Zutavern A, von Mutius E, Harris J, et al. The introduction of solids in relation to asthma and eczema. Arch Dis Child 2004;89:303–8.
74. Koplin JJ, Osborne NJ, Wake M, et al. Can early introduction of egg prevent egg allergy in infants? A population-based study. J Allergy Clin Immunol 2010;126: 807–13.
75. Kajosaari M, Saarinen UM. Prophylaxis of atopic disease by six months' total solid food elimination. Evaluation of 135 exclusively breast-fed infants of atopic families. Acta Paediatr Scand 1983;72:411–4.
76. Prescott SL, Smith P, Tang M, et al. The importance of early complementary feeding in the development of oral tolerance: concerns and controversies. Pediatr Allergy Immunol 2008;19:375–80.
77. Prescott SL, Bouygue GR, Videky D, et al. Avoidance or exposure to foods in prevention and treatment of food allergy? Curr Opin Allergy Clin Immunol 2010;10:258–66.
78. Allen CW, Campbell DE, Kemp AS. Food allergy: is strict avoidance the only answer? Pediatr Allergy Immunol 2009;20:415–22.
79. Kim JS, Sicherer S. Should avoidance of foods be strict in prevention and treatment of food allergy? Curr Opin Allergy Clin Immunol 2010;10:252–7.
80. Zeiger RS, Heller S. The development and prediction of atopy in high-risk children: follow-up at age seven years in a prospective randomized study of

combined maternal and infant food allergen avoidance. J Allergy Clin Immunol 1995;95:1179–90.

81. Saloga J, Renz H, Larsen GL, et al. Increased airways responsiveness in mice depends on local challenge with antigen. Am J Respir Crit Care Med 1994;149: 65–70.
82. Hsieh KY, Tsai CC, Wu CH, et al. Epicutaneous exposure to protein antigen and food allergy. Clin Exp Allergy 2003;33:1067–75.
83. Strid J, Hourihane J, Kimber I, et al. Disruption of the stratum corneum allows potent epicutaneous immunization with protein antigens resulting in a dominant systemic Th2 response. Eur J Immunol 2004;34:2100–9.
84. Simonte SJ, Ma S, Mofidi S, et al. Relevance of casual contact with peanut butter in children with peanut allergy. J Allergy Clin Immunol 2003;112:180–2.
85. Frank L, Marian A, Visser M, et al. Exposure to peanuts in utero and in infancy and the development of sensitization to peanut allergens in young children. Pediatr Allergy Immunol 1999;10:27–32.
86. Strid J, Thomson M, Hourihane J, et al. A novel model of sensitization and oral tolerance to peanut protein. Immunology 2004;113:293–303.
87. Strid J, Hourihane J, Kimber I, et al. Epicutaneous exposure to peanut protein prevents oral tolerance and enhances allergic sensitization. Clin Exp Allergy 2005;35:757–66.
88. Frossard CP, Tropia L, Hauser C, et al. Lymphocytes in Peyer patches regulate clinical tolerance in a murine model of food allergy. J Allergy Clin Immunol 2004; 113:958–64.
89. Levy Y, Broides A, Segal N, et al. Peanut and tree nut allergy in children: role of peanut snacks in Israel? Allergy 2003;58:1206–7.
90. Hill DJ, Hosking CS, Heine RG. Clinical spectrum of food allergy in children in Australia and South-East Asia: identification and targets for treatment. Ann Med 1999;31:272–81.
91. Dalal I, Binson I, Reifen R, et al. Food allergy is a matter of geography after all: sesame as a major cause of severe IgE-mediated food allergic reactions among infants and young children in Israel. Allergy 2002;57:362–5.
92. Husby S, Mestecky J, Moldoveanu Z, et al. Oral tolerance in humans. T cell but not B cell tolerance after antigen feeding. J Immunol 1994;152:4663–70.
93. EAT Study. 2010. Available at: http://www.eatstudy.co.uk/. Accessed February 24, 2011. [Internet Communication].
94. Poole JA, Barriga K, Leung DY, et al. Timing of initial exposure to cereal grains and the risk of wheat allergy. Pediatrics 2006;117:2175–82.
95. Ivarsson A. The Swedish epidemic of coeliac disease explored using an epidemiological approach–some lessons to be learnt. Best Pract Res Clin Gastroenterol 2005;19:425–40.
96. Prevent Celiac Disease Study. 2010. Available at: http://www.preventceliacdisease.com/. Accessed February 24, 2011. [Internet Communication].
97. Eggesbo HB, Sovik S, Dolvik S, et al. Proposal of a CT scoring system of the paranasal sinuses in diagnosing cystic fibrosis. Eur Radiol 2003;13:1451–60.
98. Bager P, Wohlfahrt J, Westergaard T. Caesarean delivery and risk of atopy and allergic disease: meta-analyses. Clin Exp Allergy 2008;38:634–42.
99. Dioun AF, Harris SK, Hibberd PL. Is maternal age at delivery related to childhood food allergy? Pediatr Allergy Immunol 2003;14:307–11.
100. Waser M, Michels KB, Bieli C, et al. Inverse association of farm milk consumption with asthma and allergy in rural and suburban populations across Europe. Clin Exp Allergy 2007;37:661–70.

101. Perkin MR, Strachan DP. Which aspects of the farming lifestyle explain the inverse association with childhood allergy? J Allergy Clin Immunol 2006;117: 1374–81.
102. Arslanoglu S, Moro GE, Schmitt J, et al. Early dietary intervention with a mixture of prebiotic oligosaccharides reduces the incidence of allergic manifestations and infections during the first two years of life. J Nutr 2008;138:1091–5.
103. Lee J, Seto D, Bielory L. Meta-analysis of clinical trials of probiotics for prevention and treatment of pediatric atopic dermatitis. J Allergy Clin Immunol 2008; 121:116–21.
104. Martindale S, Janssen K, van Schadewijk A, et al. Antioxidant intake in pregnancy in relation to wheeze and eczema in the first two years of life. Am J Respir Crit Care Med 2005;171:121–8.
105. Ram FS, Rowe BH, Kaur B. Vitamin C supplementation for asthma. Cochrane Database Syst Rev 2004;(3):CD000993.
106. Calvani M, Alessandri C, Sopo SM, et al. Consumption of fish, butter and margarine during pregnancy and development of allergic sensitizations in the offspring: role of maternal atopy. Pediatr Allergy Immunol 2006;17:94–102.
107. Sausenthaler S, Koletzko S, Schaaf B, et al. Maternal diet during pregnancy in relation to eczema and allergic sensitization in the offspring at 2 y of age. Am J Clin Nutr 2007;85:530–7.
108. Salam MT, Li YF, Langholz B, et al. Maternal fish consumption during pregnancy and risk of early childhood asthma. J Asthma 2005;42:513–8.
109. Newson RB, Shaheen SO, Henderson AJ, et al. Umbilical cord and maternal blood red cell fatty acids and early childhood wheezing and eczema. J Allergy Clin Immunol 2004;114:531–7.
110. Dunstan JA, Giliani S, Gu Y, et al. Fish oil supplementation in pregnancy modifies neonatal allergen-specific immune responses and clinical outcomes in infants at high risk of atopy: a randomized, controlled trial. J Allergy Clin Immunol 2003; 112:1178–84.
111. Dunstan JA, Mori TA, Barden A, et al. Maternal fish oil supplementation in pregnancy reduces interleukin-13 levels in cord blood of infants at high risk of atopy. Clin Exp Allergy 2003;33:442–8.
112. Peat JK, Mihrshahi S, Kemp AS, et al. Three-year outcomes of dietary fatty acid modification and house dust mite reduction in the Childhood Asthma Prevention Study. J Allergy Clin Immunol 2004;114:807–13.
113. Kull I, Bergstrom A, Lilja G, et al. Fish consumption during the first year of life and development of allergic diseases during childhood. Allergy 2006;61:1009–15.
114. Marks GB. Environmental factors and gene-environment interactions in the aetiology of asthma. Clin Exp Pharmacol Physiol 2006;33:285–9.
115. Simpson A, Custovic A. Allergen avoidance in the primary prevention of asthma. Curr Opin Allergy Clin Immunol 2004;4:45–51.
116. Field CJ, Van Aerde JE, Robinson LE, et al. Effect of providing a formula supplemented with long-chain polyunsaturated fatty acids on immunity in full-term neonates. Br J Nutr 2008;99(1):91–9.
117. Long KZ, Santos JI. Vitamins and the regulation of the immune response. Pediatr Infect Dis J 1999;18:283–90.
118. Hypponen E, Laara E, Reunanen A, et al. Intake of vitamin D and risk of type 1 diabetes: a birth-cohort study. Lancet 2001;358:1500–3.
119. Hollingsworth JW, Maruoka S, Boon K, et al. In utero supplementation with methyl donors enhances allergic airway disease in mice. J Clin Invest 2008; 118:3462–9.

120. Haberg SE, London SJ, Stigum H, et al. Folic acid supplements in pregnancy and early childhood respiratory health. Arch Dis Child 2009;94:180–4.
121. Matsui EC, Matsui W. Higher serum folate levels are associated with a lower risk of atopy and wheeze. J Allergy Clin Immunol 2009;123:1253–9.
122. Milner JD, Stein DM, McCarter R, et al. Early infant multivitamin supplementation is associated with increased risk for food allergy and asthma. Pediatrics 2004; 114:27–32.
123. Kull I, Bergström A, Melén E, et al. Early-life supplementation of vitamins A and D, in water-soluble form or in peanut oil, and allergic diseases during childhood. J Allergy Clin Immunol 2006;118:1299–304.
124. Sidbury R, Sullivan AF, Thadhani RI, et al. Randomized controlled trial of vitamin D supplementation for winter-related atopic dermatitis in Boston: a pilot study. Br J Dermatol 2008;159:245–7.
125. Ginde AA, Mansbach JM, Camargo CA Jr. Vitamin D, respiratory infections, and asthma. Curr Allergy Asthma Rep 2009;9:81–7.
126. Camargo CA Jr, Clark S, Kaplan MS, et al. Regional differences in EpiPen prescriptions in the United States: the potential role of vitamin D. J Allergy Clin Immunol 2007;120:131–6.
127. Mullins RJ, Clark S, Camargo CA Jr. Regional variation in infant hypoallergenic formula prescriptions in Australia. Pediatr Allergy Immunol 2010;21:e413–20.
128. Mullins RJ, Clark S, Camargo CA Jr. Regional variation in epinephrine autoinjector prescriptions in Australia: more evidence for the vitamin D-anaphylaxis hypothesis. Ann Allergy Asthma Immunol 2009;103:488–95.
129. Rudders SA, Espinola JA, Camargo CA Jr. North-south differences in US emergency department visits for acute allergic reactions. Ann Allergy Asthma Immunol 2010;104:413–6.
130. Sheehan WJ, Graham D, Ma L, et al. Higher incidence of pediatric anaphylaxis in northern areas of the United States. J Allergy Clin Immunol 2009;124:850–2.
131. Green TD, LaBelle VS, Steele PH, et al. Clinical characteristics of peanut-allergic children: recent changes. Pediatrics 2007;120:1304–10.
132. Sicherer SH, Furlong TJ, Munoz-Furlong A, et al. A voluntary registry for peanut and tree nut allergy: characteristics of the first 5149 registrants. J Allergy Clin Immunol 2001;108:128–32.
133. Vassallo MF, Banerji A, Rudders SA, et al. Season of birth and food allergy in children. Ann Allergy Asthma Immunol 2010;104:307–13.
134. Lagunova Z, Porojnicu AC, Lindberg F, et al. The dependency of vitamin D status on body mass index, gender, age and season. Anticancer Res 2009; 29:3713–20.
135. Wortsman J, Matsuoka LY, Chen TC, et al. Decreased bioavailability of vitamin D in obesity. Am J Clin Nutr 2000;72:690–3.
136. Visness CM, London SJ, Daniels JL, et al. Association of obesity with IgE levels and allergy symptoms in children and adolescents: results from the National Health and Nutrition Examination Survey 2005–2006. J Allergy Clin Immunol 2009;123:1163–9, 1169.e1–4.
137. Branum AM, Lukacs SL. Food allergy among children in the United States. Pediatrics 2009;124:1549–55.
138. Vassallo MF, Camargo CA Jr. Potential mechanisms for the hypothesized link between sunshine, vitamin D, and food allergy in children. J Allergy Clin Immunol 2010;126:217–22.
139. Heinrich J, Holscher B, Bolte G, et al. Allergic sensitization and diet: ecological analysis in selected European cities. Eur Respir J 2001;17:395–402.

140. Forastiere F, Pistelli R, Sestini P, et al. Consumption of fresh fruit rich in vitamin C and wheezing symptoms in children. SIDRIA Collaborative Group, Italy (Italian Studies on Respiratory Disorders in Children and the Environment). Thorax 2000;55:283–8.
141. Okoko BJ, Burney PG, Newson RB, et al. Childhood asthma and fruit consumption. Eur Respir J 2007;29:1161–8.
142. Nagel G, Nieters A, Becker N, et al. The influence of the dietary intake of fatty acids and antioxidants on hay fever in adults. Allergy 2003;58:1277–84.
143. Bodner C, Godden D, Brown K, et al. Antioxidant intake and adult-onset wheeze: a case-control study. Aberdeen WHEASE Study Group. Eur Respir J 1999;13:22–30.
144. Shaheen SO, Newson RB, Henderson AJ, et al. Umbilical cord trace elements and minerals and risk of early childhood wheezing and eczema. Eur Respir J 2004;24:292–7.
145. Fukuie T, Nomura I, Horimukai K, et al. Proactive treatment appears to decrease serum immunoglobulin-E levels in patients with severe atopic dermatitis. Br J Dermatol 2010;163:1127–9.
146. Berth-Jones J, Arkwright PD, Marasovic D, et al. Killed *Mycobacterium vaccae* suspension in children with moderate-to-severe atopic dermatitis: a randomized, double-blind, placebo-controlled trial. Clin Exp Allergy 2006;36:1115–21.
147. Turcanu V, Maleki SJ, Lack G. Characterization of lymphocyte responses to peanuts in normal children, peanut-allergic children, and allergic children who acquired tolerance to peanuts. J Clin Invest 2003;111:1065–72.

Food Allergy Therapy: Is a Cure Within Reach?

Anna Nowak-Węgrzyn, MD[a,*], Antonella Muraro, MD, PhD[b]

KEYWORDS

• Food allergy • Immunotherapy • Oral immunotherapy
• Oral desensitization • Milk allergy • Peanut allergy
• Egg allergy • Food allergy therapy

Food allergy is a growing public health problem.[1] In the United States, it is estimated that 3.9% of general population under 18 years of age is affected by food allergies; the prevalence increased by 18% from 1997 to 2007.[2] Currently, the only treatment of food allergy relies on strict food avoidance, dietary management to avoid nutritional deficiencies, and prompt emergency treatment of acute reactions. There is an unmet medical need for an effective food allergy therapy; thus, development of therapeutic interventions for food allergy is a top research priority. Studies concentrate on the foods most commonly implicated in severe IgE-mediated anaphylactic reactions (peanut, tree nuts, and shellfish) and the most common food allergens, such as cow's milk and hen's egg.[3] The promising therapies under investigation can be classified as food allergen-nonspecific and food allergen-specific.[4] The food allergen-nonspecific therapies for food-induced anaphylaxis include monoclonal anti-IgE antibodies, which increase the threshold dose for peanut in peanut-allergic individuals, and Chinese herbs, which prevent peanut anaphylaxis in an animal model and are currently being evaluated in human studies (**Table 1**). The food allergen-specific therapies include oral immunotherapy (OIT), sublingual immunotherapy (SLIT), and epicutaneous immunotherapy (EPIT) with native food allergens (**Table 2**) and mutated recombinant proteins, which have decreased IgE-binding activity, coadministered within heat-killed *Escherichia coli* to generate maximum immune response (**Table 3**).

The authors have nothing to disclose.

[a] Department of Pediatrics, Jaffe Food Allergy Institute, Mount Sinai School of Medicine, Box 1198, One Gustave L. Levy Place, New York, NY 10029, USA
[b] Department of Pediatrics, Food Allergy Centre, Veneto Region, University of Padua, Via Giustiniani 3, 35128 Padua, Italy
* Corresponding author.
E-mail address: anna.nowak-wegrzyn@mssm.edu

Pediatr Clin N Am 58 (2011) 511–530
doi:10.1016/j.pcl.2011.02.010 **pediatric.theclinics.com**
0031-3955/11/$ – see front matter

Table 1
Allergen-nonspecific therapy for food allergy

Therapy	Mechanism of Action	Effects	Comments
Monoclonal anti-IgE	Binds to circulating IgE, prevents IgE deposition on mast cells, and blocks degranulation. Interferes with the facilitated antigen presentation by B-cell and dendritic cells.	Improves symptoms of asthma and allergic rhinitis; provides protection against peanut anaphylaxis in 75% of treated patients.	Subcutaneous at monthly or 2-week intervals, unknown long-term consequences of IgE elimination; food nonspecific; ongoing studies of combined anti-IgE and milk OIT in children
Traditional TCM	Down-regulation of T_H2 cytokines (IL-4, IL-5, and IL-13), up-regulation of T_H1 cytokines (IFN-γ and IL-12), decreased allergen IgE, decreased T-cell proliferation to peanut.	Reverses allergic inflammation in the airways, affords prolonged protection from peanut anaphylaxis (for ~half of mouse lifespan).	Oral, generally safe and well tolerated; current studies focus on identification of the crucial active herbal components in the multiherb formulas and establishing optimal dosing in phase I and II clinical trials

WHO NEEDS FOOD ALLERGY THERAPY?

Subjects at high risk for severe anaphylaxis and those unlikely to outgrow food allergy spontaneously are most in need of food allergy therapy. Traditional allergy tests (measurement of food allergen-specific IgE antibodies in serum or skin prick test) do not reliably predict the severity of future reactions or the spontaneous development of tolerance. The severity of food-allergic reactions may relate to the diversity of the immune response to IgE-binding epitopes on food allergens (**Fig. 1**). In a peptide microarray-based immunoassay, children with severe reactions to peanut and milk had IgE antibodies that bound to higher number of epitopes than children with mild reactions.[5–7] Persistent milk-allergic children had increased epitope diversity compared with those who outgrew their allergy.[7] Using a competitive peptide microarray assay, allergic patients demonstrated a combination of high-affinity and low-affinity IgE binding whereas those who had outgrown their milk allergy had primarily low-affinity binding.[7] Similarly, persistent egg allergy was associated with recognition of the sequential epitopes on ovomucoid, the major egg white allergen. Subjects who generated IgE antibody responses against both the conformational and sequential epitopes of ovomucoid were likely to have persistent egg allergy. In contrast, subjects who generated IgE antibody responses predominantly against the conformational epitopes of ovomucoid were more likely to have transient egg allergy.[8] Recognition of the specific casein epitopes might identify children at risk for more persistent milk allergy.[9] Persistence of food allergy might be related to high lifetime peak values of food-specific serum IgE antibodies. Two reports describing the natural history of milk and egg allergy in children with multiple food allergies observed that few children with peak milk-specific or egg white–specific IgE antibody levels greater than or equal to 50 kilounits of antibody (kU_A)/L (UniCAP, Phadia, Uppsala, Sweden) outgrew their respective allergy by teenage years.[10,11]

Table 2
Native allergen immunotherapy for food allergy

Therapy	Mechanism of Action	Effects	Comments
Subcutaneous			
Conventional peanut immunotherapy	Altered T-cell responses, up-regulation of suppressor cells	Increased oral peanut tolerance	Subcutaneous injections of gradually increasing doses of allergen; unacceptably high rate of serious adverse events
Birch pollen immunotherapy for oral allergy to apple	Marked reduction in skin test reactivity to raw apple; effect of immunotherapy inversely correlated with baseline skin reactivity but not with serum apple or birch IgE	Significant reduction or total resolution of oral allergy symptoms to raw Golden Delicious apple in a subset of patients receiving immunotherapy for at least 12 months	Clinical effect lasting for up to 30 months after discontinuation in >50% of patients
Oral/Sublingual			
OIT	Decreased: skin test reactivity, food IgE, and IL-4 production by food-specific PBMCs Increased: food IgG, IgA, $CD4^{+}CD23$ high T cells; IL-10	Oral food desensitization or increased threshold dose of food for clinical reactions up to 6 months; short-term success rate approximately 75%	No long-term follow-up data; many patients experience recurrence of symptoms if food not ingested on a daily basis. Significant rate of moderate to severe adverse reactions; convenience of home administration of maintenance doses
SLIT	Serum hazelnut IgG4 and total IL-10 increased in treated group; no change in hazelnut IgE	Oral food desensitization or increased threshold dose on oral hazelnut challenge	Systemic side effects rate 0.2% during rush buildup phase; adverse reaction rate less than with OIT; no long-term follow-up

Abbreviation: PBMCs; peripheral blood mononuclear cells.

Table 3
Engineered allergen immunotherapy for food allergy

	Mechanism of Action	Effects	Comments
Approaches Actively Investigated			
Engineered recombinant peanut IT	Binding to mast cells eliminated or markedly decreased, T-cell responses comparable to native peanut allergens	Protection against peanut anaphylaxis in mice	Improved safety profile compared with conventional IT, requires identification of IgE-binding sites
Heat-killed bacteria mixed with or expressing modified peanut proteins	Upregulation of T_H1 and T-regulatory cytokine responses	Protection against peanut anaphylaxis in mice, lasting up to 10 weeks after treatment	Concern for toxicity of bacterial adjuvants, excessive T_H1 stimulation, and potential for autoimmunity; heat-killed *E coli* expressing modified peanut allergens administered rectally viewed as the safest approach for future human studies. Human studies in adults ongoing
Approaches No Longer Actively Investigated[a]			
Peptide immunotherapy[68]	Overlapping peptides (10–20 amino acids long) that represent the entire sequence of allergen. Binding to mast cells eliminated, T-cell responses preserved	Protection against peanut anaphylaxis in mice	Improved safety profile compared with conventional IT, does not require identification of IgE-binding epitopes; not feasible because the Food and Drug Administration requires quantification of each peptide within the peptide mixture; too expensive.
Plasmid DNA-based immunotherapy[69–71]	Induces prolonged humoral and cellular responses due to CpG motifs in the DNA backbone	Protection against peanut anaphylaxis in sensitized AKR/J mice but induction of anaphylaxis in C3H/HeJ ($H\text{-}2^K$) mice; no effect on peanut-IgE antibody levels	Serious concerns regarding safety in view of strain-dependent effects in mice, concern for excessive T_H1 stimulation and autoimmunity
Immunostimulatory sequences (ISS-ODN)[72]	Potent stimulation of T_H1 via activation of antigen-presenting cells, natural killer cells, and B cells; increased T_H1 cytokines	Protection against peanut sensitization in mice	Not shown to reverse established peanut allergy, concern for excessive T_H1 stimulation, and potential for autoimmunity

Abbreviations: ISS-ODN, immunostimulatory sequences-oligodeoxynucleotides; IT, immunotherapy.

[a] These three additional immunomodulatory approaches to peanut allergy were explored in the animal studies but subsequently were abandoned in favor of other treatments due to practical considerations. It is possible that the peptide immunotherapeutic approach will be revisited when the most relevant epitopes for T cells on major peanut allergens are identified and the vaccine contains only the selected peptides that represent T-cell epitopes.

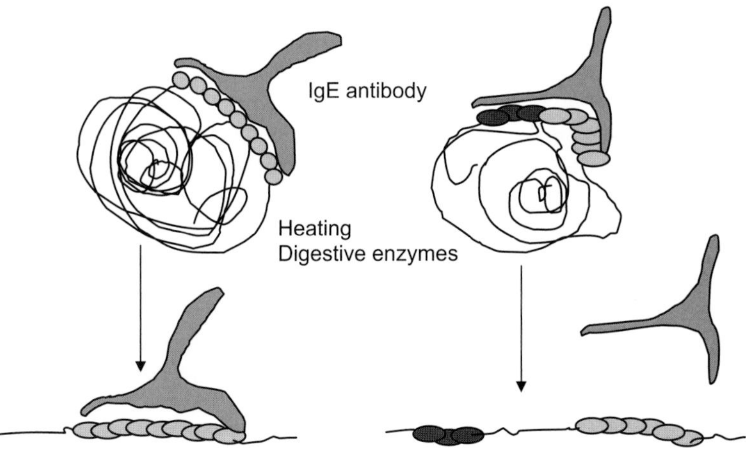

Fig. 1. Allergenic IgE antibody–binding epitopes. Children who generate IgE antibodies predominantly directed at conformational epitopes are more likely to have transient egg allergy. Children who generate IgE antibodies also against sequential epitopes are more likely to have persistent milk and egg allergy. Children who generate IgE antibodies against a large number of sequential epitopes are more likely to have more severe reactions.

FOOD ALLERGEN-NONSPECIFIC THERAPY

Humanized Monoclonal Anti-IgE

Humanized monoclonal anti-IgE antibodies bind to the constant region of IgE antibody molecules and prevent the IgE molecules from binding to high-affinity receptors, Fc_{ϵ}-RIs, expressed on the surface of mast cells and basophils, and low-affinity receptors, Fc_{ϵ}RIIs, expressed on B cells, dendritic cells, and intestinal epithelial cells. Anti-IgE cannot interact with IgE molecules when they are bound to IgE receptors and, therefore, cannot induce mast cell or basophil degranulation by cross-linking IgE; thus, the risk of immediate allergic reactions is reduced.[12] A multicenter randomized trial evaluated humanized monoclonal anti-IgE mouse IgG1 antibody (TNX-901) in 84 patients with a history of peanut allergy.[13] Baseline threshold dose of peanut protein necessary to elicit objective symptoms was established. Subjects were randomized to receive four doses of either humanized monoclonal antibody TNX-901 (150, 300, or 450 mg) or placebo subcutaneously every 4 weeks. They underwent a second oral peanut challenge within 2 to 4 weeks after the fourth dose. The mean amount of peanut flour that elicited objective symptoms and resulted in stopping of the food challenge (the sensitivity threshold) increased in all groups, with an apparent dose response, but was statistically significant only in the highest anti-IgE dose (450 mg) group. In this group, the sensitivity threshold increased from approximately one-half of a peanut kernel (178 mg) to almost 9 peanut kernels (2805 mg). Approximately 25% of subjects treated even with the highest dose of TNX-901, however, showed no change in their sensitivity threshold. A clinical trial of a different anti-IgE humanized IgG1 antibody (omalizumab) in peanut-allergic children older than 6 years of age was discontinued prematurely due to safety concerns related to severe anaphylactic reactions that occurred during the initial peanut challenge.

Combined treatment with anti-IgE and specific food allergen OIT may be a safer option because of the potential ability of anti-IgE to decrease immediate side effects of allergen OIT.[14] Studies of a combination therapy are ongoing in children and adults with milk allergy.

Traditional Chinese Medicine

Herbal remedies have been successfully used in China for centuries, although not for food allergies. The mechanism of action of traditional Chinese medicine (TCM) is unknown and TCM has not been systematically evaluated in randomized clinical trials. Food allergy herbal formula (FAHF)-1, a mixture of 11 herbs that has been used by TCM for treatment of parasitic infections, gastroenteritis, and asthma, was tested in a mouse model of peanut allergy.[15] Mouse models of food allergy were essential in the early stages of development of novel therapies for food allergy because human studies were considered unsafe due to the risk for anaphylaxis. Mouse models of peanut allergy mimicked human peanut allergy by the oral route of sensitization, symptoms of anaphylaxis after ingestion, generation of peanut-specific IgE antibodies, and release of allergic mediators (histamine) during the peanut challenge. FAHF-1 protected peanut-allergic mice against peanut-induced anaphylaxis and reduced mast cell degranulation and histamine release. Peanut-specific serum IgE levels decreased significantly after 2 weeks of treatment and remained lower 4 weeks after discontinuation of treatment. FAHF-1 had no toxic effects on liver or kidneys even at the doses that significantly exceeded the therapeutic dose.

A modified formula, FAHF-2, composed of 9 herbs, completely blocked anaphylaxis to peanut challenge up to 5 months after therapy.[16] A phase I clinical safety trial in adults 12 to 45 years of age with peanut and tree nut allergy was recently completed. FAHF-2 was found to be safe and well tolerated.[17] A phase II extended safety and efficacy trial is currently enrolling subjects 12 to 45 years of age with peanut, tree nut, sesame, fish, or shellfish allergy. FAHF-2 is expected to exert a similar protective effect against a variety of unrelated foods. The individual active substances in each herb are being identified, their mechanism of action characterized, and potency standardized. Each individual herb exerts some protective effect, but none offers equivalent protection from anaphylaxis compared with the complete FAHF-2 mixture of 9 herbs. The therapeutic effect of FAHF-2 seems to be in large part mediated by $CD8^+$ T cells producing interferon (IFN)-γ.[18,19]

ALLERGEN-SPECIFIC IMMUNOTHERAPY

Immunotherapy involves administration of allergens with or without adjuvants that skew the immune responses away from T_H2 proallergic responses. In traditional environmental allergen immunotherapy, the dose escalation (also referred to as buildup phase) may be rushed over 1 to a few days (typically done in the hospital) or may last 4 to 6 months (typically done in the office). The maintenance phase begins when the highest tolerated dose has been reached. Maintenance dose is continued for extended periods of time; in subcutaneous allergen immunotherapy, maintenance dose is administered in the office; in OIT and SLIT, maintenance dose is administered at home.

Desensitization Versus Permanent Oral Tolerance

Desensitization is distinct from permanent oral tolerance. In a desensitized state, the protective effect depends on daily, uninterrupted exposure to the allergen; however, when the dosing is interrupted or discontinued, the protective effect may be lost or significantly reduced. Oral desensitization is likely due to increased food-specific IgG4 and decreased food-specific IgE antibodies, and decreased reactivity of effector cells (mast cells and basophils). In contrast, permanent oral tolerance is not affected by prolonged periods of food abstinence. The mechanism of persistent oral tolerance likely involves the initial development of regulatory T cells and immunologic deviation away from the proallergic T_H2 response and, in later stages, anergy. The permanence of protection may be tested with intentional interruption of dosing for at least 4 to 8 weeks followed by a supervised oral food challenge.

Subcutaneous Peanut Immunotherapy

The first evidence that immunotherapy may decrease the threshold of reactivity (desensitize) to a food allergen was provided by two controlled studies of subcutaneous peanut immunotherapy. In the initial study, 3 subjects treated with peanut extract had 67% to 100% symptom reduction during double-blind, placebo-controlled peanut challenges and a 2-log to 5-log reduction in endpoint skin prick skin test reactivity to peanut.[20] One placebo-treated subject completed the study and had no change in peanut challenge symptoms or skin prick test sensitivity to peanut. In a follow-up study of 12 subjects, 6 were treated with a maintenance dose of 0.5 mL of 1:100 wt/vol peanut extract for 12 months.[21] All treated subjects were able to ingest increased quantities of peanut during oral challenges and had decreased sensitivity on titrated peanut skin prick test, whereas untreated controls experienced no changes. Anaphylaxis after subcutaneous dose administration, however, occurred a mean of 7.7 times during 12 months in the 6 patients who received maintenance, with an average of 9.8 epinephrine injections per study subject. Only 3 subjects (50%) were able to achieve the maintenance dose due to adverse events. This important study demonstrated that injected peanut allergen could be successfully used to induce desensitization, but the significant risk for anaphylaxis precluded this treatment from being further evaluated in clinical studies.

Birch Pollen Immunotherapy for the Pollen-Food Allergy Syndrome

Individuals sensitized to airborne pollen proteins may develop oral-pharyngeal pruritus from ingestion of raw fruits and vegetables that contain proteins homologous to the proteins in pollen. The classic pollen-food allergy syndrome (PFAS) or oral allergy syndrome is due to sensitization to the birch pollen major allergen, Bet v 1. Oropharyngeal symptoms occur on contact with the pollen cross-reactive apple allergen Mal d 1. Subcutaneous immunotherapy is an established treatment of pollen allergic rhinitis and, theoretically, could also benefit PFAS. An open trial of subcutaneous birch pollen immunotherapy in 49 adults with birch pollen allergic rhinitis and oral symptoms induced by raw apple reported a significant reduction (50%–95%) or complete resolution of apple-induced oral allergy symptoms ($P<.001$) in 41 (84%) compared with no improvement in controls.[22] In a follow-up study, symptoms and skin test reactivity were compared after the 12-month immunotherapy course and 30 months after discontinuation of immunotherapy.[23] More than 50% of subjects still tolerated apple at the 30-month follow-up visit, although the majority showed a return of pretreatment sensitization by skin test. Subsequent clinical trials, in which oral allergy symptoms to apple were diagnosed with double-blind, placebo-controlled food challenges, confirmed a beneficial effect of subcutaneous birch pollen immunotherapy in a subset of subjects.[24,25] Similar findings were reported from an observational study of 16 adult subjects suffering from PFAS (hazelnut, walnut, lettuce, peach, and cherry) and plane tree pollen allergic rhinitis who were treated with plane tree pollen immunotherapy.[26] Doses of immunotherapy higher than those typically required to induce improvement in seasonal birch pollen rhinitis may be necessary to improve birch-related PFAS. The most beneficial effects on PFAS were observed in the studies that included adults monosensitized to birch tree. In addition, the T-cell immune responses to birch pollen cross-reactive food allergens, such as apple (Mal d 1), hazelnut (Cor a 1), and carrot (Dau c 1), might be at least in part Bet v 1 independent. In that case, vaccines based on modified recombinant food allergens would represent a superior approach to the treatment of PFAS.[27] A few case reports highlighted the possibility of inducing allergy to cross-reactive food allergens in the course of subcutaneous birch pollen immunotherapy for the environmental allergens, such as development of allergy to snails during immunotherapy to dust mites or to raw fruits during immunotherapy to pollens.

Oral Immunotherapy

The first report of successful OIT, in a boy with severe anaphylactic allergy to egg, was published in the early twentieth century.[28] OIT is currently being explored for cow's milk, peanut, and egg allergies. The oral route of administration takes advantage of cells and immune pathways involved in the induction of oral tolerance. Animal studies suggest that feeding high doses of an antigen causes nonresponsiveness due to anergy or deletion of antigen-specific T lymphocytes, whereas continuous feeding low doses of an antigen induces regulatory T cells.[3,29] In contrast, intermittent feedings or nonoral exposures (eg, cutaneous or inhalational) predispose to IgE sensitization and allergic symptoms after food ingestion.[30]

ORAL IMMUNOTHERAPY TRIALS

During OIT, food is mixed in a vehicle and ingested in gradually increasing doses. The dose escalation occurs in a controlled setting; regular ingestion of tolerated doses during the buildup phase and a maintenance dose occurs at home. Early case series and uncontrolled trials provided evidence that a subset of food-allergic subjects could be desensitized to milk, egg, fish, fruit, peanut, and celery.[31–34] In some subjects who ultimately tolerated a maintenance dose, even for a significant period of time, allergic symptoms redeveloped if the food was not ingested on a regular basis, highlighting a concern that permanent tolerance was not achieved.[35]

In the first randomized trial of OIT, children with IgE-mediated cow's milk allergy (CMA) or hen's egg allergy were randomly assigned to OIT or elimination diet as a control group.[36] OIT treatment with fresh cow's milk or lyophilized egg white protein was performed daily at home. Children were re-evaluated by food challenge after a median of 21 months. Children in the OIT group were subsequently placed on an elimination diet for 2 months before a follow-up rechallenge to test for permanent oral tolerance. At follow-up challenge, 9 of 25 children (36%) showed permanent tolerance in the OIT group, 3 of 25 (12%) were tolerant with regular intake, and 4 of 25 (16%) were partial responders. In the control group, 7 of 20 children (35%) also developed tolerance over the study period. Although the rate of permanent tolerance was not different between the groups, some children were tolerant with regular intake and some were tolerant to a smaller maintenance dose (desensitized) and were protected from inadvertent exposures as they continued to ingest the daily dose of the food.

In the first placebo-controlled trial of OIT, 20 children with IgE-mediated milk allergy were randomized 2:1 to milk or placebo OIT.[37] The buildup occurred during an in-office day (initial dose, 0.4 mg of milk protein; final dose, 50 mg), followed by daily dosing at home with 8 weekly in-office dose increases to a maximum of 500 mg. Home daily maintenance doses were continued for 3 to 4 months. Double-blind, placebo-controlled milk challenges, skin prick tests, and milk protein serologic studies were performed before and after OIT. Nineteen patients, 6 to 17 years of age, completed the treatment: 12 in the active group and 7 in the placebo group. The median milk cumulative dose inducing a reaction in both groups was 40 mg at the baseline challenge. After OIT, the median cumulative dose in the active treatment group was 5140 mg (range 2540–8140 mg), whereas all patients in the placebo group reacted at 40 mg (P = .0003). Among 2437 active OIT doses and 1193 placebo doses, there were 1107 (45.4%) and 134 (11.2%) total reactions, respectively, most commonly local symptoms (**Table 4**). Milk-specific IgE levels did not change significantly in either group. Milk-IgG levels increased significantly in the active treatment group, with a predominant milk-IgG_4 level increase.

Safety and efficacy of OIT were investigated in 60 children with a history of severe milk-induced anaphylaxis and milk-specific IgE greater than 85 kU_A/L, who reacted to less than or equal to 0.8 mL of milk during a baseline oral milk challenge.[38] Children were randomly divided into two groups: 30 children received OIT with a 10-day rush phase, including 3 to 10 daily doses up to 20 mL of undiluted milk in the hospital, followed by a slow dose-escalation phase at home (increasing by 1 mL every second day); the remaining 30 comparison subjects continued on a milk-free diet. After 1

Table 4
Benefits and risks of food oral immunotherapy

Success Rate[a]	% of Treated Subjects
Peanut	~77[40]
Milk	~37–70[37,38,43]
Egg	~55[39]
Side Effects	**% of the doses of immunotherapy associated with side effects**
Peanut[40,42,44]	Buildup Mild oral and pharyngeal symptoms: 69 Mild or moderate skin symptoms: 62 Mild to moderate nausea or abdominal pain: 44 Diarrhea/emesis: 21 Mild wheezing: 18 Maintenance Upper respiratory symptoms: 29 Cutaneous: 24 Treatment of adverse reactions given for 0.7 of home doses, 2 subjects received one dose epinephrine
Milk[36,41]	Blinded, randomized, placebo-controlled study[37] Local (oral pruritus) median: 16% of doses per child Gastrointestinal median: 2% of doses per child Epinephrine was used in 0.2% of total doses; 4 doses of epinephrine were used to treat 4 subjects: 2 doses during buildup and 2 doses during home maintenance Open-label home study[43] 2.5%–96.4% of Doses per subject in the first 3 months compared with 0%–79% in the subsequent months Total percentages of doses with reactions: Local reactions (oral pruritus): 17 Gastrointestinal: 3.7 Respiratory: 0.9 Cutaneous: 0.8 Multisystem: 5.5 Epinephrine was used for 6 reactions: 0.2% (4 subjects)

[a] Defined as ability to ingest the significant amount food on a regular basis for at least 6 months which is equivalent to desensitized state.

year, 11 of 30 (36%) subjects in the OIT group were able to ingest a daily dose of milk equal or greater than 150 mL; 16 subjects (54%) were able to ingest from 5 mL to less than 150 mL. Three children (10%) were unable to complete the OIT because of the frequent adverse reactions. In the comparison group, all 30 children reacted to less than 5 mL of milk during the repeated oral food challenge at 12 months. Adverse reactions were common in both groups but no child had severe anaphylaxis. During the rush phase, intramuscular epinephrine was administered 4 times; 1 dose per child in 4 children. During the home phase, 2 children required treatment, including epinephrine in the emergency department.

Egg OIT

Another study reported preliminary results on 7 children with nonanaphylactic egg allergy treated with egg OIT.[39] These children underwent a 24-month egg OIT protocol involving modified rush buildup and maintenance phases. Double-blind, placebo-controlled food challenges were performed at the end of the study and all children tolerated significantly more egg protein than at study onset. Two subjects remained tolerant to egg after a period of strict egg avoidance. Egg-specific IgG concentrations increased significantly, whereas there was no significant change in egg-specific IgE concentrations.

Peanut OIT

Peanut OIT trials conducted in young children with peanut allergy have attracted significant attention.[40,41] In a US study, 39 subjects were enrolled (64% boys). The median age at enrollment was 57.5 months (range, 12–111 months).[40] All children completed the initial day escalation phase, during which the starting dose of 0.1-mg peanut protein was doubled every 30 minutes, up to 50 mg. During the buildup phase, children ingested peanut flour with other safe food every day. Doses were increased by 25 mg every 2 weeks until 300 mg was reached. During the maintenance phase, the dose of 300 mg was continued daily until the follow-up food challenge was performed. After the food challenge, the daily dose was increased to 1800 mg. Children were evaluated every 4 months while on continued maintenance dosing (a total of 36 months). Ten (25%) children subsequently withdrew after the initial day escalation phase. Six discontinued for personal reasons, including transportation issues, parental anxiety, and failure to perform home dosing. The other 4 subjects discontinued because of allergic reactions to the OIT that did not resolve with continued treatment or dose reduction. Three had gastrointestinal complaints, and 1 had symptoms of asthma. Twenty-nine subjects completed all 3 phases of the study and peanut challenges.

During the initial day escalation, 36 patients (92%) experienced some symptoms; most common were upper respiratory symptoms, with 27 patients (69%) reporting mild sneezing/itching and mild laryngeal symptoms. No patients experienced severe upper respiratory or laryngeal symptoms; 17 patients (44%) reported mild to moderate nausea or abdominal pain; 8 patients (21%) had diarrhea/emesis; and 24 subjects (62%) had mild or moderate skin symptoms. A total of 6 patients experienced chest symptoms during the initial escalation day; all 6 had mild wheezing, and 2 progressed to moderate wheezing. Three of the subjects with chest symptoms during the initial day escalation also had a previous diagnosis of asthma. During the final food challenge, 27 of the 29 children who completed the protocol ingested 3.9 g of peanut flour (approximate equivalent of 11 peanut kernels). By 6 months, titrated skin prick tests and activation of basophils decreased significantly. Peanut-specific IgE antibody concentrations decreased by 12 to 18 months whereas peanut-specific IgG4 increased significantly.

Among the children who participated in the trial of peanut OIT, 20 of 39 completed all phases of the study.[40,42] Risk of mild wheezing was 15% (6/39) during the initial escalation. The risk of any symptoms after the buildup phase doses was 46%, with a risk of 29% for upper respiratory tract and 24% for skin symptoms. The risk of an adverse reaction with any home dose was 3.5%: upper respiratory tract (1.2%) and skin (1.1%) symptoms. Treatment was given for 0.7% of home doses. Two subjects received epinephrine after 1 home dose each. Allergic reactions during home dosing were significantly more common in the milk OIT, from 2.55 to 96.4% of doses per subject in the first 3 months compared with 0% to 79.8% in the subsequent 3 months.[43] Local and multisystem reactions decreased whereas all other reactions remained unchanged during the maintenance phase of OIT. Systemic reactions occurred at previously tolerated doses in the setting of exercise or viral illness. As recently highlighted, the risk of an allergic reaction to a previously tolerated dose of food is associated with physical exertion after dosing, dosing on empty stomach, dosing during menses, concurrent febrile illness, and suboptimally controlled asthma (see **Table 4**).[36,43,44]

SUBLINGUAL IMMUNOTHERAPY

SLIT with food represents an alternative approach to desensitization or oral tolerance and was first reported using fresh kiwifruit pulp extract in a 29-year-old woman with a history of kiwifruit-induced anaphylaxis.[45] The extract or kiwifruit cube was kept under the tongue for 1 minute before swallowing (combined SLIT and OIT). Five years into kiwifruit-modified SLIT, treatment was interrupted for 4 months and then resumed without any problems.[46]

In a randomized, double-blind, placebo-controlled trial, adults with hazelnut allergy (54.5% with a history of oral allergy symptoms) confirmed by double-blind placebo-controlled food challenge were randomly assigned to 1 of 2 groups, hazelnut immunotherapy (n = 12) or placebo (n = 11).[47] Subjects kept the hazelnut extract solution in the mouth for at least 3 minutes and then spat it out. All treated subjects reached the planned maximum dose with a 4-day rush protocol, followed by a daily maintenance dose (containing 188.2 μg of Cor a 1 and 121.9 μg of Cor a 8, major hazelnut allergens). Systemic reactions were observed in 0.2% of the total doses administered during the rush buildup phase and were treated with oral antihistamines. Local reactions, mainly immediate oral pruritus, were observed in 7.4% (109 reactions/1466 doses). Four patients in the active group reported abdominal pain several hours after dosing on one occasion each during the buildup phase. All local reactions during the maintenance phase were limited to oral pruritus and occurred in a single patient. After 5 months of SLIT, the mean threshold dose of ingested hazelnut-provoking allergic symptoms increased from 2.3 g to 11.6 g in the active group (P = .02) compared with 3.5 g to 4.1 g in placebo (non-significant). Almost 50% of treated subjects tolerated the highest dose (20 g) of hazelnut during follow-up, double-blind, placebo-controlled food challenge compared with 9% in the placebo group. Levels of serum hazelnut-specific IgG4 antibody and total serum interleukin (IL)-10 increased only in the active group, but there were no differences in hazelnut-specific IgE antibody levels preimmunotherapy and postimmunotherapy.

Another study evaluated SLIT in 8 children with CMA.[48] A day after an initial positive oral milk challenge, children started SLIT with 0.1 mL of milk for the first 2 weeks, increasing by 0.1 mL every 15 days until 1 mL per day was given. Milk was kept in the mouth for 2 minutes and then discharged. Seven subjects completed the protocol; one subject withdrew due to oral symptoms. After 6 months of treatment, the threshold dose of milk increased from a mean of 39 mL at baseline to 143 mL (P<.01).

Preliminary data on OIT and SLIT are encouraging; however, at this time, these treatments are considered experimental and additional studies must address many issues, including the optimal dose; ideal duration of OIT/SLIT; degree of protection, safety, and efficacy for different ages; severity and type of food allergies responsive to treatment; and the need for patient protection during home administration. In view of the recent reports of reactions to the tolerated doses of OIT at home, it may be necessary to hold doses during acute febrile illness, avoid exercise within 2 hours after dosing, and take the daily OIT dose with a meal or snack.[44] Rhinitis and asthma should be maintained under optimal control. Finally, because a subset of children with food allergies develops tolerance spontaneously, future studies must address diagnostic tests that distinguish among those with transient and persistent food allergies to identify the subjects who will benefit from therapy.

EPICUTANEOUS IMMUNOTHERAPY

Epicutaneous patches that solubilize the allergen by perspiration and disseminate it into the thickness of the stratum corneum represent an alternative delivery route of immunotherapy.[49] Epicutaneous delivery is less invasive than subcutaneous injection and may have a lower risk for systemic reactions than subcutaneous, oral, or sublingual food allergen delivery. A proof-of-concept study on the efficacy of EPIT on intact skin was done in mice sensitized to aeroallergens or food allergens.[50] Mice were sensitized to pollen (n = 18), house dust mite (n = 24), ovalbumin (n = 18), or peanut (n = 18) and allocated to 1 of 3 groups: EPIT, subcutaneous immunotherapy, and no treatment. In addition, control animals not sensitized and not treated were followed as a fourth group. After 8 weeks of treatment, lung function testing by plethysmography was performed after aerosol provocation with appropriate allergens and showed reduced airway responsiveness to methacholine in EPIT mice. IgG2a for pollen, house dust mite, ovalbumin, and peanuts was significantly increased in the EPIT group versus not treated mice. In mice sensitized to the 4 allergens tested, EPIT was as efficacious as subcutaneous immunotherapy, considered the reference immunotherapy. EPIT may represent a more convenient route with a superior safety profile compared with subcutaneous immunotherapy, OIT, or SLIT.

In a pilot study, 18 children (mean age 3.8 years, range 10 months to 7.7 years) with CMA were randomized 1:1 to receive active EPIT or placebo.[51] CMA was confirmed by a clinician-supervised oral food challenge at baseline and the cumulative tolerated dose of milk was established. Children received three 48-hour applications (1 mg skimmed milk powder or 1 mg glucose as placebo) via the skin patch per week for 3 months. Treated children showed a trend toward increased cumulative tolerated dose at the follow-up oral milk challenge after 3 months of EPIT, from a mean 1.8 mL at baseline to 23.6 mL at 3 months. The mean cumulative tolerated dose did not change in the placebo-treated group. There were no significant changes in cow's milk–specific IgE levels from baseline to 3 months in either group. The most common side effects were local pruritus and eczema at the site of application. There were no severe systemic adverse reactions; however, one subject in the active group had repeated episodes of diarrhea after EPIT with milk. Reports from earlier mouse studies have demonstrated increased potential for the development of IgE sensitization to peanut via the epicutaneous route compared with ingestion, raising concerns as to whether epicutaneous delivery might worsen food allergy.[30] It is impossible to fully understand the effect of EPIT on milk allergy from this small pilot study due to the small sample size and short duration of the study as well as limited information about immunologic parameters. This preliminary report suggests, however, that further investigation of the novel epicutaneous antigen delivery for food allergy immunotherapy is warranted.

DIET CONTAINING EXTENSIVELY HEATED COW'S MILK AND EGG

Two large clinical trials investigated the tolerance of extensively heated (baked into other products) milk and egg in children with milk (n = 100) and egg (n = 117) allergy.[52,53] Thermal processing largely destroys IgE-binding epitopes but not sequential IgE-binding epitopes (see **Fig. 1**). Prior studies determined that children with persistent milk and egg allergy generated IgE antibodies directed primarily against sequential epitopes of egg ovomucoid and milk casein.[8,9] These observations suggested that at least a subset of children might tolerate extensively heated (eg, baked) products with milk and egg. In each study, more than 80% of children were tolerant to milk and egg baked into muffins and waffles during an initial oral challenge and incorporated these foods into their daily diet at home. Children were being followed every 3 to 6 months and tolerated the baked diet well. There was no increase in acute allergic reactions and no increase in severity of underlying atopic diseases, such as asthma, atopic dermatitis, or eczema. There was no increase in the intestinal permeability of carbohydrate markers (lactulose and mannitol) over the first year on the diet and children had no growth impairment. Commercially available tests for food-specific IgE levels did not reliably identify subjects tolerant to extensively heated milk and egg, and oral food challenge was indispensable. Children tolerant to unheated milk, however, had the lowest basophil reactivity to milk whereas children who reacted to extensively heated milk had significantly higher basophil reactivity to stimulation with milk protein.[54] In the milk study, the majority of children who reacted to extensively heated milk had milk-specific IgE antibody levels greater than 35 kU_A/L (UniCAP, Phadia) and, therefore, in a subsequent study, subjects with milk-specific IgE antibody levels greater than 35 kU_A/L were excluded. In the milk study, severe reactions that required treatment with epinephrine occurred only in children who reacted to the extensively heated milk products. All of the subjects who tolerated the extensively heated milk products and subsequently reacted to unheated milk had milder reactions and none received epinephrine. This suggests that tolerance to extensively heated milk products is a marker of a milder milk allergy that is likely to be outgrown. In contrast, in the egg study, there were equal proportions of children who received epinephrine during the heated and unheated egg challenges.

The immunologic changes observed during the ingestion of baked goods with milk and egg included increasing food-specific IgG4 antibodies, decreasing wheal sizes from prick skin tests, and no consistent changes in the food-specific IgE antibodies. There was a significantly higher percentage of casein-specific regulatory T cells in extensively heated milk–tolerant children compared with children with allergy to extensively heated milk. A higher frequency of casein-specific regulatory T cells correlated with a phenotype of mild clinical disease and favorable prognosis.[55]

These findings suggest that large subsets of children with milk and egg allergy might include extensively heated products in their diets. Furthermore, the immunologic changes induced by the diet containing baked milk and egg products are similar to the changes observed during OIT trials. Tolerance to extensively heated milk and egg might identify subjects with favorable prognosis. The diet containing extensively heated milk and egg might represent a safer and more natural approach to oral immunomodulation. Until further studies have been completed to establish the overall safety and efficacy of this method, however, baked milk and egg diet should be approached with caution and introduction of heated foods done under physician supervision.

IMMUNOTHERAPY WITH RECOMBINANT ENGINEERED FOOD PROTEINS

Alteration of the IgE antibody–binding sites (epitopes) can decrease the risk of an acute allergic reaction during immunotherapy. Point mutations introduced by site-directed mutagenesis in the known IgE epitopes of major food allergens and polymerization of proteins result in decreased IgE binding during immunotherapy. In vivo efficacy of engineered recombinant peanut proteins was first tested in a mouse model of peanut anaphylaxis.[56,57] Mice were sensitized to whole peanut and then desensitized by intranasal administration of engineered recombinant Ara h 2 (3 doses per week for 4 weeks). Desensitization with the engineered recombinant Ara h 2 protein significantly decreased severity of anaphylactic reactions after oral peanut challenge compared with a control group.

Modified food allergens may be combined with bacterial adjuvants to further reduce food-specific IgE production. Initially, heat-killed *Listeria moncytogenes* combined with engineered peanut allergens (mAra h 1–3) was shown effective in preventing peanut anaphylaxis.[58] Safety concerns about using whole-cell pathogenic bacteria in humans were raised, however, due to the risk of inducing adverse inflammatory reactions. In subsequent studies, a nonpathogenic strain of *Escherichia coli* was used as an adjuvant and vaccine was delivered orally and rectally. Oral delivery was not effective, presumably due to breakdown of the peanut-containing *E coli*. Peanut-allergic C3H/HeJ mice treated with 3 different doses of heat-killed *E coli* expressing modified proteins Ara h 1–3 (HKE-MP123) per rectum had reduced severity of anaphylaxis ($P<.01$) compared with the sham-treated group.[59] Only the medium-dose and high-dose HKE-MP123–treated mice, however, remained protected for up to 10 weeks after treatment. Peanut-specific IgE levels were significantly lower in all HKE-MP123–treated groups ($P<.001$); they were most reduced in the high-dose HKE-MP123–treated group at the time of each challenge. A phase I clinical safety study is currently enrolling adult subjects with peanut allergy. In the future, probiotic bacteria might be used as adjuvants to avoid the concerns of excessive T-helper cell type 1 (T_H1) stimulation by killed pathogenic bacteria.

PROBIOTICS FOR PREVENTION AND TREATMENT OF FOOD ALLERGY

The concept of probiotic foods was introduced more than a century ago by Fuller. Probiotics are live bacteria or their components that have beneficial effect on the health of the host presumably by improving intestinal microbial balance. The major sources of probiotics are dairy products that contain *Lactobacillus* and *Bifidobacterium* species.

Probiotics generate increasing interest as a potential approach to food allergy prevention and therapy (**Table 5**). In one trial, 159 expectant mothers who had at least one first-degree relative (or partner) with history of atopic disease (atopic dermatitis, asthma, or allergic rhinitis) were randomized to either receive *Lactobacillus* GG supplementation or placebo.[60] Treatment was continued during breastfeeding and was given to the infants for 6 months, starting on the first day of life. At age 2 years, 23% of children had atopic dermatitis in the probiotic-treated group compared with 46% in the placebo group ($P = .008$), relative risk of 0.51 (95% CI, 0.32–0.84), indicating that *Lactobacillus* GG had some effect on the prevention of early atopic disease in infants at high risk. This study, however, raised several questions. The prevalence of atopic dermatitis in the placebo-treated group was very high but the severity of atopic dermatitis was very low (geometric mean scoring atopic dermatitis [SCORAD] index of 10.4 out of maximum 103) and not different from the probiotic-treated group (geometric mean SCORAD index of 9.8). Furthermore, there was no difference between the two study groups in any of the objective markers, such as the prevalence

Table 5
Probiotics for food allergy prevention and treatment

	Mechanism of Action	Effects	Comments
Prevention			
Lactobacillus GG randomized human trial (N = 159), mother supplemented before delivery and infants supplemented for 6 months[60,61]	Unclear; there was no difference between the two study groups in number of positive prick skin tests to selected food and environmental allergens, total serum IgE as well as serum allergen-specific IgE levels to milk, egg, cat, and house dust mite.	At age 2 years, 23% of children had atopic dermatitis in the probiotic-treated group compared with 46% in the placebo group ($P = .008$); the protective effect persisted up to 7 years of age.	The prevalence of atopic dermatitis in the placebo-treated group was very high but the severity of atopic dermatitis was very low (geometric mean SCORAD index of 10.4 out of maximum 103) and not different from the probiotic-treated group (geometric mean SCORAD index of 9.8).
Cow's milk–based formula with prebiotics[62]	Prebiotics enhance gut colonization with healthy commensal (probiotic) bacteria.	Cumulative incidence of atopic dermatitis at 1 year of age was significantly lower in the prebiotic group (5.7%) than in the control group (9.7%, $P = .04$).	There was no effect on the IgE-sensitization to egg white and cow's milk. The number needed to prevent 1 case of atopic dermatitis by supplementation of prebiotics was 25 infants.
Lactococcus lactis transfected with murine IL-10[67]	Decreased serum IgE and IgG1, increased IgA in the gut, increased gut and serum IL-10.	Pretreatment of young mice before sensitization with β-lactoglobulin in the presence of cholera toxin protected against anaphylaxis on the oral food challenge.	This approach was only tested in the mouse model; however, the concept of probiotic bacteria may be applied to delivery of engineered allergens in human studies.
Treatment			
Lactobacillus rhamnosus GG and Bifidobacterium lactis[63]	Symptomatic improvement was associated with the increase in IgA and the suppression of TNF-α synthesis.	2-Month treatment with Lactobacillus rhamnosus GG and Bifidobacterium lactis in addition to a milk elimination diet decreased the severity of atopic dermatitis symptoms in infants and young children with established cow's milk hypersensitivity.	

of positive prick skin tests to selected food and environmental allergens, total serum IgE, and serum allergen-specific IgE levels to milk, egg, cat, and house dust mite. Nevertheless, the 7-year follow-up data confirmed the long-lasting protective effect of early *Lactobacillus* GG supplementation.[61] Risk of eczema was significantly reduced in the *Lactobacillus* GG group compared with the placebo group, odds ratio 0.58 (95% CI, 0.35–0.94; $P = .03$). The effect of prebiotics-oligosaccharides shown to promote probiotic colonization of the gastrointestinal tract on primary prevention of atopic dermatitis was investigated in 830 healthy term infants at low risk for atopy (no history of allergic disease, such as atopic dermatitis, asthma, or hay fever, in any parent or sibling).[62] Infants were randomized 1:1 to feeding with cow's milk–based formula containing prebiotics (a mixture of neutral and pectin-derived acidic oligoscharides) or with cow's milk–based formula without prebiotics. Up to the first birthday, atopic dermatitis occurred in 5.7% infants in the prebiotic group compared with 9.7% infants in the control group ($P = .04$).

In another study, 2-month treatment with *Lactobacillus rhamnosus* GG and *Bifidobacterium lactis* in addition to a milk elimination diet decreased the severity of atopic dermatitis symptoms infants and young children with established cow's milk hypersensitivity.[63] Symptomatic improvement was associated with the increase in IgA and the suppression of tumor necrosis factor (TNF)-α synthesis. The exact mechanisms by which probiotics may affect atopic disease remain speculative. Possible mechanisms of probiotic immunomodulation include increased synthesis of IgA and IL-10, suppression of TNF-α, inhibition of casein-induced T-cell activation and circulating soluble CD4, and Toll-like receptor 4 signaling.[64–66]

Probiotic Bacteria Expressing IL-10

Lactococcus lactis was transfected to secrete murine IL-10 and then given to young mice before oral sensitization with β-lactoglobulin, a whey protein in cow's milk.[67] Symptoms during oral challenge and serum and fecal β-lactoglobulin–specific antibody concentrations were measured. Antibody titers were correlated with numbers of cells secreting IL-10 in the spleen and Peyer patches. Pretreatment with IL-10–transfected *Lactococcus lactis* reduced anaphylaxis symptoms and inhibited β-lactoglobulin–specific serum IgE and IgG1 concentrations. It also increased the production of β-lactoglobulin–specific IgA in the gut. These results suggest that a probiotic bacteria engineered to deliver IL-10 in the gut might be able to decrease food-induced anaphylaxis and provide an option to prevent IgE-type sensitization in a murine model of milk allergy. These findings need to be validated in human studies for prevention of food allergy.

SUMMARY

Food allergy is an increasingly prevalent problem in westernized societies. A variety of promising immunomodulatory approaches are under investigation for treatment and prevention of food allergy.

REFERENCES

1. Sicherer SH, Sampson HA. Food allergy: recent advances in pathophysiology and treatment. Annu Rev Med 2009;60:261–77.
2. Branum AM, Lukacs SL. Food allergy among children in the United States. Pediatrics 2009;124(6):1549–55.
3. Skripak JM, Sampson HA. Towards a cure for food allergy. Curr Opin Immunol 2008;20(6):690–6.

4. Scurlock AM, Burks AW, Jones SM. Oral immunotherapy for food allergy. Curr Allergy Asthma Rep 2009;9(3):186–93.
5. Shreffler WG, Beyer K, Chu TH, et al. Microarray immunoassay: association of clinical history, in vitro IgE function, and heterogeneity of allergenic peanut epitopes. J Allergy Clin Immunol 2004;113(4):776–82.
6. Flinterman AE, Knol EF, Lencer DA, et al. Peanut epitopes for IgE and IgG4 in peanut-sensitized children in relation to severity of peanut allergy. J Allergy Clin Immunol 2008;121(3):737–43.
7. Wang J, Lin J, Bardina L, et al. Correlation of IgE/IgG4 milk epitopes and affinity of milk-specific IgE antibodies with different phenotypes of clinical milk allergy. J Allergy Clin Immunol 2010;125(3):695–702.
8. Cooke SK, Sampson HA. Allergenic properties of ovomucoid in man. J Immunol 1997;159(4):2026–32.
9. Chatchatee P, Jarvinen KM, Bardina L, et al. Identification of IgE- and IgG-binding epitopes on alpha(s1)-casein: differences in patients with persistent and transient cow's milk allergy. J Allergy Clin Immunol 2001;107(2):379–83.
10. Savage JH, Matsui EC, Skripak JM, et al. The natural history of egg allergy. J Allergy Clin Immunol 2007;120(6):1413–7.
11. Skripak JM, Matsui EC, Mudd K, et al. The natural history of IgE-mediated cow's milk allergy. J Allergy Clin Immunol 2007;120(5):1172–7.
12. MacGlashan DWJ, Bochner BS, Adelman DC, et al. Down-regulation of Fc (epsilon)RI expression on human basophils during in vivo treatment of atopic patients with anti-IgE antibody. J Immunol 1997;158:1438–45.
13. Leung DY, Sampson HA, Yunginger JW, et al. Effect of anti-IgE therapy in patients with peanut allergy. N Engl J Med 2003;348(11):986–93.
14. Kuehr J, Brauburger J, Zielen S, et al. Efficacy of combination treatment with anti-IgE plus specific immunotherapy in polysensitized children and adolescents with seasonal allergic rhinitis. J Allergy Clin Immunol 2002;109(2):274–80.
15. Li XM, Zhang TF, Huang CK, et al. Food allergy herbal formula -1 (FAHF-1) blocks peanut-induced anaphylaxis in a murine model. J Allergy Clin Immunol 2001;108: 639–46.
16. Srivastava KD, Kattan JD, Zou ZM, et al. The Chinese herbal medicine formula FAHF-2 completely blocks anaphylactic reactions in a murine model of peanut allergy. J Allergy Clin Immunol 2005;115(1):171–8.
17. Wang J, Patil SP, Yang N, et al. Safety, tolerability, and immunologic effects of a food allergy herbal formula in food allergic individuals: a randomized, double-blinded, placebo-controlled, dose escalation, phase 1 study. Ann Allergy Asthma Immunol 2010;105(1):75–84.
18. Qu C, Srivastava K, Ko J, et al. Induction of tolerance after establishment of peanut allergy by the food allergy herbal formula-2 is associated with up-regulation of interferon-gamma. Clin Exp Allergy 2007;37(6):846–55.
19. Srivastava KD, Qu C, Zhang T, et al. Food Allergy Herbal Formula-2 silences peanut-induced anaphylaxis for a prolonged posttreatment period via IFN-gamma-producing CD8+ T cells. J Allergy Clin Immunol 2009;123(2):443–51.
20. Oppenheimer JJ, Nelson HS, Bock SA, et al. Treatment of peanut allergy with rush immunotherapy. J Allergy Clin Immunol 1992;90(2):256–62.
21. Nelson HS, Lahr J, Rule R, et al. Treatment of anaphylactic sensitivity to peanuts by immunotherapy with injections of aqueous peanut extract. J Allergy Clin Immunol 1997;99(6 Pt 1):744–51.
22. Asero R. Effects of birch pollen-specific immunotherapy on apple allergy in birch pollen-hypersensitive patients. Clin Exp Allergy 1998;28:1368–73.

23. Asero R. How long does the effect of birch pollen injection SIT on apple allergy last? Allergy 2003;58(5):435–8.
24. Bucher X, Pichler WJ, Dahinden CA, et al. Effect of tree pollen specific, subcutaneous immunotherapy on the oral allergy syndrome to apple and hazelnut. Allergy 2004;59(12):1272–6.
25. Bolhaar ST, Tiemessen MM, Zuidmeer L, et al. Efficacy of birch-pollen immunotherapy on cross-reactive food allergy confirmed by skin tests and double-blind food challenges. Clin Exp Allergy 2004;34(5):761–9.
26. Alonso R, Enrique E, Pineda F, et al. An observational study on outgrowing food allergy during non-birch pollen-specific, subcutaneous immunotherapy. Int Arch Allergy Immunol 2007;143(3):185–9.
27. Kinaciyan T, Jahn-Schmid B, Radakovics A, et al. Successful sublingual immunotherapy with birch pollen has limited effects on concomitant food allergy to apple and the immune response to the Bet v 1 homolog Mal d 1. J Allergy Clin Immunol 2007;119(4):937–43.
28. Schofield AT. A case of egg poisoning. Lancet 1908;1:716.
29. Chehade M, Mayer L. Oral tolerance and its relation to food hypersensitivities. J Allergy Clin Immunol 2005;115(1):3–12.
30. Strid J, Hourihane J, Kimber I, et al. Epicutaneous exposure to peanut protein prevents oral tolerance and enhances allergic sensitization. Clin Exp Allergy 2005;35(6):757–66.
31. Patriarca C, Romano A, Venuti A, et al. Oral specific hyposensitization in the management of patients allergic to food. Allergol Immunopathol (Madr) 1984; 12(4):275–81.
32. Patriarca G, Schiavino D, Nucera E, et al. Food allergy in children: results of a standardized protocol for oral desensitization. Hepatogastroenterology 1998; 45(19):52–8.
33. Patriarca G, Nucera E, Roncallo C, et al. Oral desensitizing treatment in food allergy: clinical and immunological results. Aliment Pharmacol Ther 2003;17(3): 459–65.
34. Patriarca G, Nucera E, Pollastrini E, et al. Oral rush desensitization in peanut allergy: a case report. Dig Dis Sci 2006;51(3):471–3.
35. Rolinck-Werninghaus C, Staden U, Mehl A, et al. Specific oral tolerance induction with food in children: transient or persistent effect on food allergy? Allergy 2005; 60(10):1320–2.
36. Staden U, Rolinck-Werninghaus C, Brewe F, et al. Specific oral tolerance induction in food allergy in children: efficacy and clinical patterns of reaction. Allergy 2007;62(11):1261–9.
37. Skripak JM, Nash SD, Rowley H, et al. A randomized, double-blind, placebo-controlled study of milk oral immunotherapy for cow's milk allergy. J Allergy Clin Immunol 2008;122(6):1154–60.
38. Longo G, Barbi E, Berti I, et al. Specific oral tolerance induction in children with very severe cow's milk-induced reactions. J Allergy Clin Immunol 2008;121(2): 343–7.
39. Buchanan AD, Green TD, Jones SM, et al. Egg oral immunotherapy in nonanaphylactic children with egg allergy. J Allergy Clin Immunol 2007;119(1):199–205.
40. Jones SM, Pons L, Roberts JL, et al. Clinical efficacy and immune regulation with peanut oral immunotherapy. J Allergy Clin Immunol 2009;124(2):292–300.
41. Clark AT, Islam S, King Y, et al. Successful oral tolerance induction in severe peanut allergy. Allergy 2009;64(8):1218–20.

42. Hofmann AM, Scurlock AM, Jones SM, et al. Safety of a peanut oral immunotherapy protocol in children with peanut allergy. J Allergy Clin Immunol 2009; 124(2):286–91.
43. Narisety SD, Skripak JM, Steele P, et al. Open-label maintenance after milk oral immunotherapy for IgE-mediated cow's milk allergy. J Allergy Clin Immunol 2009;124(3):610–2.
44. Varshney P, Steele PH, Vickery BP, et al. Adverse reactions during peanut oral immunotherapy home dosing. J Allergy Clin Immunol 2009;124(6):1351–2.
45. Mempel M, Rakoski J, Ring J, et al. Severe anaphylaxis to kiwi fruit: immunologic changes related to successful sublingual allergen immunotherapy. J Allergy Clin Immunol 2003;111(6):1406–9.
46. Kerzl R, Simonowa A, Ring J, et al. Life-threatening anaphylaxis to kiwi fruit: protective sublingual allergen immunotherapy effect persists even after discontinuation. J Allergy Clin Immunol 2007;119(2):507–8.
47. Enrique E, Pineda F, Malek T, et al. Sublingual immunotherapy for hazelnut food allergy: a randomized, double-blind, placebo-controlled study with a standardized hazelnut extract. J Allergy Clin Immunol 2005;116(5):1073–9.
48. De Boissieu D, Dupont C. Sublingual immunotherapy for cow's milk protein allergy: a preliminary report. Allergy 2006;61(10):1238–9.
49. Senti G, Graf N, Haug S, et al. Epicutaneous allergen administration as a novel method of allergen-specific immunotherapy. J Allergy Clin Immunol 2009; 124(5):997–1002.
50. Mondoulet L, Dioszeghy V, Ligouis M, et al. Epicutaneous immunotherapy on intact skin using a new delivery system in a murine model of allergy. Clin Exp Allergy 2010;40(4):659–67.
51. Dupont C, Kalach N, Soulaines P, et al. Cow's milk epicutaneous immunotherapy in children: a pilot trial of safety, acceptability, and impact on allergic reactivity. J Allergy Clin Immunol 2010;125(5):1165–7.
52. Nowak-Wegrzyn A, Bloom KA, Sicherer SH, et al. Tolerance to extensively heated milk in children with cow's milk allergy. J Allergy Clin Immunol 2008; 122(2):342–7 347.
53. Lemon-Mule H, Sampson HA, Sicherer SH, et al. Immunologic changes in children with egg allergy ingesting extensively heated egg. J Allergy Clin Immunol 2008;122(5):977–83.
54. Wanich N, Nowak-Wegrzyn A, Sampson HA, et al. Allergen-specific basophil suppression associated with clinical tolerance in patients with milk allergy. J Allergy Clin Immunol 2009;123(4):789–94.
55. Shreffler WG, Wanich N, Moloney M, et al. Association of allergen-specific regulatory T cells with the onset of clinical tolerance to milk protein. J Allergy Clin Immunol 2009;123(1):43–52.
56. Bannon GA, Cockrell G, Connaughton C, et al. Engineering, characterization and in vitro efficacy of the major peanut allergens for use in immunotherapy. Int Arch Allergy Immunol 2001;124(1–3):70–2.
57. Srivastava KD, Li XM, King N, et al. Immunotherapy with modified peanut allergens in a murine model of peanut allergy [abstract]. J Allergy Clin Immunol 2002;109:S287.
58. Li XM, Srivastava K, Huleatt JW, et al. Engineered recombinant peanut protein and heat-killed Listeria monocytogenes coadministration protects against peanut-induced anaphylaxis in a murine model. J Immunol 2003;170(6): 3289–95.

59. Li XM, Srivastava K, Grishin A, et al. Persistent protective effect of heat-killed Escherichia coli producing "engineered," recombinant peanut proteins in a murine model of peanut allergy. J Allergy Clin Immunol 2003;112(1):159–67.
60. Kalliomaki M, Salminen S, Arvilommi H. Probiotics in primary prevention of atopic disease: a randomised placebo-controlled trial. Lancet 2001;357:1076–9.
61. Gruber C, van SM, Mosca F, et al. Reduced occurrence of early atopic dermatitis because of immunoactive prebiotics among low-atopy-risk infants. J Allergy Clin Immunol 2010;126(4):791–7.
62. Kalliomaki M, Salminen S, Poussa T, et al. Probiotics during the first 7 years of life: a cumulative risk reduction of eczema in a randomized, placebo-controlled trial. J Allergy Clin Immunol 2007;119(4):1019–21.
63. Majamaa H, Isolauri E. Probiotics: a novel approach in the management of food allergy. J Allergy Clin Immunol 1997;99:179–85.
64. Isolauri E, Juntunen M, Sillanaukee P, et al. A human Lactobacillus strain (Lactobacillus GG) promotes recovery from acute diarrhea in children. Pediatrics 1989; 88:90–7.
65. Pessi T, Sutas Y, Hurme M, et al. Interleukin-10 generation in atopic children following oral *Lactobacillus rhamnosus* GG. Clin Exp Allergy 2000;30:1804–8.
66. Sutas Y, Hurme M, Isolauri E. Downregulation of antiCD3 antibody-induced IL-4 production by bovine caseins hydrolysed with *Lactobacillus* GG-derived enzymes. Scand J Immunol 1996;43:687–9.
67. Frossard CP, Steidler L, Eigenmann PA. Oral administration of an IL-10-secreting Lactococcus lactis strain prevents food-induced IgE sensitization. J Allergy Clin Immunol 2007;119(4):952–9.
68. Li S, Li XM, Burks AW, et al. Modulation of peanut allergy by peptide-based immunotherapy [abstract]. J Allergy Clin Immunol 2001;107:S233.
69. Horner AA, Nguyen MD, Ronaghy A, et al. DNA-based vaccination reduces the risk of lethal anaphylactic hypersensitivity in mice. J Allergy Clin Immunol 2000; 106(2):349–56.
70. Roy K, Mao HQ, Huang SK, et al. Oral gene delivery with chitosan–DNA nanoparticles generates immunologic protection in a murine model of peanut allergy. Nat Med 1999;5(4):387–91.
71. Nguyen MD, Cinman N, Yen J, et al. DNA-based vaccination for the treatment of food allergy. Allergy 2001;56(Suppl 67):127–30.
72. Srivastava K, Li XM, Bannon GA, et al. Investigation of the use of ISS-linked Ara h2 for the treatment of peanut-induced allergy [abstract]. J Allergy Clin Immunol 2001;107:S233.

Index

Note: Page numbers of article titles are in **boldface** type.

Pediatr Clin N Am 58 (2011) 531–542
doi:10.1016/S0031-3955(11)00039-3

F

H

I

L

M

N

O